Epilepsy

Guest Editor

STEVEN C. SCHACHTER, MD

NEUROLOGIC CLINICS

www.neurologic.theclinics.com

Consulting Editor
RANDOLPH W. EVANS, MD

November 2009 • Volume 27 • Number 4

SAUNDERS an imprint of ELSEVIER, Inc.

W.B. SAUNDERS COMPANY
A Division of Elsevier Inc.

1600 John F. Kennedy Boulevard • Suite 1800 • Philadelphia, Pennsylvania 19103-2899

http://www.theclinics.com

NEUROLOGIC CLINICS Volume 27, Number 4
November 2009 ISSN 0733-8619, ISBN-13: 978-1-4377-1245-2, ISBN-10: 1-4377-1245-2

Editor: Donald Mumford

Neurologic Clinics (ISSN 0733-8619) is published quarterly by Elsevier Inc., 360 Park Avenue South, New York, NY 10010–171. Months of issue are February, May, August, and November. Periodicals postage paid at New York, NY, and additional mailing offices. Subscription prices are $247.00 per year for US individuals, $401.00 per year for US institutions, $124.00 per year for US students, $310.00 per year for Canadian individuals, $482.00 per year for Canadian institutions, $344.00 per year for international individuals, $482.00 per year for international institutions, and $175.00 for Canadian and foreign students/residents. To receive student/resident rate, orders must be accompanied by name of affiliated institution, date of term, and the *signature* of program/residency coordinator on institution letterhead. Orders will be billed at individual rate until proof of status is received. Foreign air speed delivery is included in all *Clinics* subscription prices. All prices are subject to change without notice. **POSTMASTER:** Send address changes to *Neurologic Clinics*, Elsevier Health Sciences Division, Subscription Customer Service, 3251 Riverport Lane, Maryland Heights, MO 63043. **Customer Service: Telephone: 1-800-654-2452 (U.S. and Canada); 314-447-8871 (outside U.S. and Canada). Fax: 314-447-8029. E-mail: journalscustomerservice-usa@elsevier.com (for print support); journalsonlinesupport-usa@elsevier.com (for online support).**

Reprints. For copies of 100 or more of articles in this publication, please contact the Commercial Reprints Department, Elsevier Inc., 360 Park Avenue South, New York, New York, 10010-1710; Tel.: (+1) 212-633-3812; Fax: (+1) 212-462-1935, and E-mail: reprints@elsevier.com.

Neurologic Clinics is also published in Spanish by Nueva Editorial Interamericana S.A., Mexico City, Mexico.

Neurologic Clinics is covered in *Current Contents/Clinical Medicine, MEDLINE/PubMed (Index Medicus), EMBASE/Excerpta Medica, and PsycINFO, and ISI/BIOMED.*

Printed and bound by CPI Group (UK) Ltd, Croydon, CR0 4YY

Transferred to Digital Print 2011

Contributors

CONSULTING EDITOR

RANDOLPH W. EVANS, MD
Professor of Neurology, Distinguished Chair in Movement Disorders Director,
Parkinson's Disease Center and Movement Disorders Clinic; Department of Neurology,
Baylor College of Medicine, Houston, Texas

GUEST EDITOR

STEVEN C. SCHACHTER, MD
Professor of Neurology, Departments of Neurology, Harvard Medical School and Beth
Israel Deaconess Medical Center; Chief Academic Officer, Center for Integration
of Medicine and Innovative Technology Boston, Boston, Massachusetts

AUTHORS

GUS A. BAKER, FBPsS, PhD
Division of Neurosciences, University of Liverpool, United Kingdom

DINA BATTINO, MD
Department Of Neurophysiopathology, Fondazione I.R.C.C.S. Istituto Neurologico
"Carlo Besta", Italy

MICHEL BAULAC, MD
Center for Epilepsy, AP-HP, Hôpital de la Pitié-Salpêtrière, Paris, France

STEPHANIE BAULAC, PhD
UPMC/Inserm, Hôpital de la Pitié-Salpêtrière, Paris, France

ANNE T. BERG, PhD
Research Professor, Department of Biology, Northern Illinois University,
DeKalb, Illinois

MARTIN J. BRODIE, MBChB, MD
Professor of Medicine and Clinical Pharmacology, Department of Medicine and
Therapeutics; Director, Epilepsy Unit, Western Infirmary, Scotland

ROBERT S. FISHER, MD, PhD
Maslah Saul MD Professor, Department of Neurology and Neurological Sciences,
Stanford University School of Medicine, Stanford, California

SHERYL R. HAUT, MD
Department of Neurology, Montefiore Medical Center, Albert Einstein College of Medicine,
Bronx, New York

BRUCE P. HERMANN, PhD
Professor, Department of Neurology, University of Wisconsin School of Medicine and Public Health, Madison, Wisconsin

ANN JACOBY, PhD
Professor, Division of Public Health, University of Liverpool, Liverpool, United Kingdom

JANA E. JONES, PhD
Assistant Professor, Department of Neurology, University of Wisconsin School of Medicine and Public Health, Madison, Wisconsin

ANDRES M. KANNER, MD
Professor of Departments of Neurological Sciences and Psychology, Rush Medical College at Rush University; Director, Laboratory of Electroencephalography and Video-EEG-Telemetry, Rush University Medical Center; Associate Director, Section of Epilepsy and Rush Epilepsy Center, Rush University Medical Center, Chicago, Illinois

JACK J. LIN, MD
Assistant Professor, Department of Neurology, University of California, Irvine, California

RICHARD B. LIPTON, MD
Department of Neurology, Montefiore Medical Center, Albert Einstein College of Medicine and Department of Epidemiology and Population Health, Albert Einstein College of Medicine, Bronx, New York

JULIANA LOCKMAN, MD
Epilepsy Fellow, Department of Neurology and Neurological Sciences, Stanford University School of Medicine, Stanford, California

LINA NASHEF, MBCHB, MD, FRCP
Consultant Neurologist and Honorary Senior Lecturer, Neurology Department, King's College Hospital, London, United Kingdom

PAGE B. PENNELL, MD
Director of Research, Department of Neurology, Division of Epilepsy, Brigham and Women's Hospital, Harvard Medical School, Boston, Massachusetts

DIMITRIS G. PLACANTONAKIS, MD, PhD
Department of Neurological Surgery, Weill Medical College of Cornell University, New York-Presbyterian Hospital, New York

MARKUS REUBER, MD, PhD, FRCP
Senior Clinical Lecturer in Neurology, Genomic Division of Medicine, Academic Neurology Unit, University of Sheffield, Royal Hallamshire Hospital, United Kingdom

PHILIPPE RYVLIN, MD, PhD
Professor of Neurology, Department of Functional Neurology and Epileptology, Institut Des Epilepsies de l'Enfant et de l'Adolescent, Hospices Civils de Lyon, Lyon, France

THEODORE H. SCHWARTZ, MD
Department of Neurological Surgery, Weill Medical College of Cornell University, New York-Presbyterian Hospital, New York

MICHAEL SEIDENBERG, PhD
Professor, Department of Psychology, Rosalind Franklin School of Medicine and Science, Chicago, Illinois

DEE SNAPE, RGN, MA
Division of Public Health, University of Liverpool, Liverpool, United Kingdom

LINDA J. STEPHEN, MBChB, MRCGP
Associate Specialist, Epilepsy Unit, Division of Cardiovascular and Medical Sciences, Western Infirmary, Scotland

TORBJÖRN TOMSON, MD, PhD
Departments of Neurology and Clinical Neuroscience, Karolinska Institutet, Stockholm, Sweden

Contents

This article reviews evidence of quality of life (QOL) determinants in people affected by epilepsy, including detractors and promoters. Emerging factors of particular significance for QOL are highlighted, including seizure frequency, medication side effects, psychological comorbidity, and stigma and discrimination. This article also examines the role of resilience, interpreted in its widest sense, for promoting good QOL, even in the presence of poorly controlled seizures. The importance of addressing both clinical and wider psychosocial issues is highlighted and some possible directions for future research into QOL in epilepsy are suggested.

Depressive disorders are the most frequent psychiatric comorbidity in patients with epilepsy (PWE). Although they are typically considered a psychiatric disorder, ample data suggest that depressive disorders are a neurologic disorder with psychiatric clinical manifestations. Patients with epilepsy whose seizures originate in temporal and frontal lobes have the highest prevalence of comorbid depressive disorders. Not only are patients with epilepsy at higher risk of developing depression but also patients with depression are at higher risk of developing epilepsy. This article reviews these data, the clinical manifestations of depressive disorders in PWE, and their significant impact on the suicidal risk and quality of life.

A new literature is now under way, one linking cognitive abnormalities directly to indices of structural, functional, metabolic, and other neurobiologic markers of cerebral integrity, independent of their association with clinical epilepsy characteristics. These trends are reviewed in this article. The focus is on temporal lobe epilepsy (TLE) as a model with which to address the core points because this form of localization-related epilepsy has been very carefully studied from both a cognitive and imaging standpoint. Some pertinent historical issues are touched on first, followed by more detailed reviews of the cognitive and neuroimaging abnormalities that have been found in TLE, followed by an overview of studies examining direct structure-function relationships in TLE and other epilepsies.

Psychogenic non-epileptic seizures (PNES) are one of the most common differential diagnoses of epilepsy. PNES are poorly understood and often sub-optimally treated. This article summarizes current knowledge about the etiology of PNES. Through describing the interactions of predisposing, precipitating, perpetuating, and triggering factors, an integrated biopsychosocial model of a complex disorder is developed. PNES emerge as a dissociative response to a range of different stressors in vulnerable individuals. Once established, maintaining factors turn a temporary disturbance into a chronically disabling disorder.

This article reviews the clinical evidence for seizure prediction. The epilepsy cycle is considered, including the interictal, preictal, ictal, and postictal phases. Evidence suggesting that the preictal phase can sometimes be identified based on neurophysiologic signals, premonitory features, the presence of trigger factors, or self-report is discussed. Diary studies have shown that seizures are not randomly distributed in time and that a subgroup of persons with epilepsy can predict an impending seizure. Paper diary data and preliminary analysis of electronic diary data suggest that seizure prediction is feasible.

The interactions between hormones, epilepsy, and the medications used to treat epilepsy are complex, with tri-directional interactions which affect both men and women in various ways. Abnormalities of baseline endocrine status occur more commonly in people with epilepsy, and are most often described for the sex steroid hormone axis. Common symptoms include sexual dysfunction, decreased fertility, premature menopause, and polycystic ovarian syndrome. Antiepileptic drugs (AEDs) and hormones have a bidirectional interaction, with a decrease in the efficacy of hormonal contraceptive agents with some AEDs and a decrease in the concentration and efficacy of other AEDs with hormonal contraceptives. Endogenous hormones can influence seizure severity and frequency, resulting in catamenial patterns of epilepsy. However, this knowledge can be used to develop hormonal strategies to improve seizure control in people with epilepsy.

Epilepsy affects approximately 50 million people worldwide, with an annual incidence of 50 to 70 cases per 100,000 population. The condition can strike at any time of life, with an immediate impact on everyday activities and routine. Key to optimal management is swift referral to an epilepsy specialist, appropriate investigation, and timely institution of antiepileptic drug therapy. In the past 20 years, the explosion of 13 new agents into the marketplace has greatly increased the potential for therapeutic intervention. This article explores the rationale for treatment selection in adults with epilepsy.

During the last few years epilepsy and pregnancy registries and other large scale observational studies have provided new information on the teratogenic effects of the most frequently used antiepileptic drugs (AEDs). The prevalence of major congenital malformations associated with exposure to carbamazepine or lamotrigine appears to be only marginally increased from the expected, while malformation rates with valproate have been reported to be 2 to 4 times higher. Recent studies also suggest that compared with carbamazepine, lamotrigine and phenytoin, exposure to valproate *in utero* may be associated with poorer postnatal cognitive development. However, adverse outcomes with valproate appear to be dose-related, and doses below 800-1,000 mg/day might not be associated with worse outcome than with other AEDs. Information on the teratogenic potential of other newer generation AEDs than lamotrigine is still insufficient.

There is no single definition of pharmacoresistant (intractable, refractory) epilepsy. Prospective identification of pharmacoresistance is complicated by the variability of its appearance across different types of epilepsy and the variability of seizure control within a given patient over time. Failure of informative trials of two appropriate antiepileptic drugs has been recommended as a threshold that should trigger referral for evaluation at a comprehensive epilepsy center. Maximizing seizure control is imperative for reducing the risks and consequences of epilepsy, including the cognitive and psychiatric comorbidities and even sudden death.

Pharmacologic therapy represents the first line of treatment of epilepsy and is effective in most patients. However, about 20% to 30% of cases develop intractable seizures that cannot be controlled by medication alone. In such cases, surgical intervention is considered for therapeutic, often curative purposes. Dynamic spatiotemporal variability in the epileptic focus renders seizure localization a challenge to the clinician. Many diagnostic modalities have been developed to identify different aspects of the

THE CLINICS ARE NOW AVAILABLE ONLINE!

Access your subscription at:
www.theclinics.com

Preface

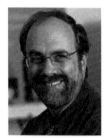

Steven C. Schachter, MD
Guest Editor

The diagnosis and management of patients who have epilepsy have greatly evolved over recent years. This issue of *Neurologic Clinics* presents state-of-the-art reviews by renowned experts of critical issues that illustrate this evolution and underscore their importance in the care of patients. The first six papers focus on the interrelationships between seizures and psychological, neuropsychological, and hormonal factors. The next five papers discuss pharmacologic treatment selection, drug resistance, approaches to localizing seizure onset, and deep brain stimulation as a possible non-pharmacological intervention. The final two papers present an update on the genetics of idiopathic epilepsies and a thought-provoking approach to sudden, unexpected death in epilepsy.

I am grateful to the contributors for their fine efforts and hope that readers find this collection of articles valuable in successfully addressing the complex problems associated with the diagnosis and treatment of epilepsy.

Steven C. Schachter, MD
Professor of Neurology
Departments of Neurology
Harvard Medical School and Beth Israel Deaconess Medical Center

Chief Academic Officer
Center for Integration of Medicine and Innovative Technology Boston
330 Brookline Avenue, K-478
Boston, MA 02215, USA

E-mail address:
sschacht@bidmc.harvard.edu (S.C. Schachter)

Neurol Clin 27 (2009) xiii
doi:10.1016/j.ncl.2009.09.017
0733-8619/09/$ – see front matter © 2009 Elsevier Inc. All rights reserved.

Determinants of Quality of Life in People with Epilepsy

Ann Jacoby, PhD[a],*, Dee Snape, RGN, MA[a], Gus A. Baker, FBPsS, PhD[b]

KEYWORDS

- Epilepsy • Quality of life • Seizure frequency • Depression
- Resilience • Stigma

All individuals have multiple determinants of quality of life (QOL).[1] In people with epilepsy, these determinants include aspects specific to their condition, which may be clinically or psychosocially based. This article describes the potential determinants of QOL for adults affected by epilepsy and the relative weightings, as shown in the current literature. Although, adults and children have some common determinants, important differences exist in what constitutes the key QOL determinants.

The determinants this article addresses include seizures, treatment and service provision, mood, personality traits, socioeconomic position, demographic characteristics, and social milieu and attitudes. For some of these, a wealth of data exists, whereas for others evidence is relatively limited. Therefore, this article highlights areas for further research and models of QOL that may help guide it.

THE COMPLEXITY OF QUALITY OF LIFE

The World Health Organization (WHO) defines QOL as an individual's "perception of their position in life in the context of the culture and value systems in which they live and in relation to their goals, expectations, standards and concerns."[2] WHO notes that QOL is a broad concept affected in a complex way by a person's physical health, psychological state, level of independence, social relationships, and personal beliefs, and their relationship to salient features of their environment. This definition provides the conceptual framework for the WHO measure (WHOQOL).

The WHOQOL consists of 100 items, incorporating six broad QOL domains, within which are nested 24 QOL facets (**Table 1**). The interrelatedness of the separate QOL domains is supported by recent analysis of the WHOQOL-100 structure, which suggested the possibility of merging domains one and three, and domains two and six,

[a] Division of Public Health, University of Liverpool, Whelan Building, 3rd Floor, The Quadrangle, Brownlow Hill, Liverpool, L69 3GB, UK
[b] Division of Neurosciences, University of Liverpool, Whelan Building, Brownlow Hill, Liverpool, L69 3GB, UK
* Corresponding author.
E-mail address: ajacoby@liv.ac.uk (A. Jacoby).

Neurol Clin 27 (2009) 843–863
doi:10.1016/j.ncl.2009.06.003
0733-8619/09/$ – see front matter © 2009 Elsevier Inc. All rights reserved.

Table 1
World Health Organization conceptual model for quality of life

Quality of Life Domain	Facets Incorporated within QOL Domains
1. Physical health	Energy and fatigue Pain and discomfort Sleep and rest
2. Psychological	Bodily image and appearance Negative feelings Positive feelings Self-esteem Thinking, learning, memory, and concentration
3. Level of independence	Mobility Activities of daily living Dependence on medicinal substances and medical aids Work capacity
4. Social relationships	Personal relationships Social support Sexual activity
5. Environment	Financial resources Freedom, physical safety, and security Health and social care: accessibility and quality Home environment Opportunities for acquiring new information and skills Participation in and opportunities for recreation/leisure Physical environment (pollution/noise/traffic/climate) Transport
6. Spirituality/religion/personal beliefs	Religion/spirituality/personal beliefs

Data from What quality of life? The WHOQOL Group. World Health Organization Quality of Life Assessment. World Health Forum 1996;17(4):354–6.

to create four domains. This merging was subsequently realized in the reduced version of WHOQOL, the 30-item WHOQOL-BREF, which assesses four major domains: physical, psychological, social relationships, and environment.

To establish whether all the relevant domains and facets are included in attempts to measure QOL, Bowling[3,4] interviewed more than 2000 people in the United Kingdom on what they considered the important things, both positive and negative, about their lives. Informants were asked to identify things that were important, rank these things in order of importance, and then rate their current status in relation to each from "as good as it possibly could be" to "as bad as it possibly could be." They were also asked to rate their life overall; and those who had limiting long-standing illness or disability were asked to define and rate the important effects of ill-health on their lives.

Bowling[3,4] reported that the priorities according to the different QOL domains/facets were different between persons in good health and those who had limiting long-standing illness or disability. Among healthy persons, the most frequently mentioned were finances and standard of living, followed by relationships with family and friends, personal health, health of close others, and social life/leisure activities. Among those who had illness or disability, priority was given, unsurprisingly, to ability to get out and about, followed by social life/leisure activities, and availability of/ability to work.

Bowling also reported considerable variation in views on area of QOL impacted by ill-health. For example, respondents who had mental health disorders, mainly depression, were most likely to report availability of/ability to work as the most important negative effect, whereas respondents who had respiratory and cardiovascular disease reported that getting out and about was the most important effect. Bowling's work thus supports the view that assessments of QOL in persons who have health problems should be disease-specific.

Regarding epilepsy, Fisher and colleagues[5] delineated a range of QOL domains and facets deemed critical by people who have epilepsy. The data were drawn from two separate surveys, one involving just more than 1000 individuals who participated in a community-based questionnaire survey, the other involving just more than 1000 callers to the U.S. Epilepsy Foundation. Considering that 50% of respondents reported incomplete control of their seizures and only a third reported an interval of greater than 6 months between seizures, they unsurprisingly listed uncertainty and fear of having seizures as the worst thing about having epilepsy, followed by the associated stigma. Major QOL facets highlighted as problematic included school, employment, and driving, with driving the most often cited lifestyle limitation. The importance of driving as a QOL facet is, of course, highly culturally specific, but aspects of QOL almost universally impacted negatively include education and employment, and psychological status and social/interpersonal relationships, including propensity to marry and have children.

WHAT IS THE EVIDENCE FOR QUALITY OF LIFE DETERMINANTS IN EPILEPSY?
The Role of Seizures

The effects on psychosocial health of active epilepsy and ongoing seizures are well documented.[6–10] For example, Baker and colleagues[7] reported findings from a European-wide study involving more than 5000 people affected by epilepsy recruited through national patient support organizations. Informants reporting at least one seizure per month also reported the greatest perceived impacts of their epilepsy and the most impaired QOL, as assessed by their scores on the SF-36 health status measure, whereas those experiencing no seizures in the past year reported the least impact and scored highest (**Fig. 1**).

Likewise, in the United States, Leidy and colleagues[8] reported that patients experiencing six or more seizures in the previous 6 months had significantly poorer QOL, as measured with the SF-36, than those experiencing one to five, who in turn had poorer profiles than the seizure-free patients. Leidy and colleagues[8] noted that score differences were substantial, suggesting that even small reductions in seizure frequency "could have a dramatic impact" on QOL.

This argument is reinforced by the work of Birbeck and colleagues,[11] who showed that reducing the number of intractable seizures only translated into meaningful improvements in QOL when complete seizure freedom was achieved (**Table 2**).

In a survey involving more than 40,000 California-dwelling respondents, Kobau and colleagues[12] reported a role for seizure frequency and recency: adults who experienced recent seizures reported poorer health overall, more mentally and physically unhealthy days, and more days on which their activities were limited than individuals who had active epilepsy but no recent seizures, who in turn fared worse than those who had inactive epilepsy or no history of seizures.

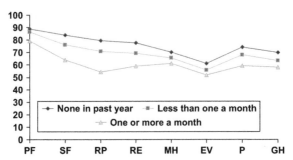

Fig. 1. Health status (SF-36 scores) according to seizure frequency. *Data from* Baker GA, Jacoby A, Buck D, et al. Quality of life of people with epilepsy: a European study. Epilepsia 1997;38(3):3537–62.

The fact that persons who have active epilepsy and ongoing seizures report impacts on QOL seems unsurprising. More surprising, perhaps, is the findings that as a whole group, people who have epilepsy have poorer QOL than those who do not, even when the seizures are distant in time. For example, Strine and colleagues[13] examined QOL in more than 31,000 adults aged 18 years and older in the United States, among whom just more than 400 (1.4% of total responders) reported having had seizures at some point in their lives. Furthermore, individuals in this group were more likely to have psychological distress, including serious mental illness; to be physically inactive; and to report physical comorbidities, and to be less likely to be married and be employed.

Another large-scale health survey involving more than 60,000 Canadians[14] also showed that QOL was significantly poorer in those identifying themselves as having had seizures at some time than in those who either had a chronic illness other than epilepsy or described themselves as healthy. These findings somewhat conflict, however, with those of other studies, which suggest that distance from seizures markedly reduces QOL impact. For example, in a study in Norway, Stavem and colleagues[15] showed SF-36 scores close to those of the normal population among the 70% of participants who reported being seizure-free in the previous year.

Table 2
Health-related quality of life across groups with different levels of change in seizure freedom

	100% Change in Seizure Freedom	75%–99% Change in Seizure Freedom	50%–74% Reduction in Seizure Freedom	0%–50% Reduction or Increase in Seizure Freedom	P Value
QOLIE-89	7.32	0.96	−0.20	−0.62	.0004
QOLIE-89 MH	6.41	1.71	−2.09	−0.52	.0003
QOLIE-89 PH	7.11	−0.67	−0.37	−1.07	.002
QOLIE-89 CF	4.29	−0.16	−0.37	−0.12	NS
QOLIE-89 EP	7.26	3.04	1.86	0.57	.007
SF-36 MH	7.11	1.92	−3.53	−0.98	.0008
SF-36 PF	3.66	−1.14	1.79	−0.98	NS

Data from Birbeck GL, Hays RD, Cui XP, et al. Seizure reduction and quality of life improvements in people with epilepsy. Epilepsia 2002;43(5):535–8.

Furthermore, in the study by Leidy and colleagues,[8] SF-36 domain and summary scale (mental and physical health) scores for patients who reported being seizure-free (in whom the median time since the last seizure was 365 days) were similar to those for the general United States population.

Jacoby[16] examined the role of seizure remission for QOL in 607 persons living in the United Kingdom. In this cohort, all of whom had been seizure-free for a minimum of 2 years and many for considerably longer, the effects on QOL were minimal. Psychological health, as measured by a six-domain profile, was good; only small percentages viewed epilepsy as a serious illness (12%), worried a lot about their epilepsy (8%), felt stigmatized by it (14%), or felt socially restricted by it (4%). Little evidence was seen of reduced social activity, and employment rates were near those of the normal United Kingdom population. Therefore, Jacoby's data suggest that any short-term impacts of seizures on QOL can be overcome with time.

Dworetzky and colleagues[17] also compared scores on the SF-36 general health measure for 30 adults experiencing a single seizure, 29 who had well-controlled epilepsy, and 24 recently diagnosed as having hypertension, finding no significant differences among the groups at baseline for overall QOL, SF-36 domain scores, or perceived impact of their condition. When SF-36 scores were compared with age-adjusted population norms, adults experiencing a single seizure had significantly lower scores for the energy/vitality and physical role functioning domains, but comparable scores for the other six, although when asked at follow-up, more than a third (38%) believed their seizure had a moderate to extreme impact. The authors concluded, therefore, that experiencing a single seizure has only a modest impact on life quality.

Some light is shed on the differential reporting of the role of seizures in QOL by the recent important work by Velissaris,[18] who mapped, quantitatively and qualitatively, the psychosocial adjustment of persons experiencing a first seizure. She found that at seizure onset, patients experienced differing degrees of sense of loss of control, which she termed either *limited* or *pervasive*, but that by rebuilding sense of control, even those whose sense of loss was initially pervasive were able to make positive adjustments. However, patients who reported a continued pervasive sense of loss of control at 12-month follow-up also showed poor psychological adjustment and high distress. In these patients who had also experienced further seizures, QOL impacts were similar in nature to those reported by patients with longstanding epilepsy.

The potentially dramatic effects of remitting seizures on QOL can also be seen in reports of outcomes of surgery for seizures unresponsive to drug treatment.[19–24] Using the QOLIE-89 measure, Spencer and colleagues[22] assessed QOL at intervals up to 5 years in a large cohort of patients undergoing surgery. QOL improved substantially across all outcome groups in the immediate postoperative period, declining again in persons experiencing persistent seizures until it reached presurgical levels, but continuing to improve in persons remaining seizure-free, until levelling off at approximately 2 years postsurgery. This study and those reported by Mikati and colleagues[23] and Wilson and colleagues[24] support these findings in the context of drug-related remissions, and suggest that when patients are rendered completely seizure-free, QOL can improve to normalization within a relatively short timeframe, roughly between 2 and 3 years.

The Role of Treatment and Service Provision

Because treatment with antiepileptic medication (AED) quickly renders most people seizure-free, and seizure freedom is strongly associated with higher quality of life, drug treatment is an important, if indirect, QOL determinant. However, the positive effects of AEDs for seizure control are counterbalanced by their potential adverse effects, which reduce QOL in individuals subject to them, and patients commonly report more than one AED-related side effect.[25] Only limited research, however, has investigated the relative contribution of specific adverse effects to impaired health-related QOL.[26]

Adverse side effects may be the most clinically relevant determinant, aside from seizure frequency, of QOL in patients who have resistant epilepsy. A large survey of more than 5000 patients from 15 different European countries found that approximately 50% reported fatigue and 40% concentration problems associated with each of the investigated AEDs.[7]

More recently, using the validated Adverse Events Profile (AEP) measure,[27] Perucca and colleagues[25] reported that the mean number of patient-reported adverse effects in 200 patients experiencing refractory seizures on AEDs was 6.5, and the effects could be segregated into five distinct classes: cognition/coordination, mood/emotion, sleep, weight/cephalgia, and tegument/mucosa. High scores for each AEP class were associated with impaired QOL, as assessed using the QOLIE-89, with the strongest relationship in the cognition/coordination class, followed by mood/emotion and then sleep. Together, cognition/coordination score, scores on a validated depression scale, and weight/cephalgia scores accounted for 71% of the variance on QOL scores.

In a subgroup of 62 patients enrolled in a clinical trial, improvements in three of the five classes (cognition/coordination, mood/emotion, and tegument/mucosa) were significantly associated with improvements in QOL scores, although in a multivariate analysis only cognition/coordination remained important, identifying this as the most deleterious.

Several studies have shown that people affected by epilepsy commonly report impaired memory and learning, attention and concentration problems, slower information processing and psychomotor speed, and language deficits as side effects of their AED. More than half of the adults in a recent survey conducted by the International Bureau for Epilepsy (IBE) reported that cognitive impairment significantly affected their ability to engage in work, education, and leisure activities, and had a negative impact on family and relationships.[28] Respondents highlighted several side effects they would most like to avoid, if possible, among which sleepiness/tiredness and memory problems were the most common (**Fig. 2**).

Similar results were reported in a study involving both parents and children, who expressed significant concerns about how epilepsy and its treatment affected their day-to-day functioning, particularly their cognitive functioning.[29] An interesting finding from both studies is the degree to which respondents attributed their cognitive difficulties to their AED treatment, despite evidence that several other important factors appear to contribute to cognitive dysfunction in people affected by epilepsy, including the underlying etiology of their epilepsy, psychosocial issues, and the effects of recurrent seizures.[30] Undoubtedly a complex interactive relationship exists among AED medication side effects, psychological well-being, and quality of life. However, Gilliam and colleagues[31] suggest that direct clinical intervention to reduce reported side effects is likely to result in QOL improvements.

Withdrawal from AEDs has been shown to promote QOL improvements, although whether this is because of the reduction on existing treatment-associated adverse effects or patient concerns about possible long-term treatment effects and social labelling is not entirely clear. In the United Kingdom MRC Antiepileptic Drug Withdrawal Study, taking AEDs was associated with QOL decrements.[32] At 2 years

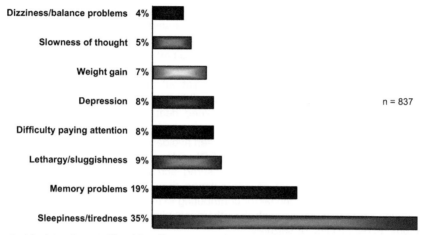

Fig. 2. Ideal treatment. The side effects respondents would most like to avoid. *Data from* International Bureau for Epilepsy. Epilepsy and Cognitive Function Survey. Heemstede, Netherlands: IBE, 2004.

postrandomization, those remaining on AEDs and experiencing side effects had significantly poorer QOL according to a range of indicators than those not experiencing any (**Table 3**).[33] Likewise, Hessen and colleagues[34] reported that discontinuation of AEDs resulted in improvements in symptoms of depression and irritability. The role of AEDs for QOL is also apparent in the longitudinal study by Sillanpaa and colleagues,[35] in which QOL decrements were found to persist into adulthood among a group with childhood-onset uncomplicated epilepsy. These authors noted that the major impact was for those still on medication as adults, despite whether they were in seizure remission, concluding that, "even if medications do not have a direct adverse effect...[they] may be a marker for a variety of other adverse effects, including stigma."[35]

In addition to treatment-specific effects, QOL is likely to be somewhat affected by the quality of care received, although the amount of potential "noise" in the system is large and differences may therefore be difficult to show. Recent surveys of services for people affected by epilepsy[36] suggest that the treatment gap in its broadest sense

Table 3		
Influence of antiepileptic medication side effects on quality of life outcomes		
Outcome	Relative Risk (95% CIs)[a]	Relative Risk (95% CIs)[b]
Impaired energy[c]	3.25 (1.87, 5.66)	3.39 (2.02, 5.70)
Impaired sleep[c]	0.75 (0.40, 1.41)	0.69 (0.34, 1.27)
Self-reported health excellent/good	0.82 (0.44, 1.51)	0.77 (0.43, 1.37)
Social activities restricted	2.61 (1.35, 5.06)	3.28 (1.76, 6.13)
Currently in employment	0.94 (0.56, 1.58)	0.84 (0.52, 1.38)

[a] Analysis based on 275 subjects currently taking antiepileptic medication (AED); compares those reporting side effects with those not reporting side effects.
[b] Analysis based on 403 subjects; compares those on AEDs and reporting side effects with those on AEDS not reporting side effects and those not on AEDs as a single group.
[c] Assessed using the Nottingham Health Profile.
Courtesy of Ann Jacoby, PhD, Liverpool, UK.

is not a feature only of developing countries but manifests worldwide. In the study in the United Kingdom, Jacoby and colleagues[37] found that few patients underwent regular review of their condition or had been counselled about its QOL implications.

Knowledge gaps and negative attitudes on the part of health professionals treating people affected by epilepsy may also contribute to QOL impairments through poor clinical management of seizures and coaching about stigma.[38,39] At its most extreme, poor quality care can lead to the worst possible outcome for a patient. In a recent United Kingdom audit of sudden unexplained deaths among people affected by epilepsy, poor seizure control was identified as a major risk factor and approximately half of the deaths were believed to have been avoidable with optimal care.[40]

At a less extreme level, but still key for QOL, DiIorio and colleagues[41] showed that patient satisfaction with their care (measured across six domains: interpersonal manner, communication, technical competence, time spent with the doctor, financial aspects, and access) was one factor contributing to the variance in scores on a scale measuring perceived stigma, with the others including seizure activity and negative outcome expectancies for seizures.

The Role of Comorbidities

Rapidly expanding literature addresses the role of comorbidities as determinants of QOL of people affected by epilepsy. In the 2005 California Health Survey,[42] 604 of 43,020 respondents to a telephone survey reported a history of epilepsy, and this group also reported significantly higher rates of asthma, emphysema/chronic obstructive pulmonary disease, heart disease, stroke, arthritis, and cancer than the population with no history of epilepsy (**Table 4**). The group with epilepsy was also significantly more likely to report themselves as generally, physically, or mentally unhealthy on more than 14 of the previous 30 days, and to rate their health as only fair or poor.

Pulsipher and colleagues[43] studied QOL in 93 patients who had temporal lobe epilepsy, half of whom reported presence of a medical comorbidity, a psychiatric comorbidity, or both. Most common among the medical comorbidities were cerebrovascular or respiratory disease and endocrine disorders; most common among the

Table 4
Comorbid health condition characteristics of persons affected and not affected by epilepsy in the 2005 California Health Interview Survey

Comorbid Condition	History of Epilepsy/Seizure Disorder	
	Yes (% [n])	No (% [n])
Type 2 diabetes	7.7 [52]*	5.7 [2831]
Asthma	21.9 [143]	12.6 [5758]
Emphysema/chronic obstructive pulmonary disorder	5.2 [48]	1.9 [1258]
High blood pressure	28.8 [204]	24.8 [12,695]
Heart disease	9.7 [85]	6.2 [3596]
Stroke	9.4 [79]	2.2 [1249]
Arthritis/gout	32.3 [242]	18.9 [10,900]
Cancer	11.1 [102]	7.9 [4896]

Data from Elliott JO, Lu B, Shneker B, et al. Comorbidity, health screening, and quality of life among persons with a history of epilepsy. Epilepsy Behav 2009;14(1):127.

psychiatric comorbidities were anxiety and mood disorders. These authors reported that increasing numbers of comorbid conditions was significantly associated with decreasing overall QOL and life satisfaction, and that comorbid medical and psychiatric conditions together accounted for almost 14% of the variance in QOL scores.

The differential effects of different comorbidities was also highlighted, with the number of comorbid psychiatric conditions better predictive of scores for psychosocial satisfaction, epilepsy-related effects, and cognition, and the number of comorbid medical conditions better predictive of role limitations and physical performance. The message that "recognition and identification of co-morbid medical and psychiatric conditions are important"[43] is strongly reinforced by the work of many other authors, particularly with reference to the psychiatric conditions.

The prevalence of the two most common psychiatric comorbidities among people affected by epilepsy—anxiety and depression—is high, estimated at between 10% and 25% for anxiety[44] and 10% and 60% for depression.[45] In a large sample of adults completing the United States 2004 HealthStyles Survey,[46] those self-reporting epilepsy were twice as likely to self-report anxiety or depression in the previous year than those not affected by epilepsy; and those who had active epilepsy (defined as seizures in the past 3 months or on AED medication) were three times more likely.

Although greater research attention to date has been given to the role of depression for QOL, Hesdorffer[47] notes that this psychiatric comorbidity remains poorly understood. She highlights that contrary to what might be expected, the associations between epilepsy and depression are not necessarily confined to individuals who experience frequent seizures. For example, in a cross-sectional study involving patients affected by epilepsy, those with less-severe epilepsy[48] were 11 times more likely to have experienced moderate to severe depression than a comparator group of blood donors.

In line with this finding, Attarian and colleagues[49] found no relationship between seizure intractability and severity of depression, which was as prevalent in patients seizure-free for 6 months or longer as in patients experiencing continuing seizures. The complexity of the epilepsy–depression association is further highlighted by the community-based study reported by Mensah and colleagues,[50] in which factors predictive of depression included not only seizure activity but also the presence of drug side effects, other chronic health problems, and lack of paid employment.

Hesdorffer[47] suggests several possible explanations for the increased prevalence of depression among people affected by epilepsy compared with those who are not, including the idea that depression is a precursor of epilepsy, epilepsy is a cause of depression, and epilepsy and depression share a common set of underlying mechanisms and risk factors. Despite the nature of their relationship, their combined and independent impacts on QOL are becoming increasingly clear. Reduced QOL is commonly reported among people affected by epilepsy who have depression, compared with those who are depression-free.[51–53]

Zeber and colleagues[53] found QOLIE-89 scores to be significantly reduced by comorbid depression for all types of seizures. Likewise, Senol and colleagues[10] reported that depression, alongside seizure frequency and fatigue, was a key influencing factor for reduced QOL. Loring and colleagues[52] reported that symptoms of depression, along with worry about seizures, were the most important factors affecting QOL in persons who had intractable epilepsy, as measured by the epilepsy-specific QOLIE-89 scale. Similarly, Boylan and colleagues[54] note that in their study of patients who had refractory epilepsy, depression was common, severe, underdiagnosed, largely untreated, and a powerful determinant of QOL, whereas seizure-related factors were not.

So strong was the association between depression and QOL in the study by Tracy and colleagues[55] that its authors posit that, "any therapeutic intervention observed to improve 'quality of life'... must at least consider the possibility that the outcome is strongly related to alteration in mood, not betterment of the underlying neurologic or medical condition." However, the emphasis on depression should not eclipse the important role of the frequent concomitant anxiety because, as noted by Johnson and colleagues,[56] anxiety exerts its own independent effects on QOL in people affected by epilepsy. In their study, self-reported anxiety accounted for more than 30% of the variance in QOL scores (similar to the variance accounted for by depression) and independently predicted scores on the epilepsy, cognitive, physical health, and mental health subscales of the QOLIE-89 measure.

However, anxiety disorders often go untreated.[57] Salas-Puig and colleagues[58] have reported that self-reported memory impairments in just more than 600 patients completing a self-rated memory efficiency scale were largely explainable by the presence of depressive or anxiety symptoms. The degree to which pharmacotherapy or psychotherapy interventions can reduce anxiety and depression in this population are an important area for future research.[56,57]

The Role of Psychological Predisposition and Resilience

The concept of resilience focuses on the means through which individuals manage to fare better than expected in the face of adversity. In its broadest interpretation, resilience refers not simply to individual psychological traits, but to a triad of personal, family, and wider social context factors, and to a process whereby confronting a serious adverse life event can lead to positive adaptation trajectories.[59] Research has explored the usefulness of the concept in contexts as diverse as childhood adversity, poverty, aging, and ill-health.[60]

Experts have suggested that resilience is the most common outcome after a traumatic event, including the diagnosis of a chronic illness.[61] This argument is supported in the context of epilepsy by the findings of several authors that, after a sudden dip in QOL immediately after the onset of seizures, most people who have newly diagnosed epilepsy experience a fairly quick return (generally suggested as somewhere between 1 and 2 years) to (almost) normal functioning (compared with the general population) and a life quality comparable to that which preceded the event.

Regardless of how pervasive their reported sense of loss of control at point of diagnosis, few patients (16%) in the study by Velarissis[18] reported high loss of control by 12-month follow-up. Most seemed to have been able, through a range of coping strategies and adaptations, to restore some sense of control over their lives and therefore achieved a state of psychological equilibrium. Velarissis[18] notes that further research is needed to identify medical and wider psychosocial factors promoting resilience in people who have newly diagnosed epilepsy. Although recent studies have reported on the role of family resilience in coping with the onset of epilepsy in children,[62] its role for promoting good QOL in adulthood has yet to be fully explored.

Nonetheless, current epilepsy-focused research supports the broad-based concept of resilience proposed here. For example, in the study by Amir and colleagues,[63] the negative effects of disease severity were clearly mediated by a high sense of mastery and high levels of social support. Pais-Ribeiro and colleagues[64] report that an optimistic orientation to the condition and a perception of cognitive function as good were strongly predictive of the physical and mental health and overall QOL in patients affected by epilepsy, whereas clinical factors, including seizure frequency and severity, emerged as unimportant. The authors conclude that interventions with "an epilepsy-specific optimistic orientation" can therefore have a profound effect on the lives of individuals affected by epilepsy, and that patient support groups should have the goal of fostering positive expectations of life with epilepsy among their members. Although perhaps not yet directly addressed in the context of epilepsy, the concept of happiness also deserves attention, because it has been shown to be another important psychological attribute predictive of life success and of positive clinical outcomes in individuals who have neurologic disorders.[65]

Other factors contributing to resilience, and hence good QOL among people affected by epilepsy, include what has been described as *cerebral reserve* (as indicated by higher educational level or occupational attainment or increased participation in mindful activities) and spirituality. For example, Oyegbile and colleagues[66] showed that although degree of generalized cognitive impairment, which is a major contributor to disease burden, was associated with duration of epilepsy, this association was attenuated by having more years of formal education (and ceased to be significant). The authors suggest that years of education may, in fact, be a marker "for those who, at the outset of the disorder, are on different trajectories" regarding educational attainment and lifespan cognition and, by implication, QOL.

Other studies reporting educational level as a predictor of QOL in adults include those by Loring and colleagues[52] and Pulsipher and colleagues.[43] Wakamoto and colleagues[67] examined long-term outcomes in individuals who had childhood-onset epilepsy now aged 20 years and older, and concluded that patients who had normal intelligence had favorable prognosis.

Although rarely referred to in the epilepsy literature, Giovagnoli and colleagues[68] explored the contribution of spirituality to QOL. These authors documented significant correlations between aspects of spirituality and overall QOL (using the WHOQOL Spirituality, Religiousness and Personal Beliefs Field-Test Instrument and WHOQOL-100, respectively).

On a less positive note, Hermann[69] highlighted the tendency for people affected by epilepsy to have a more external locus of control than individuals who have other medical disorders or the general population, and that "such a general outlook is associated with a more passive stance and depressogeneic thinking." His own research supports this thesis, because he showed a significant relationship between locus of control and psychiatric distress in patients who had intractable seizures being considered for seizure surgery.[70,71]

Some further sense of how this psychological disposition may impact on QOL can be derived from the study by Asadi-Pooya and colleagues,[72] who examined health locus of control in 200 patients attending an epilepsy outpatient clinic. These patients were found to have weak perceptions of internal control and strong perceptions of external control, and for those who had high scores on one of the locus of control subscales, *powerful others*, these were highly correlated with anxiety levels, although not with depression.

In a study by Gramstad and colleagues,[73] 101 patients heterogeneous in epilepsy severity were assessed for positive and negative affect, self-efficacy, and health-related locus of control, and their scores on these measures were correlated with scores on the Washington psychosocial seizure inventory (WPSI). Locus of control emerged as unimportant, a finding the authors tentatively attribute to weaknesses in the measure used, but large correlations were found between negative affect and WPSI emotional adjustment, overall psychological adjustment, and QOL (all greater than 0.45). The implications of these various study findings about the role of locus of control for patient self-management need careful consideration.

The Role of Sociodemographic Characteristics

That there will be differential impacts of epilepsy and treatment on quality of life at different stages of the life cycle is self-evident.[74] In brief summary, children and adolescents who have epilepsy seem to have a relatively more compromised QOL than those who have other chronic conditions or their healthy peers,[75,76] and those in late adolescence may be at greater risk than are those at earlier developmental stages.

Kim[77] comments that identity formation may be a particularly difficult task for adolescents who have epilepsy who "have not been able to build up competencies in the earlier developmental stages." Williams and colleagues[78] have documented the role of parental anxiety in compromising QOL of children who have epilepsy, reinforcing that interventions and support should target the family holistically.

In terms of its impact on older people's QOL, epilepsy can represent a watershed, with both immediate and less-immediate deleterious consequences, often embodying a process of "marginalization and disempowerment."[79] However, most formal QOL assessment instruments have been developed and tested in adults younger than 65 years[80] and may not properly address these issues.

Furthermore, although many commonalities in QOL concerns exist among younger and older adults who have epilepsy,[81] differences have been seen between "younger" and "older" old people in the perceived QOL impacts.[82] In one of the few reported studies that focuses on age in adults who have epilepsy, Pugh and colleagues[83] report that older adults (≥ 65 years) seemed to have less-compromised QOL (as measured using a generic health status measure, the SF-36) and seemed more resilient in coping with it than young (18–40 years) and middle-aged (41–64 years) adults. They suggest that these findings may be explained by work showing that older people reappraise negative events in a more positive light than do their younger counterparts.

The role of other sociodemographic factors, such as gender and socioeconomic status, although rarely the main foci of descriptive studies of QOL of people affected by epilepsy, is also addressed in the literature. Educational level was found to be a predictor of overall QOL and three of five QOL domains in the study cited earlier by Pulsipher and colleagues.[43] Socioeconomic status, classified according to a range of indicators, including household income and amenities, was an important predictor of QOL in the study by Alanis-Guevara and colleagues,[84] as was female gender. Senol and colleagues[10] investigated association of QOL with clinical and sociodemographic characteristics in 103 adults aged 18 years and older diagnosed with epilepsy for at least a year and on medication. They found no QOL effects for gender, marital status, or occupation, but a univariate analysis showed that lower educational level and income were significantly associated with lower QOLIE-89 overall and subscale scores.

Income, although not education, remained a significant predictor of overall QOL and of mental and physical health and cognitive function scores in a multiple regression analysis. In this study, age was also an important QOL predictor, with advanced age significantly associated with lower QOL, in contrast to the studies cited earlier. In a large community sample,[85] sociodemographic characteristics, such as gender, education, and income level, were found to be highly predictive of resilience, with poorer resilience manifested by women and individuals who had lower levels of education and lower income. However, the authors recognize that the relatively low amount of the variance in resilience scores, 11%, means that other unexplored variables played an important role.

Low socioeconomic status has been shown to be a risk factor for developing epilepsy[86,87] and the cause of more epilepsy-linked hospital admissions.[88] It is also implicated as a cause of disparities in health care,[89] including discontinuation of treatment,[90] with obvious QOL implications.

The Role of Social Milieu and Attitudes

A much reiterated message in the literature is that epilepsy is not just a clinical condition, but also a social label. Temkin[91] shows the tension between medical and mythical conceptions of the condition, positioning epilepsy as a discredited disorder through time and place. However, despite western medicalization of epilepsy and the relative success of clinical treatment regimes, this legacy of misconception continues to shape present-day attitudes and beliefs about epilepsy.[92]

Epilepsy has long evoked the application of both formal and informal sanctions that remain evident even today.[93] Although in many countries individuals affected by epilepsy are seen as having a prescribed disability, and as such an entitlement to protection under the law, the limitations imposed by statute, prejudice, fear, and lack of understanding sometimes operate without supportive evidence and have major implications for social functioning and life choices. These limitations show that the issue of stigma remains "real and serious."[94]

Health-related stigma arises, according to Weiss and Ramakrishna,[95] when a medically unwarranted adverse judgement is made about a person. For persons affected by epilepsy, the attribution of medically unwarranted judgements in relation to education,[96] employment,[97] insurance,[98] and health care provision[99] has been shown in the research literature. Not surprisingly, the ensuing disruption of these judgments place the everyday, "taken-for-granted" world of those affected by epilepsy into relief, and are easier for some individuals to cope with than others.

Research focusing on affected individuals' perception of stigma indicates its positive association with impaired self-esteem, self-efficacy, and sense of mastery; perceived helplessness; increased rates of anxiety and depression; increased somatic symptomology; and reduced life satisfaction.[71,100–102] Overall QOL seems poorer in persons affected by epilepsy who report higher perceived levels of stigma, and in a study conducted in the Netherlands, Suurmeijer and colleagues[103] identified perceived stigma as the fourth most important factor in determining QOL after psychological distress, loneliness, and adjustment. These authors also note stigma accounted for twice the amount of variance in QOL scores as did clinical variables such as seizure frequency and antiepileptic drug side-effects. Although a cultural element to epilepsy stigma is evidenced in this work, the social issues arising from a diagnosis of epilepsy and the repercussions for QOL will be very important to people during their lifetime, often presenting a greater challenge than the medical management of the condition.

Trostle[104] shifts the focus of social stigma investigation from that of the stigmatized individual to those who do the stigmatizing, commenting that, "to have epilepsy is to open oneself to the full force of past and contemporary social prejudice and misunderstanding." Substantial evidence about the attitudes of others toward people affected by epilepsy comes from a series of five yearly studies conducted in the United States from 1949 to 1979.[105]

In this study, public responses suggested that although levels of knowledge about epilepsy in the United States had stayed approximately the same over the period in question, attitudes toward it had improved steadily and significantly.

For example, in respondents who said "yes" to whether they would object to their child playing with another child affected by epilepsy, their work identified a significant decline in negative opinion from 24% in 1949 to only 6% in 1979. Parallel studies conducted in Europe from the early 1980s reported wide variations in level of public affirmation in response to the question about children affected by epilepsy, ranging from 27% for Italy in the 1980s[106] to 6% for the Czech Republic in the early 2000s.[107]

An investigation into the effectiveness of national initiatives to promote the integration of people affected by epilepsy over a 6-year period in Hungary[108] found improvements in expressed public attitudes regarding association with a child affected by epilepsy, marriage to a person affected by epilepsy, and employment of a person affected by epilepsy. Similarly, changes in public attitudes to epilepsy in the Czech Republic[107] showed that over a 16-year period, familiarity with epilepsy was significantly higher in 1997 than 1981, intolerance toward people with epilepsy had declined, and knowledge about epilepsy had risen.

Despite these findings, the authors of both studies emphasize a less-than-satisfactory social outcome for people affected by epilepsy. Most recently, a public survey of attitudes to epilepsy, conducted as part of a national omnibus survey in the United Kingdom,[109] found that most participants were well informed about and held positive attitudes toward epilepsy, although important gaps in knowledge and attitudes were also identified, with clear potential for discriminatory behavior. In the same year, Spatt and colleagues[110] found that nearly a tenth of Austrian respondents expressed negative attitudes toward people affected by epilepsy, which these authors believe is a sufficiently large proportion to suggest that "most patients will be confronted with them on a regular basis."

This pattern of inconsistency in public attitudes across time and place suggests that globally, much work still remains to reduce the impact of stigma, requiring both personal and public adaptation. Several possible strategies have been highlighted, including educating people affected by epilepsy and their families to address the relationship among knowledge, stigma, and adjustment;[111,112] developing and implementing public education initiatives[113,114] to promote increased awareness of epilepsy as a social and medical disorder; advocating and increasing the level of contact between people affected by epilepsy and those who are not to create an environment that can influence legislative and policy change[115,116]; and launching worldwide strategies, such as the current Global Campaign against Epilepsy initiative, Epilepsy: Out of the Shadows.[117] Central to any intervention, however, is the need to focus on reducing the misconceptions and misinformation about epilepsy that present such a threat to the identity and QOL of persons affected by epilepsy.

HIGH QUALITY OF LIFE IS NOT INCOMPATIBLE WITH HAVING EPILEPSY

Some clear detractors exist for QOL of patients affected by epilepsy, as do some clear promoters. Current research suggests that seizure frequency and psychological co-morbidities are frontrunners among the detractors, but stigma and discrimination are also high on the list and likely contributors to psychological comorbidities. Tackling the negative impacts for QOL of patients affected by epilepsy therefore requires patient-focused inputs from health and social care, and public-focused ones at the wider societal level. As shown in an earlier review by Jacoby and Baker,[118] QOL impacts are clearly linked to the clinical trajectory of epilepsy, but are also intimately linked to the psychosocial contexts in which this trajectory is negotiated, and the relevance and importance of particular QOL issues vary accordingly. This fact highlights a need for interventions aimed at improving QOL of patients affected by epilepsy to be targeted on both sets of determining factors.

Although the two terms have often been used interchangeably by QOL researchers, QOL is a separate and distinct construct from the more confined one of *health status*. In a meta-analysis of 12 chronic illness studies, Smith and colleagues[119] used structural equation modelling to examine the relationship between these constructs. They concluded that they are distinct, with patients giving much greater emphasis to mental health than physical function when rating overall QOL, and vice versa when rating health status.

Buck[120] examined the same interrelationship in the context of stroke. Her informants were asked to rate both health and QOL overall on a five-point scale from excellent to poor. The responses were then correlated with scores on a stroke-specific measure, the NEWSQOL, which comprises 11 domains. Across two separate time points (two points in the stroke trajectory), scores for overall QOL were found to correlate most highly with the domains of sleep, cognition, feelings, and interpersonal relationships, whereas scores for overall health correlated most highly with sleep, cognition, mobility, and fatigue.

In a multiple regression analysis, the strongest QOL predictor was feelings and the strongest health status predictor was sleep. If, as these authors' research supports, QOL and health status are two separate constructs to which aspects of functioning contribute differentially, it is unsurprising that some patients affected by epilepsy are able to report high QOL despite having impaired health status, even very poorly controlled seizures. This article's authors own work and that of others has shown that the two are not inevitably mutually exclusive. Further exploration of the constituent ingredients of high QOL, through research focusing on what has broadly been termed as *resilience*, will be important in defining future interventions aimed at its maximization.

REFERENCES

1. Katz S. The science of quality of life. J Chronic Dis 1987;40(6):459–63.
2. World Health Organisation Quality of Life Group. What quality of life? World Health Organisation quality of life assessment. World Health Forum 1996; 17(4):354–6.
3. Bowling A. What things are important in people's lives? A survey of the public's judgements to inform scales of health related quality of life. Soc Sci Med 1995; 41(10):1447–62.
4. Bowling A. The effects of illness on quality of life: findings from a survey of households in Great Britain. J Epidemiol Community Health 1996;50(2):149–55.
5. Fisher RS, Vickrey B, Gibson P. The impact of epilepsy from the patient's perspective I. Descriptions and subjective perceptions. Epilepsy Res 2000; 41(1):39–51.
6. Jacoby A, Baker GA, Steen N, et al. The clinical course of epilepsy and its psychosocial correlates: findings from a UK Community study. Epilepsia 1996; 37(2):148–61.
7. Baker GA, Jacoby A, Buck D, et al. Quality of life of people with epilepsy: a European study. Epilepsia 1997;38(3):353–62.
8. Leidy NK, Elixhauser A, Vickrey B, et al. Seizure frequency and the health-related quality of life of adults with epilepsy. Neurology 1999;53:162–6.

9. Djibuti M, Shakarishvili R. Influence of clinical, demographic, and socioeconomic variables on quality of life in patients with epilepsy: findings from Georgian study. J Neurol Neurosurg Psychiatr 2003;74(5):570–3.

10. Senol V, Soyuer F, Arman F, et al. Influence of fatigue, depression, and demographic, socioeconomic, and clinical variables on quality of life of patients with epilepsy. Epilepsy Behav 2007;10(1):96–104.

11. Birbeck GL, Hays RD, Cui XP, et al. Seizure reduction and quality of life improvements in people with epilepsy. Epilepsia 2002;43(5):535–8.

12. Kobau R, Zahran H, Grant D, et al. Prevalence of active epilepsy and health-related quality of life among adults with self-reported epilepsy in California: California Health Interview Survey, 2003. Epilepsia 2007;48(10):1904–13.

13. Strine TW, Kobau R, Chapman DP, et al. Psychological distress, comorbidities, and health behaviors among US adults with seizures: results from the 2002 National Health Interview Survey. Epilepsia 2005;46(7):1133–9.

14. Wiebe S, Bellhouse DR, Fallahay C, et al. Burden of epilepsy: the Ontario Health Survey. Can J Neurol Sci 1999;26(4):263–70.

15. Stavem K, Loge JH, Kaasa S. Health status of people with epilepsy compared with a general reference population. Epilepsia 2000;41(1):85–90.

16. Jacoby A. Epilepsy and the quality of everyday life: findings from a study of people with well-controlled epilepsy. Soc Sci Med 1992;34(6):657–66.

17. Dworetzky BA, Hoch DB, Wagner AK, et al. The impact of a single seizure on health status and health care utilization. Epilepsia 2000;41(2):170–6.

18. Velissaris SL. The psychosocial effects of a newly diagnosed seizure in adulthood [PhD Thesis]. Melbourne, Australia: University of Melbourne; 2009.

19. Bien CG, Schulze-Bonhage A, Soeder BM, et al. Assessment of the long-term effects of epilepsy surgery with three different reference groups. Epilepsia 2006;47(11):1865–9.

20. Jones JE, Berven NL, Ramirez T, et al. Long-term psychosocial outcomes of anterior temporal lobectomy. Epilepsia 2002;43(8):896–903.

21. Tellez-Zenteno JF, Dhar R, Hernandez-Ronquillo L, et al. Long-term outcomes in epilepsy surgery: antiepileptic drugs, mortality, cognitive and psychosocial aspects. Brain 2007;130(2):334–45.

22. Spencer SS, Berg AT, Vickrey B, et al. Health-related quality of life over time since resective epilepsy surgery. Ann Neurol 2007;62(4):327–34.

23. Mikati MA, Comair YG, Rahi A. Normalization of quality of life three years after temporal lobectomy: a controlled study. Epilepsia 2006;47(5):928–33.

24. Wilson SJ, Bladin PF, Saling MM, et al. The longitudinal course of adjustment after seizure surgery. Seizure 2001;10(3):165–72.

25. Perucca P, Carter J, Vahle V, et al. Adverse antiepileptic drug effects: towards a clinically and neurobiologically relevant taxonomy. Neurology 2009;72(14): 1223–9.

26. Perucca P, Gilliam FG, Schmidt B. Epilepsy treatment as a pre-determinant of psychosocial ill-health. Epilepsy Behav 2009;15(2):S31–5.

27. Baker GA, Frances P, Middleton E. Initial development, reliability, and validity of a patient-based adverse events scale. Epilepsia 1994;35(Suppl 7):80.

28. International Bureau for Epilepsy. Epilepsy and cognitive function survey. Heemstede, Netherlands: IBE; 2004.

29. Baker GA, Hargis E, Hish M, et al. Perceived impact of epilepsy in teenagers and young adults: an international survey. Epilepsy Behav 2008;12(3):395–401.

30. Baker GA, Taylor J, Hermann B. How can cognitive status predispose to psychological impairment? Epilepsy Behav 2009;15:S31–5.

31. Gilliam FG, Fessler AJ, Baker G, et al. Systematic screening allows reduction of adverse antiepileptic drugs: a randomized trial. Neurology 2004;62(1):23–7.
32. Jacoby A, Johnson AL, Chadwick DW. Psychosocial outcomes of antiepileptic drug discontinuation. Epilepsia 1992;33(6):1123–31.
33. Jacoby A. Psychosocial functioning in people with epilepsy in remission and the outcomes of antiepileptic drug withdrawal [PhD Thesis]. Newcastle Upon Tyne, United Kingdom: University of Newcastle Upon Tyne; 1995.
34. Hessen E, Lossius MI, Reinvang I, et al. Slight improvement in mood and irritability after antiepileptic drug withdrawal: a controlled study in patients on monotherapy. Epilepsy Behav 2007;10(3):449–55.
35. Sillanpaa M, Haataja L, Shinnar S. Perceived impact of childhood onset epilepsy on quality of life as an adult. Epilepsia 2004;45(8):971–7.
36. Global Campaign Against Epilepsy. Atlas: epilepsy care in the World 2005. Geneva: WHO; 2005.
37. Jacoby A, Graham-Jones S, Baker GA, et al. A general practice records audit of the process of care for people with epilepsy. Br J Gen Pract 1996;46(411): 595–9.
38. Scambler G. Coping with epilepsy. In: Laidlaw J, Richens A, Chadwick DW, editors. A textbook of epilepsy. Edinburgh: Churchill Livingston; 1993. p. 733–47.
39. Chomba EN, Haworth A, Atadzhanov M, et al. Zambian health care workers knowledge, attitudes, beliefs, and practices regarding epilepsy. Epilepsy Behav 2007;10(1):111–9.
40. Hanna NJ, Black M, Sander JW, et al. The national sentinel audit of epilepsy-related death. London (England): The Stationery Office; 2002.
41. DiIorio C, Shafer PO, Letz R, et al. The association of stigma with self-management and perceptions of health care among adults with epilepsy. Epilepsy Behav 2003;4(3):259–67.
42. Elliot JO, Lu B, Shneker B, et al. Comorbidity, health screening and quality of life among persons with a history of epilepsy. Epilepsy Behav 2009;14(1): 125–9.
43. Pulsipher DT, Seidenberg M, Jones J, et al. Quality of life and comorbid medical and psychiatric conditions in temporal lobe epilepsy. Epilepsy Behav 2006;9(3): 510–4.
44. Gaitatzis A, Trimble MR, Sander JW. The psychiatric comorbidity of epilepsy. Acta Neurol Scand 2004;110(4):207–20.
45. Gilliam F, Kanner AM. Treatment of depressive disorders in epilepsy patients. Epilepsy Behav 2002;3(5):S2–9.
46. Kobau R, Gilliam F, Thurman DJ. Prevalence of self-reported epilepsy or seizure disorder and its associations with self-reported depression and anxiety: results from the 2004 Health Styles survey. Epilepsia 2006;47(11):1915–21.
47. Hesdorffer DC, Lee P. Health, wealth and culture as predominant factors in psychosocial morbidity. Epilepsy Behav 2009;15(2):S36–40.
48. Beghi E, Spagnoli P, Airoldi L, et al. Emotional and affective disturbances in patients with epilepsy. Epilepsy Behav 2002;3(3):255–61.
49. Attarian H, Vahle V, Carter J, et al. Relationship between depression and intractability of seizures. Epilepsy Behav 2003;4(3):298–301.
50. Mensah SA, Beavis JM, Thapar AK, et al. The presence and clinical implications of depression in a community population of adults with epilepsy. Epilepsy Behav 2006;8(1):213–9.
51. Ettinger A, Reed M, Cramer J. Depression and comorbidity in community-based patients with epilepsy or asthma. Neurology 2004;63(6):1008–14.

52. Loring DW, Meador KJ, Lee GP. Determinants of quality of life in epilepsy. Epilepsy Behav 2004;5(6):976–80.
53. Zeber JE, Copeland LA, Amuan M, et al. The role of comorbid psychiatric conditions in health status in epilepsy. Epilepsy Behav 2007;10(4):539–46.
54. Boylan LS, Flint LA, Labovitz DL. Depression but not seizure frequency predicts quality of life in treatment-resistant epilepsy. Neurology 2004;62(2): 258–61.
55. Tracy JI, Dechant V, Sperling MR, et al. The association of mood with quality of life ratings in epilepsy. Neurology 2007;68(14):1101–7.
56. Johnson EK, Jones JE, Seidenberg M. The relative impact of anxiety, depression, and clinical seizure features on health-related quality of life in epilepsy. Epilepsia 2004;45(5):544–50.
57. Beyenburg S, Mitchell AJ, Schmidt D, et al. Anxiety in patients with epilepsy: systematic review and suggestions for clinical management. Epilepsy Behav 2005;7(2):161–71.
58. Salas-Puig J, Gil-Nagel A, Serratosa JM, et al. Self-reported memory problems in everyday activities in patients with epilepsy treated with antiepileptic drugs. Epilepsy Behav 2009;14(4):622–7.
59. Luthar SS, Cicchetti D. The construct of resilience: implications for interventions and social policies. Dev Psychopathol 2000;12(4):857–85.
60. Bartlet M, editor. Capability and resilience: beating the odds. London, England: University College London; 2006.
61. Bonanno GA. Loss, trauma, and human resilience: have we underestimated the human capacity to thrive after extremely aversive events? Am Psychol 2004; 59(1):20–8.
62. Pei-Fan M. Transition experience of parents caring for children with epilepsy: a phenomenological study. Int J Nurs Stud 2008;45(4):543–51.
63. Amir M, Roziner I, Knoll A, et al. Self-efficacy and social support as mediators in the relation between disease severity and quality of life in patients with epilepsy. Epilepsia 1999;40(2):216–24.
64. Pais-Ribeiro J, da Silva AM, Meneses RF, et al. Relationship between optimism, disease variables, and health perception and quality of life in individuals with epilepsy. Epilepsy Behav 2007;11(1):33–8.
65. Barak Y, Achiron A. Happiness and neurological diseases. Expert Rev Neurother 2009;9(4):445–59.
66. Oyegbile TO, Dow C, Jones J, et al. The nature and course of neuropsychological morbidity in chronic temporal lobe epilepsy. Neurology 2004;62(10):1736–42.
67. Wakamoto H, Nagao H, Hayashi M, et al. Long-term medical, educational, and social prognoses of childhood-onset epilepsy: a population-based study in a rural district of Japan. Brain Dev 2000;22(4):246–55.
68. Giovagnoli AR, Meneses RF, da Silva AM. The contribution of spirituality to quality of life in focal epilepsy. Epilepsy Behav 2006;9(1):133–9.
69. Hermann B, Jacoby A. The psychosocial impact of epilepsy in adults. Epilepsy Behav 2009;15(2):S11–6.
70. Hermann BP, Wyler AR. Depression, locus of control and the effects of epilepsy surgery. Epilepsia 1989;30(3):332–8.
71. Hermann BP, Whitman S, Wyler AR, et al. Psychosocial predictors of psychopathology in epilepsy. Br J Psychiatry 1990;156(1):98–105.
72. Asadi-Pooya AA, Schiling CA, Glosser D, et al. Health locus of control in patients with epilepsy and its relationship to anxiety, depression and seizure control. Epilepsy Behav 2007;11(3):347–50.

73. Gramstad A, Iversen E, Engelsen BA. The impact of affectivity dispositions, self-efficacy and locus of control on psychosocial adjustment in patients with epilepsy. Epilepsy Res 2001;46(1):53–61.
74. Jacoby A. Quality of life: age-related considerations. In: Engel J, Pedley TA, editors, Epilepsy: a comprehensive textbook, vol. 2. Philadelphia: Lippincott-Raven; 1998. p. 1121–30.
75. Austin JK, Shelton Smith M, Risinger MW, et al. Childhood epilepsy and asthma: comparison of quality of life. Epilepsia 1994;35(3):608–15.
76. Miller V, Palermo TM, Grewe SD. Quality of life in pediatric epilepsy: demographic and disease-related predictors and comparison with healthy controls. Epilepsy Behav 2003;4(1):36–42.
77. Kim WJ. Psychiatric aspects of epileptic children and adolescents. J Am Acad Child Adolesc Psychiatry 1991;30(6):874–86.
78. Williams J, Steel C, Sharp GB, et al. Parental anxiety and quality of life in children with epilepsy. Epilepsy Behav 2003;4(5):483–6.
79. Tallis R. Epilepsy in old age. Epilepsy: a Lancet review. Lancet 1990;336:519–20.
80. Devinsky O. Quality of life in the elderly. Epilepsy Behav 2005;6(1):1–3.
81. Martin R, Vogtle L, Gilliam F, et al. What are the concerns of older adults living with epilepsy? Epilepsy Behav 2005;7(2):297–300.
82. Baker GA, Jacoby A, Buck D, et al. Quality of life of older people with epilepsy: findings from a UK community study. Seizure 2001;10(2):92–9.
83. Pugh MJV, Copeland LA, Zeber JE, et al. The impact of epilepsy on health status among younger and older adults. Epilepsia 2005;46(11):1820–7.
84. Alanis-Guevara I, Pena E, Corona T, et al. Sleep disturbances, socioeconomic status, and seizure control as main predictors of quality of life in epilepsy. Epilepsy Behav 2005;7(3):481–5.
85. Campbell-Sills L, Forde DR, Stein MB. Demographic and childhood environmental predictors of resilience. J Psychiatr Res, in press.
86. Hesdorffer D, Tian H, Anand K, et al. Socioeconomic status is a risk factor for epilepsy in Icelandic adults but not in children. Epilepsia 2005;46(8):1297–303.
87. Heaney DC, MacDonald BK, Everitt A, et al. Socioeconomic variation in incidence of epilepsy: a prospective community based study in southeast England. BMJ 2002;325:1013–6.
88. Li X, Sundquist J, Sundquist K. Socioeconomic and occupational risk factors for epilepsy: a nationwide epidemiological study in Sweden. Seizure 2008;17(3):254–60.
89. Begley CE, Basu R, Reynolds T, et al. Sociodemographic disparities in epilepsy care: results from the Houston/New York City health care use and outcomes study. Epilepsia 2009;50(5):1040–50.
90. Das K, Banerjee M, Mondal GP, et al. Evaluation of socio-economic factors causing discontinuation of epilepsy treatment resulting in seizure recurrence: a study in an urban epilepsy clinic in India. Seizure 2007;16(7):601–7.
91. Temkin O. The falling sickness. Baltimore (MD): John Hopkins Press; 1971.
92. McLin WM, de Boer HM. Public perceptions about epilepsy. Epilepsia 1995;36(10):957–9.
93. Jacoby A. Stigma, epilepsy and quality of life. Epilepsy Behav 2002;3(6):S10–20.
94. Dell JL. Social dimensions of epilepsy, stigma and response. In: Whitman S, Hermann BP, editors. Psychopathology in epilepsy, social dimensions. New York: Oxford University Press; 1986. p. 185–210.

95. Weiss MG, Ramakrishna J. Interventions: research on reducing stigma. Presented at Stigma and Global Health: Developing a Research Agenda. An International Conference, Bethesda. Available at: www.stigmaconference.nih.gov. September 5–7, 2001. Accessed: July 10th, 2008.

96. Gallhofer B. Epilepsy and its prejudice: teachers' knowledge and opinions—are they a response to psychopathological phenomena? Psychopathology 1984; 17(4):187–212

97. Ratsepp M, Oun A, Haldre S, et al. Felt stigma and impact of epilepsy on employment status among Estonian people: exploratory study. Seizure 2000; 9(6):394–401.

98. Jacoby K, Jacoby A. Epilepsy and insurance in the UK: an exploratory survey of the experiences of people with epilepsy. Epilepsy Behav 2004;5(6):884–93.

99. Chadwick DW. Quality of life and quality of care in epilepsy. RSM round table series No.23. London, England: Royal Society of Medicine; 1990.

100. Collings J. Psychosocial well-being and epilepsy: an empirical study. Epilepsia 1990;31(4):418–26.

101. Jacoby A. Felt versus enacted stigma: a concept revisited. Evidence from a study of people with epilepsy in remission. Soc Sci Med 1994;38(2):269–74.

102. Baker GA, Brooks J, Buck D, et al. The stigma of epilepsy: a European perspective. Epilepsia 2000;41(4):98–104.

103. Suurmeijer TPBM, Reuvekamp MF, Aldenkamp BP. Social functioning, psychological functioning, and quality of life in epilepsy. Epilepsia 2001;42(9):1160–8.

104. Trostle J. Social aspects: stigma, beliefs and measurement. In: Engel J, Pedley TA, editors, Epilepsy: a comprehensive textbook, vol. 2. Philadelphia: Lippincott-Raven; 1998. p. 2183–9.

105. Caveness WF, Gallup GH Jr. A survey of public attitudes towards epilepsy in 1979 with an indication of trends over the past thirty years. Epilepsia 1980; 21(5):509–18.

106. Canger JR, Cornaggia C. Public attitudes towards epilepsy in Italy: results of a survey and comparison with USA and West German data. Epilepsia 1985; 26(3):221–6.

107. Novotna I, Rektor I. The trend in public attitudes in the Czech Republic towards persons with epilepsy. Eur J Neurol 2002;9(5):535–40.

108. Mirnics Z, Czikora G, Zavecz T, et al. Changes in public attitudes towards epilepsy in Hungary: results of a survey conducted in 1994 and 2000. Epilepsia 2001;42(1):86–93.

109. Jacoby A, Gorry J, Gamble C, et al. Public knowledge, private grief: a study of public attitudes to epilepsy in the United Kingdom and implications for stigma. Epilepsia 2004;45(11):1405–15.

110. Spatt J, Bauer G, Baumgartner C, et al. Predictors for negative attitudes toward subjects with epilepsy: a representative survey in the general public in Austria. Epilepsia 2005;46(5):736–42.

111. Al Adawi S, Al Salmy H, Martin RG, et al. Patient's perspective on epilepsy: self knowledge among Omanis. Seizure 2003;12(1):11–8.

112. Doughty J, Baker GA, Jacoby A, et al. Cross-cultural differences in levels of knowledge about epilepsy. Epilepsia 2003;44(1):115–23.

113. JilekAall L, Jilek M, Kaaya J, et al. Psychosocial study of epilepsy in Africa. Soc Sci Med 1997;45(5):783–95.

114. Gutteling JM, Seydel ER, Wiegman O. Previous experiences with epilepsy and effectiveness of information to change public perception of epilepsy. Epilepsia 1986;27(6):739–45.

115. de Boer H, Aldenkamp AP, Bullivant F, et al. Horizon: the trans-national epilepsy training project. Int J Adolesc Med Health 1994;7(4):325–35.
116. The Epilepsy Foundation [editorial]. Epilepsy Behav 2004;5(3):275–6.
117. Global Campaign Against Epilepsy. Out of the shadows. Available at: http://www.WHO.int. Accessed: July 10th, 2008.
118. Jacoby A, Baker GA. Quality of life trajectories in epilepsy. Epilepsy Behav 2008;12(4):557–71.
119. Smith KW, Avis NE, Assmann SF. Distinguishing between quality of life and health status in quality of life research: a meta-analysis. QOL Research 1999; 8(5):447–59.
120. Buck D. Development and validation of a stroke-specific quality of life measure [PhD Thesis]. Newcastle Upon Tyne, United Kingdom: University of Newcastle Upon Tyne; 2001.

Depression and Epilepsy: A Review of Multiple Facets of Their Close Relation

Andres M. Kanner, MD[a,b,c,d,*]

KEYWORDS

- Major depressive disorder
- Hippocampal atrophy • Temporal lobe epilepsy
- Frontal lobe epilepsy • Anxiety disorders

Today, the study of depressive disorders in epilepsy no longer is restricted to an understanding of psychosocial causes but includes an incorporation of the recent advances in research of the neurobiologic bases of mood disorders and epilepsy, which are providing important answers to the mechanisms mediating the complex relation between these two conditions. Thus, the cause of depressive disorders in epilepsy is multifactorial, including neurochemical and electrophysiologic changes related to the actual seizure disorder, iatrogenic causes, genetic predisposition for mood disorders, and psychosocial causes.

Following an overview, this article reviews the common pathogenic mechanisms operant in mood disorders and epilepsy that explain their relatively high comorbidity. This is followed by a brief review of the clinical manifestations and consequences of depressive disorders in these patients and to suggest practical strategies for their identification by non-psychiatrists.

OVERVIEW

Three-week-old Wistar rats underwent a rapid kindling to the ventral hippocampus.[1] Two to 4 weeks later, the rats were subjected to two tests developed to assess the

[a] Department of Neurological Sciences, Rush University Medical Center, 1653 West Congress Parkway, Chicago, IL 60612, USA
[b] Department of Psychiatry, Rush University Medical Center, Armour Academic Center, 600 South Paulina Street, Suite 202 Chicago, IL 60612, USA
[c] Laboratory of Electroencephalography and Video-EEG-Telemetry, Rush University Medical Center, 1653 West Congress Parkway, Chicago, IL 60612, USA
[d] Section of Epilepsy and Rush Epilepsy Center, Rush University Medical Center, 1653 West Congress Parkway, Chicago, IL 60612, USA
* Department of Neurological Sciences, Rush University Medical Center, 1653 West Congress Parkway, Chicago, IL 60612.
E-mail address: akanner@rush.edu

Neurol Clin 27 (2009) 865–880
doi:10.1016/j.ncl.2009.08.002   neurologic.theclinics.com
0733-8619/09/$ – see front matter © 2009 Elsevier Inc. All rights reserved.

presence of depression-equivalent phenomena in animal models: the forced swim test (FST) and the taste preference toward calorie-free saccharin or sucrose solutions. In the FST, a rat is placed in a situation of despair, which allows for assessment of its ability to adopt active strategies in an inescapable stressful situation. Failure to do so, as evidenced by increased immobility time during the FST, is interpreted as equivalent to a depression-like state. The second test tries to replicate the loss of an animal's ability to experience pleasure, as evidenced by loss of taste preference. Normal animals prefer sweetened to regular water; animals with suspected equivalent symptoms of depression do not exhibit such a preference. Kindled animals exhibited a sustained increase in immobility time in the FST and loss of taste preference toward calorie-free saccharin, as compared with controls.

A decade previously, a different group of investigators reported on an animal model of epilepsy using the genetic epilepsy prone rat (GEPR), with its two strains, GEPR-3 and GEPR-9; they are characterized by genetically determined predisposition to sound-induced generalized tonic/clonic seizures.[2] These animals exhibit symptomatology and endocrinologic changes reminiscent of mood disorders in humans, which are attributed to innate pre- and postsynaptic noradrenergic and serotonergic transmission deficits. The noradrenergic abnormalities result from deficient arborization of neurons arising from the locus coeruleus coupled with excessive presynaptic suppression of stimulated norepinephrine (NE) release in the terminal fields and lack of postsynaptic compensatory upregulation.[2] GEPR-9 rats have a more pronounced NE transmission deficit and exhibit more severe seizures than GEPR-3 rats.[3] The serotonergic abnormalities are attributed to abnormal serotonergic arborization coupled with deficient postsynaptic serotonin$_{1A}$-receptor density in the hippocampus.[4] Both strains have increased corticosterone serum levels, deficient secretion of growth hormone, and hypothyroidism, all of which are commonly found in humans with major depressive disorder.[5] Increments of NE or serotonin transmission with the selective serotonin reuptake inhibitor (SSRI), sertraline, can result in a dose-dependent seizure-frequency reduction in the GEPR, which correlates with extracellular thalamic serotonergic thalamic concentrations.[6] In addition, the serotonin precursor, 5-hydroxytryptamine, has anticonvulsant effects in GEPRs when combined with a monoamine oxidase inhibitor, whereas SSRIs and monoamine oxidase inhibitors exert anticonvulsant effects in genetically prone epilepsy mice and baboons and in nongenetically prone cats, rabbits, and rhesus monkeys.[6–10] High serum corticosterone levels and evidence of overactive hypothalamic-pituitary-adrenal axis are demonstrated in animal models of epilepsy and depression using Wistar rats; the extent of the hypothalamic-pituitary-adrenal hyperactivity was independent of recurrent seizures but positively correlated with the severity of equivalent symptoms of depressive mood as assessed with the tests (discussed previously).[11]

These data provide evidence of a close relation between epilepsy and phenomena associated with depressive disorders and suggest the existence of common pathogenic mechanisms operant in animal models of epilepsy and depression. Studies carried out in humans with epilepsy support such a complex relation between the two conditions: several population-based studies have established that PWE have a 5- to 20-fold higher risk of developing mood disorders,[12,13] whereas patients with a history of mood disorders have a four- to sevenfold higher risk of developing epilepsy.[14–16] These data seem to suggest a bidirectional relation between depression and epilepsy.

Another expression of this complex relation is illustrated by the impact that a history of depression has on the response of seizures to pharmacologic and surgical treatment. For example, in a study of 780 patients with newly diagnosed epilepsy, patients with a psychiatric history, in particular a history of depression preceding the onset of epilepsy, were 2.2 times more likely to develop pharmacoresistant epilepsy than those without.[17] Likewise, in a recent study, Kanner and colleagues[18,19] demonstrated that a lifetime history of depression was a predictor of failure to reach a postsurgical seizure outcome free of auras and disabling seizures after an anterotemporal lobectomy in 100 consecutive patients followed for a mean period of 8.3 ± 3.3 years. These two studies raise the question of whether patients with a history of depression who go on to develop epilepsy are at greater risk of having a more severe form of seizure disorder.

Depressive disorders are common in PWE. For example, in a study of 36,984 subjects, Tellez-Zenteno and colleagues[12] reported a 17.4% lifetime prevalence of major depressive disorders in epilepsy patients (95% CI, 10.0–24.9) versus 10.7% (95% CI, 10.2–11.2) in the general population. Furthermore, PWE had a 24.4% (95% CI, 16.0–32.8) lifetime prevalence for any type of mood disorder versus 13.2% (95% CI, 12.7–13.7). Other community-based studies have generally reported overall rates of major depression (diagnosed by interview or scores from questionnaires indicating clinical major depression) of 10% to 30%[13,20] whereas clinic/hospital-based studies reported rates of 20% to 50%.[21] Despite the high co-morbidity of depressive disorders in epilepsy, they remain under-recognized and undertreated.[22-24]

DEPRESSION: A NEUROLOGIC DISORDER WITH PSYCHIATRIC SYMPTOMS

What are the bases for this assumption? A review of the literature of the neurobiologic aspects of mood disorders supports this point: first, primary neuronatomic abnormalities presenting as structural, functional, and neuropathologic abnormalities have been reported in many studies of humans with primary mood disorders. Similar abnormalities in the same structures have been reported in PWE, in particular limbic structures in frontal and temporal lobes and subcortical structures, such as basal ganglia and thalamic nuclei. Following is a summary of the evidence available.

Structural Abnormalities

Hippocampal atrophy

In 75% to 80% of patients with temporal lobe epilepsy (TLE), mesial structures (amygdala, hippocampal formation, entorhinal cortex, and parahippocampal gyrus) are the site of the epileptogenic area[25] and hippocampal atrophy caused by mesial temporal sclerosis is the most frequent cause of TLE. By the same token, the prevalence of depression is significantly higher in PWE who have involvement of mesial temporal structures. Furthermore, bilateral hippocampal atrophy has been demonstrated by several investigators in patients with recurrent major depressive disorders without epilepsy, including patients whose mood disorder is in remission.[26-28] In addition, a significant inverse correlation between the duration of depression and the magnitude of (left) hippocampal volume is documented, whereas lower verbal memory scores were associated with the hippocampal damage of these patients.[28]

Changes in amygdala

Bilateral atrophy of the amygdala in primary major depressive disorders, attributed to a decrease of the core volumes of amygdala nuclei, also is reported.[26] Likewise, atrophy of the amygdala is often identified in patients with TLE secondary to mesial temporal sclerosis.

Neuropathologic findings

The existence of neuropathologic abnormalities in major depressive disorders further supports the neurologic nature of this condition. Apoptosis was demonstrated in a neuropathologic study of hippocampal formations that included 15 patients with a history of major depressive disorders, 16 matched controls, and nine steroid-treated patients (because high steroids are associated with hippocampal atrophy).[29] Apoptosis was present in entorhinal cortex, subiculum, dentate gyrus, and CA1 and CA4 of 11 depressed patients, three steroid-treated patients, and one control. No apoptosis of pyramidal cells, however, in CA3 was identified.

Likewise, in a neuropathologic investigation of amygdala and entorhinal cortex, in which neuronal and glial cell counts were performed in brains from seven patients with major depressive disorders (10 with bipolar disorders and 12 control cases), there was a sizable reduction of glial cells and of the glial/neurons ratio in the left amygdala and, to a lesser degree, in the left entorhinal cortex in the specimens of patients with major depressive disorders and in those of patients with bipolar disorder not treated with lithium and valproic acid.[30] In mesial temporal sclerosis, neuropathologic findings consist of astrocytosis and neuronal cell loss, most prominently in CA1 and CA3 and to a lesser degree in the dentate gyrus and subiculum, and in the amygdala, entorhinal cortex and parahippocampal gyrus.[25]

Structural Abnormalities in Frontal Lobes

Structural changes have also been identified in the prefrontal cortex, cingulate gyrus, and their white matter. Bremner and colleagues[31] reported smaller orbitofrontal cortical volumes in 15 patients with depression compared with those of 20 controls. Similarly, Coffey[32] identified smaller frontal lobe volumes in 48 inpatients with severe depression who were referred for electroshock therapy compared with 76 control patients. Taylor and colleagues[33] reported smaller orbitofrontal cortex volumes in 41 elderly patients with major depression than in 40 controls. Additionally, these investigators reported that the decreased volumes were independently associated with cognitive impairment.[34] In a study by Kumar and colleagues,[35] the magnitude of prefrontal volume changes was related to the severity of the depression, as elderly patients with major depression had greater changes than those with minor depression.

Likewise, neuropathologic studies have noted structural cortical changes in frontal lobes of depressed patients. Rajkowska and colleagues[36] reported a decrease in cortical thickness, neuronal size, and densities in layers II, III, and IV of the rostral orbitofrontal region in brains of depressed patients. There were sizable reductions in glial densities in cortical layers V and VI in the caudal orbitofrontal cortex that were also correlated with a lessoning of neuronal sizes. Lastly, the dorsolateral prefrontal cortex showed a decrease in neuronal and glial density and size in all cortical layers.

Abnormalities Demonstrated by Functional Neuroimaging Studies

Studies using positron emission tomography (PET) have documented a decrease in serotonin transmission in patients with primary depressive disorders and in PWE. For example, studies of unmedicated and medicated depressed patients compared with healthy volunteers demonstrated a decrease of serotonin$_{1A}$ receptor binding in frontal, temporal, and limbic cortex.[37–39] Binding potential values in medicated patients were similar to those in unmedicated patients.[38]

Similar abnormalities in serotonin$_{1A}$ receptor binding also were identified in patients with TLE. For example, in a PET study of patients with TLE, reduced serotonin$_{1A}$ binding was found in mesial temporal structures ipsilateral to the seizure focus in patients with and without hippocampal atrophy.[40] In addition, a 20% binding reduction was found in the raphe as well as 34% lower binding in the ipsilateral thalamic region to the seizure focus. In a separate study, decreased binding was identified in the epileptogenic hippocampus, amygdala, anterior cingulated and lateral temporal neocortex ipsilateral to the seizure focus, and also the contralateral hippocampi, but to a lesser degree, and the raphe nuclei.[41] Other investigators reported the decrease in binding of serotonin$_{1A}$ was significantly greater in the areas of seizure onset and propagation identified with intracranial electrode recordings. As in the other studies, reduction in serotonin$_{1A}$ binding was present even when quantitative and qualitative MRI was normal.[42]

One study compared serotonin$_{1A}$ receptor binding between 37 TLE patients with and without major depressive disorder and interictal PET.[43] In addition to decreased serotonin$_{1A}$ receptor binding in the epileptic focus, patients with TLE and major depressive disorders exhibited a significantly more pronounced reduction in serotonin$_{1A}$ receptor binding, extending into nonlesional limbic brain areas outside the epileptic focus. In a second study of 45 patients with TLE, Hasler, et al[44] demonstrated an inverse correlation between severity of symptoms of depression identified on the Beck Depression Inventory and serotonin$_{1A}$ receptor binding at the hippocampus ipsilateral to the seizure focus and to a lesser degree at the contralateral hippocampus and midbrain raphe. Likewise, Gilliam and colleagues[45] correlated the severity of symptoms of depression in 31 patients with TLE with the magnitude of hippocampal abnormalities identified with ^{1}H magnetic resonance spectroscopic imaging technique at 4.1 tesla using creatine/N-acetylaspartate ratio maps.[46]

Involvement of frontal lobes in primary depression has also been demonstrated with functional neuroimaging (PET and single photon emission CT).[46–48] For example, executive abnormalities are consistently reported in studies and are more apparent in more severe depressive disorders. These neuropsychologic disturbances correlated with reduced blood flow in mesial prefrontal cortex.[48]

Frontal lobe epilepsy also is associated with a higher prevalence of depression, not unlike TLE. This is not surprising given that the inferior frontal cortex is the main target of the mesolimbic dopaminergic neurons and gives input to the serotonergic neurons of the dorsal raphe nucleus. Thus, it seems that frontal lobe dysfunction may be related to a deficit in serotonergic transmission, which can predispose to depression. Functional disturbances of frontal lobe structures have been recognized in TLE, particularly in patients with TLE and comorbid depression who have been found to have bilateral reduction in inferofrontal metabolism.[49,50] Likewise, neuropsychologic testing with the Wisconsin Card Sorting Test, which is highly sensitive to executive dysfunction, has revealed poor performance in patients with TLE and comorbid depression.[51,52]

Abnormal serotonin$_{1A}$ receptor binding is not restricted to TLE and FLE. PET studies targeting the serotonin$_{1A}$ receptors reported a decreased binding potential in the dorsolateral prefrontal cortex, raphe nuclei, and hippocampus of 11 patients with juvenile myoclonic epilepsy compared with 11 controls.[53] A high comorbidity of depression and anxiety disorders has been reported in patients with this epilepsy syndrome.

Clinical Manifestations of Depressive Disorders in Epilepsy

Depressive disorders in PWE are multifaceted and may present as clusters of depressive symptoms, such as sadness, crying bouts, and feelings of anhedonia and irritability, or may appear as well-characterized disorders that meet diagnostic criteria included in the *Diagnostic and Statistical Manual of Mental Disorders, Fourth Edition* (*DSM-IV*), such as major depressive episodes and bipolar disorders. Yet, in a significant percentage of patients, mood disorders fail to meet any of the *DSM-IV* criteria. Readers are referred to the clinical criteria included in the *DSM-IV, Text Revision (DSM-IV-TR)* classification.[54] This article focuses on the clinical characteristics that are particular to depressive episodes in PWE.

In PWE, depressive episodes and symptoms have the unique characteristic of having a temporally related occurrence with seizures. Thus, they may precede (preictal) or follow the seizure (postictal), they can be the expression of the seizure (ictal), or they can occur independently of seizures (interictal).

Preictal depressive symptoms and episodes

Blanchet and Frommer investigated mood changes in the course of 56 days in 27 PWE who rated their mood on a daily basis. Symptoms of depression were reported 3 days before a seizure in 22 patients.[55] The severity of these symptoms worsened during the 24 hours preceding the seizure.

Ictal symptoms of depression

Ictal symptoms of depression are the clinical expression of a simple partial seizure in which these symptoms constitute its predominant phenomenology. It has been estimated that psychiatric symptoms occur in 25% of auras; 15% of these involve affect or mood changes.[56,57] At times, mood changes represent the only expression of simple partial seizures, and consequently, it may be difficult to recognize them as epileptic phenomena. They typically are brief, stereotypical, occur out of context, and are associated with other ictal phenomena. The most frequent symptoms include feelings of anhedonia, guilt, and suicidal ideation. More typically, however, ictal symptoms of depression are followed by alteration of consciousness as the ictus evolves from a simple to a complex partial seizure.

Postictal symptoms of depression

Postictal symptoms of depression have been investigated in a systematic manner in a study of 100 consecutive patients with poorly controlled partial seizure disorders carried out at the Rush Epilepsy Center.[58] Only symptoms that occurred after more than 50% of seizures for the previous 3-month period were included in the study. In this study, the postictal period was defined as the 72 hours that followed a seizure. Among the 100 patients, 43 experienced a mean of 4.8 ± 2.4 postictal symptoms of depression (range 2 to 9; median 5). The median duration of two thirds of symptoms was 24 hours. Thirteen of these patients experienced a minimum of seven postictal symptoms of depression lasting 24 hours or longer. Postictal suicidal ideation was identified in 13 patients (discussed later).

Interictal depressive episodes

Interictal depressive episodes are more frequent than ictal and peri-ictal depressive episodes. As stated previously, interictal depressive disorders can mimic depressive disorders included in the *DSM-IV* classification. In 25% to 50% of PWE, however, depressive episodes fail to meet *DSM-IV* diagnostic criteria. For example, using *Diagnostic and Statistical Manual of Mental Disorders, Revised Third Edition* criteria, Mendez and colleagues[59] classified approximately 50% of depressive disorders as atypical depression. Wiegartz and colleagues[23] reported that the depressive episodes of 25% of PWE were also classified as atypical depression not otherwise specified. The atypical characteristics of depressive episodes in PWE were described by Kraepelin in 1923 and confirmed a few years later by Bleuler and Gastaut.[60–62] These three investigators separately described a pleomorphic pattern of symptoms that included affective symptoms consisting of prominent irritability intermixed with euphoric mood, fear, symptoms of anxiety, anergia, pain, and insomnia. Blumer coined the term, *inter-ictal dysphoric disorder* to refer to this type of depression in epilepsy[63] and estimated that it occurred in two thirds of depressed PWE. Kanner and colleagues[22] have also identified dysthymic-like depressive episodes in PWE in a study of 97 consecutive patients with refractory epilepsy and depressive episodes severe enough to merit pharmacotherapy: 28 (29%) met *DSM-IV* criteria for major depressive disorder. The remaining 69 patients (71%) failed to meet criteria for any of the *DSM-IV* categories and presented a clinical picture consisting of anhedonia (with or without hopeless-ness), fatigue, anxiety, irritability, poor frustration tolerance, and mood lability with bouts of crying. Some patients also reported changes in appetite and sleep patterns and problems with concentration. Most symptoms presented with a waxing and waning course, with repeated, interspersed, symptom-free periods of 1 to several days' duration. The semiology most resembled a dysthymic disorder, but the recur-rence of intermittent symptom-free periods precluded *DSM-IV* criteria for this condition.

It is important to distinguish the atypical depression in epilepsy from the atypical depression according to *DSM-IV*, which includes mood reactivity (ie, mood brightens in response to actual or potential positive events) and at least two of the following symptoms[1]: significant weight gain or increase in appetite[2]; hypersomnia (sleeping too much, as opposed to the insomnia present in melancholic depression)[3]; leaden paralysis (ie, heavy, leaden feelings in arms or legs)[4]; and long-standing pattern of interpersonal rejection sensitivity (not limited to episodes of mood disturbance). Symptoms should result in significant social or occupational impairment, and melan-cholic depression or catatonic depression should not be diagnosed during the same episode.[54]

Comorbid Occurrence of Anxiety and Depressive Episodes

In patients with depressive disorders with or without epilepsy, the evaluation is incom-plete without screening for symptoms or full episodes of anxiety. For example, in a meta-analysis of studies that investigated comorbidity between depression and anxiety disorders in patients without epilepsy, Dobson and Cheung concluded that in patients with a depressive disorder a mean of 67% (range 42% to 100%) also experienced anxiety disorders concurrently or in their lifetime; conversely, in patients with anxiety disorders, a mean of 40% (range 17% to 65%) also suffered from depression.[64] By the same token, comorbid occurrence of primary social phobia and major depression and dysthymia of up to 70% is reported.[65]

In PWE, comorbid anxiety and depressive disorders are also a common occurrence. In a study of 188 PWE from five epilepsy centers, 73% of patients with a history of depression also met *DSM-IV* criteria for an anxiety disorder.[66] In that study, the *DSM-IV-TR* diagnosis of mood or anxiety disorders was established with the Mini-International Neuropsychiatric Interview (MINI) and the Structured Clinical Interview for *DSM-IV* Axis I Diagnosis.

Subsyndromic Forms of Depression

Comorbid depressive symptoms can also occur in subclinical or subsyndromic forms, with significant clinical consequences. For example, in the study of 188 consecutive PWE, 26 (64%) failed to meet any *DSM-IV* axis I diagnosis; yet, using self-rating instru-ments (Beck Depression Inventory and the Center for Epidemiologic Studies Depres-sion Scale), 26 patients also experienced symptoms of depression of mild to moderate severity. The quality of life of these patients was significantly worse than that of asymptomatic patients (Andres M. Kanner, MD, unpublished data).

Impact of Depressive Disorders in Epilepsy

Depressive disorders have a negative impact on the lives of PWE at multiple levels. First, as discussed previously, a lifetime history of depressive disorders is a predictor of a more severe form of epilepsy.[17,18] Secondly, depressive disorders are a serious risk factor for the development of suicidal ideation, behavior, and complete suicide. Third, the presence of a depressive disorder is a strong independent predictor of poor quality of life in these patients. These points are discussed in greater detail later.

Suicidality in Epilepsy

In the general population in the United States, the lifetime prevalence rates of suicide are estimated from approximately 1.1% to 1.2%, whereas the suicide attempt rates range from 1.1% to 4.6%. Recent population-based studies have reported that PWE have a three times higher risk of committing suicide than controls.[67] The highest risk of suicide was identified in PWE and comorbid psychiatric disease, in particular those with a depressive disorder, who had a 32-fold higher risk of committing suicide. In a second population-based study (from Canada) that included a sample of 36,984 subjects, the lifetime prevalence of suicidal ideation was twice as high in PWE (25%; 95% CI, 17.4–32.5) compared with that of the general population (13.3%; 95% CI, 12.8–13.8).[12] From a review of 17 studies on suicidal behavior in PWE, Robertson suggested that the lifetime prevalence rates of suicide and suicidal attempts ranged between 5% and 14.3%.[68] Furthermore, patients with TLE had suicidal rates 6 to 25 times greater than the general population.

Variables Associated with Suicidality in Epilepsy

A bidirectional relation between suicidality and epilepsy

It would be logical to assume that suicidality is a consequence of psychiatric comorbidities. Yet, there seems to be a bidirectional relation between suicidality and epilepsy; in other words, not only are PWE at greater risk of developing suicidality but also patients with a history of suicidality are at increased risk of developing epilepsy. In a population-based study performed in Iceland, Hesdorffer and colleagues[16] reported that a prior history of suicidality was associated with a fivefold increased risk of developing epilepsy. The increased risk of suicidal patients of developing epilepsy points to common pathogenic mechanisms at play in both conditions, most likely mediated by abnormal serotonergic activity in the brain.

Suicidal ideation as a postictal phenomenon

Suicidal ideation can be a habitual postictal symptom. As stated previously, in a study of 100 consecutive patients with refractory partial epilepsy, Kanner and colleagues[58] identified postictal suicidal ideation in 13 patients (13%) after more than 50% of their seizures during the previous 3 months; their duration ranged from 0.5 to 108 hours with a median duration of 24 hours. Active and passive suicidal ideation was reported by five and eight patients, respectively. Ten of these 13 patients (77%) had a past history of major depression or bipolar disorder and this association was highly significant. Furthermore, the presence of postictal suicidal ideation was also significantly associated with a history of psychiatric hospitalization. Postictal symptoms of depression were accompanied by postictal symptoms of anxiety and postictal neurovegetative symptoms.

Suicidal ideation as a complication of an interictal psychiatric disorder

The presence of psychiatric comorbidities is significantly associated with an increased risk of suicidal behavior and ideation. For example, in a study of 205 consecutive PWE from five epilepsy centers, Jones and colleagues[69] reported a 12.2% prevalence rate of current suicidal ideation and a 20.8% lifetime prevalence rate of suicide attempts. Current major depressive (47% versus 13% in those without) or anxiety disorders (58.8% versus 30.3%) were the two psychiatric conditions predictive of current suicidal ideation. In addition, major depressive episode and a manic episode were the two predictors of a lifetime suicide attempt. Other investigators have reported similar findings.

Iatrogenic suicidality

The suicidal risk associated with antiepileptic drugs (AEDs) has been recognized for a long time and reported particularly with barbiturates (phenobarbital and primidone), and especially in patients with a family history of mood disorders.[70] Suicidal ideation also is reported with other AEDs, however, such as topiramate, zonisamide, levetiracetam, vigabatrin, and felbamate, by facilitating the development of mood and anxiety episodes.[71–73] In addition, suicidal ideation and behavior can be also be precipitated by discontinuation of AEDs with mood-stabilizing properties (eg, valproic acid, carbamazepine, oxcarbazepine, and lamotrigine) in patients with a mood disorder that had been in remission with these AEDs. Finally, a small percentage of patients with refractory epilepsy who become seizure-free may develop the phenomenon of forced normalization presenting as a major depressive episode, which can result in suicidal ideation and behavior.

In January of 2008, the Food and Drug Administration (FDA) issued an alert regarding the association between suicidality and AEDs, which was based on results of a meta-analysis that included data from 199 randomized clinical trials of 11 AEDs[74]: carbamazepine, felbamate, gabapentin, lamotrigine, levetiracetam, oxcarbazepine, pregabalin, tiagabine, topiramate, valproate, and zonisamide.[6] The meta-analysis encompassed a total of 43,892 patients treated for epilepsy, psychiatric disorders, and other disorders, predominantly pain. The FDA concluded that there was a statistically significant 1.80-fold increased risk of suicidality with exposure to AEDs. Suicidality occurred in 4.3 per 1,000 patients treated with AEDs in the active arm compared with 2.2 per 1,000 patients in the comparison arm. Of all the suicidality reported, suicidal ideation accounted for 67.6%, preparatory acts for 2.8%, attempts for 26.8%, and completed suicide for 2.8%. AEDs were associated with a greater risk for suicidality with epilepsy (odds ratio [OR] 3.53; 95% CI, 1.28–12.10) than with psychiatric disorders (OR 1.51; 95% CI, 0.95–2.45) or other disorders (OR 1.87; 95% CI, 0.81–4.76). However, the validity of the results of this meta-analysis recently has been questioned because of several methodologic problems, including[75]

1. The assessment of suicidality was not gathered in a systematic prospective manner and was based on "spontaneous" reports of patients.
2. The FDA associated the increased risk of suicide with all AEDs, despite the fact that statistical significance was found in only two drugs (topiramate and lamotrigine) of the 11 AEDs studied.
3. Most epilepsy trials (92%) include patients on adjunctive therapy (compared with 14% of psychiatric trials and 15% of other medical trials). It is unclear whether or not the higher suicidality rates in the epilepsy trials were due to drug interactions, given the high proportion of epilepsy trials designed with polytherapy.
4. Suicidal behavior was greater in certain geographic regions. For example, the OR of suicidality was 1.38 in North American studies and 4.53 in studies done elsewhere. Such differences strongly suggest serious methodologic errors in data gathering.

Impact of Depression in the Quality of Life of Patients with Epilepsy

Depressive disorders yield a significant negative impact on the quality of life of PWE. Four studies reported that the presence of symptoms of depression was the most powerful predictor for each domain of health-related quality of life[76–80] and in patients with pharmacoresistant epilepsy, depression, and not seizure frequency and severity, was an independent predictor of poor quality of life. For example, Gilliam and colleagues[76] examined the variables responsible for poor quality of life identified with the Quality of Life in Epilepsy Inventory-89 (QOLIE-89) in 194 adult patients with refractory partial epilepsy and concluded that the only independent variables significantly related to poor quality-of-life scores on the QOLIE-89 summary score were high levels of depression and neurotoxicity from AEDs. Patients had a median 9.7 seizures per month (range 0.3 to 51), but the investigators saw no relationship between the type and or the frequency of seizures and summary scores.

Likewise, the presence of comorbid depressive episodes is associated with a higher use of medical services (not related to the psychiatric conditions), leading to higher costs. For example, Cramer and colleagues[81] reported that people whose depression was untreated used significantly more health resources of all types, independent of seizure type and time since the last seizure.[80] Furthermore, people with mild to moderate depression had twofold and people with severe depression fourfold higher frequency of medical visits than nondepressed people. Also, the presence and severity of depression was a predictor of worse disability scores (Sheehan Disability Scale), independent of duration of the seizure disorder.[81,82]

Screening for Depressive and Anxiety Episodes

As discussed previously, depressive disorders remain under-recognized and under-treated. A practical way of starting to solve this serious problem is to provide neurologists with screening instruments or brief questionnaires that can begin to identify symptomatic patients. It should be emphasized, however, that these screening instruments are "suggestive" of a diagnosis of depressive or anxiety disorders but such diagnoses need to be established with a more formal evaluation by a mental health worker.

An instrument to identify major depressive episodes is a six-item, self-rating screen, called the Neurologic Disorders Depression Inventory for Epilepsy (NDDI-E), which was developed specifically for PWE.[83] None of its items can be confounded with adverse events of AEDs or cognitive symptoms associated with the seizure disorder or the underlying neurologic insult that caused the epilepsy. The NDDI-E takes less than 3 minutes to complete; a score of 15 or higher is suggestive of a major depressive episode and serves as a red-flag referral to a psychiatrist for further evaluation.

As stated previously, all evaluations of depressive disorders must be accompanied by a screening for anxiety symptoms. No self-rating instrument to identify symptoms of generalized anxiety disorder has been validated for PWE. The Patient Health Questionnaire, Generalized Anxiety Disorder-7 (GAD-7) is a seven-item, self-rating instrument that takes 3 minutes to complete and is extensively used in patients with medical disorders; a score of greater than 10 is suggestive of a generalized anxiety disorder.[84]

Similarly, there are no self-rating instruments to assess a history of suicidality. Therefore, the suicidality module of the MINI[85] is used to provide valuable information. This module inquires about the history of any suicide attempt in the past, which is a strong predictor of future completed suicides. The other five questions investigate the severity of the suicidal ideation (eg, from having passive suicidal thoughts to having a plan).

Implications for Therapy

The data reviewed in this article suggest that an increase in serotonergic and noradrenergic activity has an anticonvulsant effect in animal models of epilepsy.[2-10] Regarding treatment of depressive disorders in PWE, however, it is worth reviewing additional studies that investigate the anticonvulsant efficacy of extracellular hippocampal serotonin in an animal model of pilocarpine-induced seizures in conscious rats.[86,87] Serotonin perfusions protected the rats from experiencing seizures as long as the extracellular serotonin concentrations increased between 80% and 350% from baseline. Concentrations above 900% of baseline, however, worsened seizures. This experimental model replicates the circumstances in which SSRIs and other antidepressant drugs can cause seizures in humans. A review of the literature shows that with the exception of four drugs (bupropion, amoxapine, mianserin, and clomipramine), antidepressant drugs are safe in PWE (unless taken in overdoses).[88,89] Furthermore, one double-blind placebo-controlled study with imipramine[88,90] and three open trials with SSRIs given to PWE show a decrease in seizure frequency.[91-93] Finally, a study by Alper and colleagues[94] suggested that the occurrence of seizures in depressed patients may be an expression of the increased risk of developing epileptic seizures associated with mood disorders (discussed previously).[14-16] Their data also suggest that exposure of SSRIs and selective serotonin and NE antidepressants may have a protective effect. In a comparison of seizure incidence in multiple, randomized, multicenter, placebo-controlled studies of SSRIs, the serotonin-NE reuptake inhibitor, venlafaxine, and the α_2-antagonist, mirtazapine, carried out for regulatory purposes in patients with primary depressive disorders, patients randomized to antidepressant medication had a significantly lower seizure occurrence standardized seizure ratio: 0.48 (95% CI, 0.36–0.61). These data demonstrate that the use of antidepressant medication is safe in PWE, as long as it is prescribed at therapeutic doses. The misconception that antidepressant drugs lower the seizure threshold pertains to the use of the four antidepressants (discussed previously) or to cases of toxic doses, such as overdoses or in patients whose serum concentrations can increase to toxic levels because of a genetic predisposition to a slow hepatic metabolism of these drugs.

SUMMARY

Depressive disorders are the most frequent comorbidity of PWE. As discussed in this article, the depressive disorder is another expression of a neurologic disorder with psychiatric symptoms. The high comorbidity of both conditions can be explained by the existence of common pathogenic mechanisms whereby one condition facilitates the occurrence of the other. The negative impact of depressive disorders in the life of PWE is significant; hence, a prompt recognition should be followed by a treatment designed to yield complete symptom remission.

REFERENCES

1. Mazarati AM, Siddarth P, Baldwin RA, et al. Depression after status epilepticus: behavioural and biochemical deficits and effects of fluoxetine. Brain 2008;131: 2071–83.

2. Jobe PC, Dailey JW, Wernicke JF. A noradrenergic and serotonergic hypothesis of the linkage between epilepsy and affective disorders. Crit Rev Neurobiol 1999;13:317–56.
3. Jobe PC, Mishra PK, Browning RA, et al. Noradrenergic abnormalities in the genetically epilepsy-prone rat. Brain Res Bull 1994;35:493–504.
4. Dailey JW, Mishra PK, Ko KH, et al. Serotonergic abnormalities in the central nervous system of seizure-naive genetically epilepsy-prone rats. Life Sci 1992; 50:319–26.
5. Jobe PC. Affective disorder and epilepsy comorbidity in the genetically epilepsy prone-rat (GEPR). In: Gilliam F, Kanner AM, Sheline YI. Depression and brain dysfunction. London: Taylor & Francis; 2006. p. 121–157.
6. Yan QS, Jobe PC, Dailey JW. Thalamic deficiency in norepinephrine release detected via intracerebral microdialysis: a synaptic determinant of seizure predisposition in the genetically epilepsy-prone rat. Epilepsy Res 1993;14:229–36.
7. Meldrum BS, Anlezark GM, Adam HK, et al. Anticonvulsant and proconvulsant properties of viloxazine hydrochloride: pharmacological and pharmacokinetic studies in rodents and the epileptic baboon. Psychopharmacology (Berl) 1982; 76:212–7.
8. Polc P, Schneeberger J, Haefely W. Effects of several centrally active drugs on the sleep wakefulness cycle of cats. Neuropharmacology 1979;18:259–67.
9. Piette Y, Delaunois AL, De Shaepdryver AF, et al. Imipramine and electroshock threshold. Arch Int Pharmacodyn Ther 1963;144:293–7.
10. Yanagita T, Wakasa Y, Kiyohara H. Drug-dependance potential of viloxazine hydrochloride tested in rhesus monkeys. Pharmacol Biochem Behav 1980;12: 155–61.
11. Mazarati AM, Shin D, Kwon YS, et al. Elevated plasma corticosterone level and depressive behavior in experimental temporal lobe epilepsy. Neurobiol Dis 2009;34(3):457–61.
12. Tellez-Zenteno JF, Patten SB, Jetté N, et al. Psychiatric comorbidity in epilepsy: a population-based analysis. Epilepsia 2007;48:2336–44.
13. O'Donoghue MF, Goodridge DM, Redhead K, et al. Assessing the psychosocial consequences of epilepsy: a community-based study. Br J Gen Pract 1999; 49(440):211–4.
14. Forsgren L, Nystrom L. An incident case referent study of epileptic seizures in adults. Epilepsy Res 1999;6:66–81.
15. Hesdorffer DC, Hauser WA, Annegers JF, et al. Major depression is a risk factor for seizures in older adults. Ann Neurol 2000;47:246–9.
16. Hesdorffer DC, Hauser WA, Olafsson E, et al. Depression and suicidal attempt as risk factor for incidental unprovoked seizures. Ann Neurol 2006;59:35–41.
17. Hitiris N, Mohanraj R, Norrie J, et al. Predictors of pharmacoresistant epilepsy. Epilepsy Res 2007;75:192–6.
18. Kanner AM, Byrne R, Chicharro A, et al. A lifetime psychiatric history predicts a worse seizure outcome following temporal lobectomy. Neurology 2009;72:793–9.
19. Jacoby A, Baker GA, Steen N, et al. The clinical course of epilepsy and its psychosocial correlates: findings from a U.K. Community study. Epilepsia 1996; 37(2):148–61.
20. Ettinger A, Reed M, Cramer J, Epilepsy Impact Group. Depression comorbidity in community-based patients with epilepsy or asthma. Neurology 2004;63:1008–14.
21. Edeh J, Toone B. Relationship between interictal psychopathology and the type of epilepsy. Results of a survey in general practice. Br J Psychiatry 1987;151: 95–101.

22. Kanner AM, Kozak AM, Frey M. The use of sertraline in patients with epilepsy: is it safe? Epilepsy Behav 2000;1(2):100–5.

23. Wiegartz P, Seidenberg M, Woodard A, et al. Co-morbid psychiatric disorder in chronic epilepsy: recognition and etiology of depression. Neurology 1999; 53(Suppl 2):S3–8.

24. de Marinis A, Bustamante F, Asmad C, et al. Prevalence and underrecognition of depression in patients with epilepsy: the experience of the Chilean League Against Epilepsy [abstract]. Epilepsia 2006. Presented at the annual meeting of the American Epilepsy Society, San Diego (CA). December 2 to 5, 2006.

25. Mathern GW, Babb TL, Armstrong DL. Hippocampal sclerosis. In: Engel J, Pedley TA, editors. Epilepsy: a comprehensive textbook. Philadelphia, New York: Lippincott-Raven; 1997. p. 133–55.

26. Sheline YI. Brain structural changes associated with depression. In: Gilliam F, Kanner AM, Sheline YI. Depression and brain dysfunction. London: Taylor & Francis; 2006. p. 85–104.

27. Posener JA, Wang L, Price JL, et al. High-dimensional mapping of the hippocampus in depression. Am J Psychiatry 2003;160:83–9.

28. Bell-McGinty S, Butters MA, Meltzer CC, et al. Brain morphometric abnormalities in geriatric depression: long term neurobiological effects of illness duration. Am J Psychiatry 2002;159(8):1424–7.

29. Lucassen PJ, Muller MB, Holsboer F, et al. Hippocampal apoptosis in major depression is a minor event and absent from subareas at risk for glucocorticoid overexposure. Am J Pathol 2001;158:453–68.

30. Stockheimer CA, Mahajan GJ, Konic LC, et al. Cellular changes in the postmortem hippocampus in major depression. Biol Psychiatry 2004;56:640–50.

31. Bremner JD, Vythilingam M, Vermetten E, et al. Reduced volume of orbitofrontal cortex in major depression. Biol Psychiatry 2002;51(4):273–9.

32. Coffey CE. The role of structural brain imaging in ECT. Psychopharmacol Bull 1994;30(3):477–83.

33. Taylor WD, Steffens DC, McQuoid DR, et al. Smaller orbital frontal cortex volumes associated with functional disability in depressed elders. Biol Psychiatry 2003; 53(2):144–9.

34. Taylor WD, MacFall JR, Steffens DC, et al. Localization of age-associated white matter hyperintensities in late-life depression. Prog Neuropsychopharmacol Biol Psychiatry 2003;27(3):539–44.

35. Kumar A, Zhisong J, Warren B, et al. Depression: early evidence for common neuroanatomical substrates detected by using MRI. Proc Natl Acad Sci U S A 1998;95(13):7654–8.

36. Rajkowska G, Miguel-Hidalgo JJ, Wei J, et al. Morphometric evidence for neuronal and glial prefrontal cell pathology in major depression. Biol Psychiatry 1999;45(9):1085–98.

37. Sargent PA, Kjaer KH, Bench CJ, et al. Brain serotonin 1A receptor binding measured by positron emission tomography with [11C]WAY-100635: effects of depression and antidepressant treatment. Arch Gen Psychiatry 2000;57:174–80.

38. Drevets WC, Frank E, Price JC, et al. PET imaging of serotonin 1A receptor binding in depression. Biol Psychiatry 1999;46:1375–87.

39. Oguendo MA, Placidi GP, Malone KM, et al. Positron emission tomography of regional brain metabolic responses to a serotonergic challenge and lethality of suicide attempts in major depression. Arch Gen Psychiatry 2003;60:14–22.

40. Toczek MT, Carson RE, Lang L, et al. PET imaging of 5-HT1A receptor binding in patients with temporal lobe epilepsy. Neurology 2003;60:749–56.

41. Savic I, Lindstrom P, Gulyas B, et al. Limbic reductions of 5-HT1A receptor binding in human temporal lobe epilepsy. Neurology 2004;62:1343–51.
42. Merlet I, Ostrowsky K, Costes N, et al. 5-HT1A receptor binding and intracerebral activity in temporal lobe epilepsy: an [18F]MPPF-PET study. Brain 2004;127: 900–13.
43. Theodore WH, Giovacchini G, Bonwetsch R, et al. The effect of antiepileptic drugs on 5-HT-receptor binding measured by positron emission tomography. Epilepsia 2006;47(3):499–503.
44. Hasler G, Bonwetsch R, Giovacchini G, et al. 5-HT(1A) receptor binding in temporal lobe epilepsy patients with and without major depression. Biol Psychiatry 2007;62(11):1258–64.
45. Gilliam FG, Maton BM, Martin RC, et al. Hippocampal ^{1}H-MRSI correlates with severity of depression symptoms in temporal lobe epilepsy. Neurology 2007; 68:364–8.
46. Baxter LR, Schwartz JM, Phelps ME, et al. Reduction in the prefrontal cortex glucose metabolism common to three types of depression. Arch Gen Psychiatry 1989;46:243–50.
47. Kimbrell TA, Ketter TA, George MS, et al. Regional cerebral glucose utilization in patients with a range of severities of unipolar depression. Biol Psychiatry 2002; 51:237–52.
48. Liotti M, Mayberg H, McGinnis S, et al. Unmasking disease specific cerebral blood flow abnormalities: mood challenge in patients with remitted unipolar depression. Am J Psychiatry 2002;159:1830–40.
49. Bromfield E, Altshuler L, Leiderman D. Cerebral metabolism and depression in patients with complex partial seizures. Epilepsia 1990;31:625.
50. Jokeit H, Seitz RJ, Markowitsch HJ, et al. Prefrontal asymmetric interictal glucose hypometabolism and cognitive impairment in patients with temporal lobe epilepsy. Brain 1997;12:2283–94.
51. Seidenberg M, Hermann BP, Noe A. Depression in temporal lobe epilepsy: a possible role for associated frontal lobe dysfunction? In: Sackellares JC, Berent S, editors. Psychological disturbances in epilepsy. Newton (MA): Butterworth-Heinemann; 1996. p. 143–57.
52. Hermann BP, Wyler AR, Richey ET. Wisconsin card sorting test performance in patients with complex partial seizures of temporal-lobe origin. J Clin Exp Neuropsychol 1988;10:467–76.
53. Meschaks A, Lindstrom P, Halldin C, et al. Regional reductions in serotonin 1A receptor binding in juvenile myoclonic epilepsy. Arch Neurol 2005;62:946–60.
54. American Psychiatric Association. Diagnostic and statistical manual of mental disorders. Fourth Edition. Washington, DC: American Psychiatric Association Press; 2000.
55. Blanchet P, Frommer GP. Mood change preceding epileptic seizures. J Nerv Ment Dis 1986;174:471–6.
56. Weil A. Depressive reactions associated with temporal lobe uncinate seizures. J Nerv Ment Dis 1955;121:505–10.
57. Daly D. Ictal affect. Am J Psychother 1958;115:97–108.
58. Kanner AM, Soto A, Gross-Kanner H. Prevalence and clinical characteristics of postictal psychiatric symptoms in partial epilepsy. Neurology 2004;62:708–13.
59. Mendez MF, Cummings J, Benson D, et al. Depression in epilepsy. Significance and phenomenology. Arch Neurol 1986;43:766–70.
60. Kraepelin E. In: Psychiatrie, vol. 3. Leipzig: Johann Ambrosius Barth; 1923.
61. Bleuler E. Lehrbuch der Psychiatrie. 8th edition. Berlin: Springer; 1949.

62. Gastaut H, Roger J, Lesèvre N. Différenciation psychologique des épileptiques en fonction des formes électrocliniques de leur maladie [Psychological differentiation of epileptic according to the electroclinical forms of the disease.] Rev Psychol Appl 1953;3:237–49 [in French].

63. Blumer D, Altshuler LL. Affective disorders. In: Engel J, Pedley TA, editors, Epilepsy: a comprehensive textbook, vol. II. Philadelphia: Lippincott-Raven; 1998. p. 2083–99.

64. Dobson KS, Cheung E. Relationship between anxiety and depression: conceptual and methodological issues. In: Maser JD, Cloninger CR, editors. Comorbidity of mood and anxiety disorders. Washington (DC): American Psychiatric Press; 1990.

65. Merikangas KR, Angst J. Comorbidity and social phobia: evidence from clinical, epidemiologic and genetic studies. Eur Arch Psychiatry Clin Neurosci 1995;244: 297–303.

66. Kanner AM, Gilliam FG, Hermann B, et al. Differential effect of mood and anxiety disorders on the quality of life and perception of adverse events to antiepileptic drugs in patients with epilepsy [abstract]. Epilepsia 2007;48(6):1–118.

67. Christensen J, Vestergaard M, Mortensen P, et al. Epilepsy and risk of suicide: a population-based case–control study. Lancet Neurol 2007;6:693–8.

68. Robertson MM. Suicide, parasuicide, and epilepsy. In: Engel J, Pedley TA, editors. Epilepsy: a comprehensive textbook. Philadelphia: Lippincott–Raven; 1997. p. 2141–51.

69. Jones JE, Hermann BP, Barry JJ, et al. Rates and risk factors for suicide, suicidal ideation, and suicide attempts in chronic epilepsy. Epilepsy Behav 2003;4:S31–8.

70. Brent DA, Crumrine PK, Varma RR, et al. Phenobarbital treatment and major depressive disorder in children with epilepsy. Pediatrics 1987;80:909–17.

71. Mula M, Sander JW. Suicidal ideation in epilepsy and levetiracetam therapy. Epilepsy Behav 2007;11:130–2.

72. Mula M, Trimble MR, Yuen A, et al. Psychiatric adverse events during levetiracetam therapy. Neurology 2003;61:704–6.

73. Trimble RM, Rüsch N, Betts T, et al. Psychiatric symptoms after therapy with new antiepileptic drugs: psychopathological and seizure related variables. Seizure 2000;9:249–54.

74. U.S. Department of Health and Human Services, Food and Drug Administration, Center for Drug Evaluation and Research, Office of Translational Sciences, Office of Biostatistics (2008). Statistical review and evaluation: Antiepileptic drugs and suicidality. May 21, 2008.

75. Hesdorffer DC, Kanner AM. The FDA alert on suicidality and antiepileptic drugs: fire or false alarm? Epilepsia 2009;50(5):978–86.

76. Gilliam F, Kuzniecky R, Faught E, et al. Patient-validated content of epilepsy-specific quality-of-life measurement. Epilepsia 1997;38(2):233–6.

77. Lehrner J, Kalchmayr R, Serles W, et al. Health-related quality of life (HRQOL), activity of daily living (ADL) and depressive mood disorder in temporal lobe epilepsy patients. Seizure 1999;8(2):88–92.

78. Perrine K, Hermann BP, Meador KJ, et al. The relationship of neuropsychological functioning to quality of life in epilepsy. Arch Neurol 1995;52(10):997–1003 [see comments].

79. Gilliam F. Optimizing health outcomes in active epilepsy. Neurology 2002; 58(Suppl 5):S9–S19.

80. Boylan LS, Flint LA, Labovitz L, et al. Depression but not seizure frequency predicts quality of life in treatment-resistant epilepsy. Neurology 2004;62(2):258–61.

81. Cramer JA, Blum M, Reed M, et al. The influence of comorbid depression on quality of life for people with epilepsy. Epilepsy Behav 2003;4:515–21.
82. Cramer JA, Blum D, Fanning K, et al. Epilepsy Impact Project Group. The impact of comorbid depression on health resource utilization in a community sample of people with epilepsy. Epilepsy Behav 2004;5:337–42.
83. Gilliam FG, Barry JJ, Hermann BP, et al. Rapid detection of major depression in epilepsy: a multicentre study. Lancet Neurol 2006;5:399–405.
84. Kroenke K, Spitzer RL, Williams JB, et al. Anxiety disorders in primary care: prevalence, impairment, comorbidity, and detection. Ann Intern Med 2007;146: 317–25.
85. Sheehan BV, Lecrubier Y, Sheehan KH, et al. The Mini International Neuropsychiatric Interview (MINI): the development and validation of structured diagnostic psychiatric interview for DSM-IV and ICD-10. J Clin Psychiatry 1998;59(Suppl 20):22–33.
86. Clinckers R, Smolders I, Meurs A, et al. Anticonvulsant action of hippocampal dopamine and serotonin is independently mediated by D2 and 5-HT1A receptors. J Neurochem 2004;89:834–43.
87. Kanner AM, Balabanov A. Depression in epilepsy: how closely related are these two disorders? Neurology 2002;58(Suppl 5):S27–39.
88. Fromm GH, Rosen JA, Amores CY. Clinical and experimental investigation of the effect of imipramine on epilepsy. Epilepsia 1971;12:282.
89. Fromm GH, Wessel HB, Glass JD, et al. Imipramine in absence and myoclonic-astatic seizures. Neurology 1978;28:953–7.
90. Fromm GH, Amores CY, Thies W. Imipramine in epilepsy. Arch Neurol 1972;27: 198.
91. Favale E, Rubino V, Mainardi P, Lunardi G, et al. The anticonvulsant effect of fluoxetine in humans. Neurology 1995;45:1926–7.
92. Specchio LM, Iudice A, Specchio N, et al. Citalopram as treatment of depression in patients with epilepsy. Clin Neuropharmacol 2004;27(3):133–6.
93. Favale E, Audenino D, Cocito L, et al. The anticonvulsant effect of citalopram as an indirect evidence of serotonergic impairment in human epileptogenesis. Seizure 2003;12:316–8.
94. Alper K, Schwartz KA, Kolts RL, et al. Seizure incidence in psychopharmacological clinical trials: an analysis of Food and Drug Administration (FDA) summary basis of approval reports. Biol Psychiatry 2007;62(4):345–54.

The Emerging Architecture of Neuropsychological Impairment in Epilepsy

Bruce P. Hermann, PhD[a],*, Jack J. Lin, MD[b], Jana E. Jones, PhD[a],
Michael Seidenberg, PhD[c]

KEYWORDS

- Neuropsychology • Epilepsy • Neuroimaging
- Temporal lobe epilepsy • White matter

A rich literature dating back to the early twentieth century has characterized the cognitive morbidity associated with the epilepsies and the association of this morbidity with the cause, course, and treatment of the disorder. Critical reviews over the decades have cataloged the links between cognitive disorders and specific clinical features of the epilepsies including their etiology; seizure frequency and severity; complications of the disorder (e.g. status epilepticus); antiseizure medications; and electroencephalographic abnormalities, such as the type, frequency, and distribution of interictal epileptiform and slow wave activity.[1–6]

The understanding of the neuropsychological consequences of the epilepsies evolved in concert with advancements in the wider worlds of cognitive psychology and epilepsy. First, early studies were typically but not exclusively limited to the evaluation of intelligence. Assessment of higher cognitive functions was in its formative years[7] and with the introduction of the Binet-Simon scales, and especially their adaption for use in the United States (eg, the early Vineland translation and the later Stanford-Binet revision), characterization of intellectual status in epilepsy followed quickly.[8] As a deeper understanding of human cognition developed, and newer tests and measures became available to assess those concepts, appreciation of the cognitive correlates of epilepsy expanded apace. Second, much of the early literature came from very limited segments of the population of people with epilepsy, typically from specialized institutions (or colonies) serving

[a] Department of Neurology, University of Wisconsin School of Medicine and Public Health, 600 North Highland Avenue, Madison, WI 53792, USA
[b] Department of Neurology, University of California-Irvine, Irvine, CA 92697, USA
[c] Department of Psychology, Rosalind Franklin School of Medicine and Science, 3333 N. Green Bay Road, North Chicago, IL 60064, USA
* Corresponding author.
E-mail address: hermann@neurology.wisc.edu (B.P. Hermann).

Neurol Clin 27 (2009) 881–907
doi:10.1016/j.ncl.2009.08.001
0733-8619/09/$ – see front matter © 2009 Elsevier Inc. All rights reserved.

neurologic.theclinics.com

the more complicated and severely affected individuals.[3] Over time more representative portions of the population were sought out and investigated, which yielded a less biased but still imperfect characterization of the relationship between epilepsy and intelligence and broader cognitive status.[2,9,10] The focus of research has continued to be on persons with epilepsy presenting to specialized tertiary care medical centers, although more representative population-based studies of cognition are available, particularly among children with epilepsy.[11–14] Third, classification and taxonomy of the epilepsies developed from early rudimentary systems to the evolving and increasingly sophisticated international classification of epileptic seizures and syndromes.[15,16] The neuropsychological features of these syndromes and their primary cognitive signatures have developed accordingly.[6,11,17–20] Finally, as medical technology evolved patients with epilepsy have been studied with increasing sophistication to understand the underlying neurobiology of cognitive impairment in epilepsy, a primary focus of this article.

A critical and fundamental feature of the neuropsychology of epilepsy literature is that throughout its history a primary focus has been the relationship of cognition and cognitive disorders to core clinical features of the epilepsies including but not limited to the age of onset of epilepsy, etiology, seizure type and syndrome, medications, duration of epilepsy, and electroencephalographic features.[21–26] Unequivocal associations between these clinical characteristics and neuropsychological impairments have been reported and repeatedly replicated through the decades, but the neurobiologic mechanisms through which they exert their effects have been investigated less intensively. A new literature is now under way, one linking cognitive abnormalities directly to indices of structural, functional, metabolic, and other neurobiological markers of cerebral integrity, independent of their association with clinical epilepsy characteristics. These trends are reviewed in the material to follow. The initial focus is on temporal lobe epilepsy (TLE) as a model with which to address the core points, because this form of localization-related epilepsy has been very carefully studied from both a cognitive and imaging standpoint. Some pertinent historical issues are touched on first, followed by more detailed reviews of the cognitive and neuroimaging abnormalities that have been found in TLE, followed by an overview of studies examining direct structure-function relationships in TLE and other epilepsies.

THE UNIQUE CONTRIBUTION OF TLE

Psychomotor epilepsy or TLE has provided an especially important window into the neuropsychology of epilepsy. The term "psychomotor epilepsy" was used beginning in the 1930s to describe relatively poorly understood spells that some had called psychic equivalents.[27,28] The early electroencephalographic features were characterized in the context of clinical attacks wherein "....the patient, though he may perform apparently conscious acts, is not subject to command; he may exhibit involuntary tonic movements; he may display psychomotor disturbances....and on recovery he has complete amnesia for the events which occurred in the attack."[27,29,30] These seizures were later found to be associated with an anterior temporal lobe spike focus,[30,31] and consideration of epilepsy surgery for these "nonlesional" patients developed early on in Chicago[32] and Montreal.[33]

Early surgical centers routinely incorporated cognitive assessments in their evaluations, which were performed under the supervision of Donald Hebb[34] and Brenda Milner[35,36] at the Montreal Neurological Institute, Ward Halstead[37] at the University of Illinois, and Victor Meyer at the Maudsley Hospital.[38,39] The neuropsychology of epilepsy benefitted enormously from these early opportunities to assess patients before and after surgery and to correlate cognitive changes with detailed preoperative histories, well-characterized surgical resections, careful neuropathologic examinations of resected tissue, and eventually quantitative neuroimaging.[5]

THE PALM DESERT CONFERENCES ON EPILEPSY SURGERY AND THE NEUROPSYCHOLOGY OF EPILEPSY

Important events for the neuropsychology of TLE were the Palm Desert Conferences on Epilepsy Surgery.[40] Before these international conferences there were varying opinions regarding the operational definition of surgical candidacy. Various reasonable criteria were proposed, including seizure frequency and severity, the number of failed medications, or the degree of social and occupational disability; but consensus remained to be achieved. At the second Palm Desert Conference a focus was placed on "surgically remediable syndromes," among which mesial TLE (mTLE) was prominent.[40] If a syndrome was surgically curable, it should be identified and treated with minimal delay.[41]

This conceptualization had an important impact not only on the thinking regarding optimal patient selection and surgical timing, but it also facilitated increasingly careful characterization of mTLE.[42] At that time details regarding the neuropsychological features of mTLE were few in number and the primary cognitive correlates were viewed as largely linked to material-specific memory impairment demonstrated either through formal cognitive assessment or the Wada Test. A stated contraindication to the syndrome of mTLE was the presence of generalized cognitive compromise, all of this was a reasonable early characterization.[41] For neuropsychologists who saw a steady stream of surgical candidates with well characterized mTLE, however, the neuropsychological correlates were viewed as considerably more complex. Memory asymmetry was indeed seen in a proportion of patients, an asymmetry linked to the degree of neuronal loss and sclerosis in the affected hippocampus,[43] but this pattern often occurred in the context of more distributed cognitive impairment. Formal investigations of the ability of neuropsychological tests to localize and lateralize the ictal-onset area revealed variable discriminatory power[44] and these results were viewed by some as indicative of the limitations of neuropsychological assessment. The material to follow, however, provides an overview of the distributed nature of cognitive abnormality in mTLE in the context of the distributed nature of identified structural abnormalities in mTLE, and their important associations.

THE DISTRIBUTED NATURE OF COGNITIVE IMPAIRMENT IN MTLE

By definition the syndrome of mTLE is a disorder of childhood-adolescent onset.[45] A core finding, clear from some of the earliest cognitive studies and routinely reported through the decades, is that an early age of onset of recurrent seizures is associated with a pernicious impact on a broad array of cognitive functions. This effect was reported as early as 1924[46] and subsequently confirmed in studies of adult patients with diverse seizure types,[10,47–50] and even reported in neuropsychological studies of younger patients with complex partial and other types of seizures.[51–53]

When the comprehensive neuropsychological status of patients with mTLE with confirmed hippocampal sclerosis was examined compared with healthy controls or patients with other TLE syndromes, such as so-called "MRI-negative TLE," mTLE patients exhibited a pattern of distributed cognitive impairment affecting not only memory, but also intelligence quotient (IQ), executive functions, language, sensorimotor, and other abilities **(Fig. 1)**.[54–57]

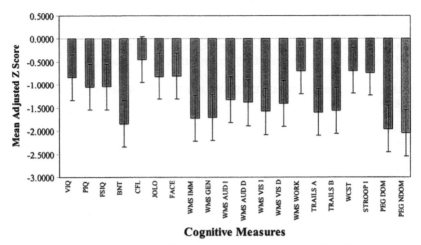

Fig. 1. Mean adjusted (age, gender, education) z scores for patients with TLE compared with healthy control subjects. (*From* Oyegbile TO, Dow C, Jones J, et al. The nature and course of neuropsychological morbidity in chronic temporal lobe epilepsy. Neurology 2004;62:1736–42.)

This average profile of distributed neuropsychological impairment in mTLE, obtained in the context of a focal epileptogenic lesion whose resection results in excellent outcome, was unexpected. The testable hypothesis was that just as memory impairment was related to neuropathology in the hippocampus, perhaps the more widespread neuropsychological abnormalities might be secondary to more diffusely existing neuroanatomic abnormality that could be detected by quantitative neuronimaging techniques, and that individual variability in neuropsychological abnormalities might be associated with individual patterns of anatomic abnormality.[54]

THE DISTRIBUTED NATURE OF ANATOMIC ABNORMALITIES IN CHRONIC TLE

The cumulative neuroimaging literature, focusing here on structural neuroimaging, has shown that anatomic abnormalities in mTLE can be extensive. For reasons that remain to be understood, mTLE seems to be associated with abnormalities in surprisingly diverse neuronal systems, a pattern consistent with the generalized and distributed average neuropsychologic profile of TLE (see **Fig. 1**).

Initial quantitative MRI volumetric and voxel-based morphometry (VBM) studies identified atrophy of the hippocampus,[58–61] along with reports of abnormalities in related structures including entorhinal cortex,[60–63] fornix,[64] parahippocampal gyrus,[61] amygdala,[60,61] basal ganglia,[65,66] and thalamus.[65,67,68] More distant extrahippocampal temporal lobe[58,69–72] and extratemporal lobe regions[69,73] were implicated including the lateral temporal cortex, frontal lobe, and the cerebellum.[74,75] With this degree of distributed atrophy, it is not surprising that reductions in overall total cerebral tissue volume were reported.[56,69,70,76–78]

With few exceptions[68,79] most of the early volumetric investigations examined one or a limited number of structures rather than characterizing a broad and diverse range of regions as to the presence and degree of abnormality. Examination of several regions in the same patient group facilitated appreciation of the distribution and relative degree of structural burden carried by many patients.[68,79] In that regard, a very helpful summary of the presence and distribution of structural abnormality associated with TLE is provided by Keller and Roberts.[80] In their review they surveyed 26 brain regions examined in VBM investigations of TLE compared with healthy controls. Their summary (**Fig. 2**) demonstrates the proportion of studies revealing abnormalities in mesial, extramesial temporal lobe, subcortical, and extratemporal lobe cortical regions. The presence and distribution of these abnormalities would suggest that cognitive abnormalities might extend beyond memory to involve diverse cognitive abilities.

DISTRIBUTED ABNORMALITIES IN CORTICAL SURFACE FEATURES IN TLE

Another example of the potential structural consequences of mTLE is provided by quantitative characterization of the cortical mantle, including indices of gyrification, cortical depth, and surface area. These indices provide important information concerning normal and abnormal brain development, the effects of normal aging, and disease impact.

Lee and colleagues[70] were among the first to examine cortical surface features (sulcal curvature) in unilateral TLE, the bulk of evidence awaiting the development of more sophisticated image processing systems. Accumulating evidence has shown that patients with unilateral TLE exhibit bilateral and diffuse abnormalities in sulcal and gyral curvature, cortical depth, and cortical complexity.[56,81–84]

Oyegbile and colleagues[56] examined cortical surface features in an initial cohort of 96 patients with TLE and 82 healthy controls. They found patients with unilateral TLE to exhibit abnormalities in whole-brain gyral and sulcal curvature with increased surface cerebrospinal fluid (CSF) volume. These cortical surface feature abnormalities were

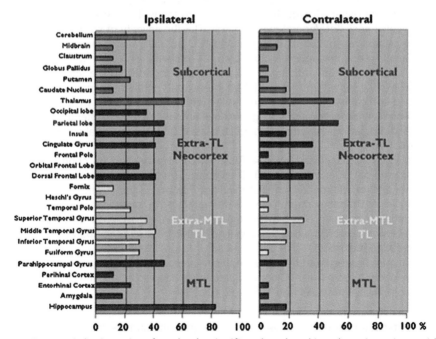

Fig. 2. Twenty-six brain regions found to be significantly reduced in volume in patients with TLE relative to healthy controls. The results are presented ipsilateral and contralateral to the epileptogenic focus. MTL, medial temporal lobe; TL, temporal lobe. (*From* Keller SS, Roberts N. Voxel-based morphometry of temporal lobe epilepsy: an introduction and review of the literature. Epilepsia 2008;49:741–57.)

generalized in nature and evident both contralateral and ipsilateral to the side of temporal lobe seizure onset.

Lin and colleagues[85] examined cortical thickness and cortical complexity in an extremely carefully defined patient cohort. Their cohort of patients exhibited at least three ictally monitored seizures demonstrating unilateral temporal lobe onset, hippocampal sclerosis demonstrated by histopathology, and class 1 outcome 2 years following surgery. Comparing 15 left and 15 right mTLE patients with 19 healthy controls, they found both left and right mTLE groups to have regions with up to 30% bilateral decrease in average cortical thickness, with significant thinning of the bilateral frontal poles, frontal operculum, orbitofrontal, lateral temporal, and occipital regions, right angular gyrus, and primary sensorimortor cortex surrounding the central sulcus (**Fig. 3**). Examining cortical complexity, the left TLE group showed significantly reduced complexity across all left and right hemisphere lobes except the right frontal lobe. The right TLE group exhibited significantly reduced cortical complexity across all lobes except the right frontal and parietal lobes. A very diffuse and bilateral pattern of abnormality was therefore evident in the cortical mantle in patients with unilateral mTLE.

Subsequent studies have elaborated and extended these findings. Bernhardt and colleagues[83] examined 110 patients with TLE (56 left, 54 right) and 45 controls, and **Fig. 4** summarizes the findings. Thinning was evident in bilateral frontocentral (superior, middle, and medial frontal gyrus; precentral gyrus; paracentral lobule); cingulate; and contralateral medial occipitotemporal regions. The most severe frontal thinning occurred in the ipsilateral precentral regions. In addition, there was severe cortical thinning in the hippocampus and parahippocampal regions ipsilateral to side of seizure onset. Contralateral to the seizure focus, there was cortical thinning in the medial occipitotemporal gyrus. In right TLE the severity of atrophy was similar and the pattern resembled that found in left TLE, but less widespread.

McDonald and colleagues[82] compared 21 patients with TLE with 21 healthy controls. Bilateral cortical thinning (5%–15%) was reported in the lateral temporal lobes (Heschl's gyrus) and frontal lobes (precentral, paracentral, pars opercularis). Unilateral cortical thinning was evident in the left superior temporal gyrus and sulcus and medial orbital cortex; and the right middle temporal gyrus and lateral orbitofrontal cortex. If analyses were restricted to mTLE patients, then the parietal cortex was also affected.

Mueller and colleagues[84] used 4-Tesla MRI and examined 35 controls and 15 patients with mTLE and 16 non-mTLE patients. Both groups exhibited widespread temporal and extratemporal cortical thinning. The mTLE group showed significant thinning in ipsilateral temporal lobe (entorhinal cortex, parahippocampal fusiform gyrus, temporopolar–anterior superior temporal region, retrosplenial region) and bilateral precentral-postcentral regions, superior frontal, transverse temporal, precuneus, and prestriate regions.

In summary, widespread temporal and extratemporal lobe abnormalities in cortical surface features seem present, both contralateral and ipsilateral to the side of seizure onset, in mTLE in particular and TLE more generally.

DISTRIBUTED ABNORMALITIES IN WHITE MATTER AND WHITE MATTER TRACTS IN TLE

In addition to gray matter abnormalities, a decrease in white matter volume is present in chronic TLE. Traditional volumetric studies have demonstrated distributed cerebral white matter abnormalities in patients with unilateral TLE, with abnormalities evident both contralateral and ipsilateral to the side of seizure onset, affecting temporal and

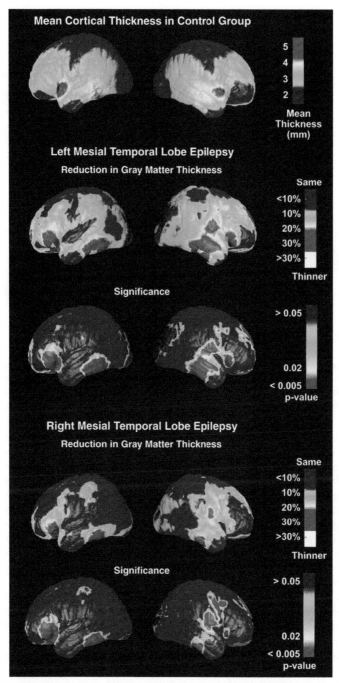

Fig. 3. Cortical thickness maps: regional reduction in mTLE groups. (*From* Lin JJ, Salamon N, Lee AD, et al. Reduced neocortical thickness and complexity mapped in mesial temporal lobe epilepsy with hippocampal sclerosis. Cereb Cortex 2007;17:2007–18.)

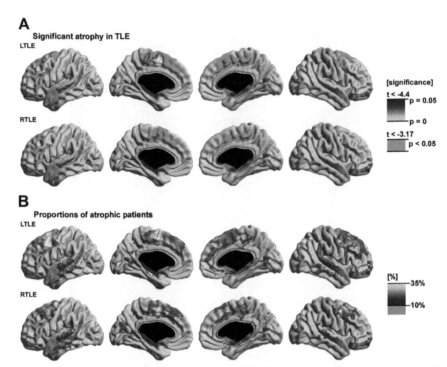

Fig. 4. Atrophy in TLE. Significant atrophy in TLE (*A*). Proportions of atrophic patients (*B*). (*From* Bernhardt BC, Worsley KJ, Besson P, et al. Mapping limbic network organization in temporal lobe epilepsy using morphometric correlations: insights on the relation between mesiotemporal connectivity and cortical atrophy. Neuroimage 2008;42:515–24.)

extratemporal regions.[86] Whole-brain VBM analyses have also demonstrated temporal and extratemporal abnormalities, although the findings are much less extensive and consistent when compared with gray matter VBM studies. McMillan and coworkers[87] found that left TLE patients had reduced white matter volume in the left temporal lobe, corpus callosum, and bilateral prefrontal cortex. In patients with right TLE, only right temporal lobe and fornix showed decreased volume. Bernasconi and colleagues[88] found that both right and left TLE individuals had reduced white matter volume in the temporal lobes, ipsilateral to side of seizure onset and the body of the corpus callosum. The right TLE individuals had additional white matter reduction in the postcentral regions. Their study did not, however, reveal frontal lobe white matter abnormalities.

Although these white matter volumetric studies further elucidate the widespread structural abnormalities in TLE, they do not provide measures of specific white matter tract coherence or the overall integrity of networks connecting different brain regions. Recent compelling evidence from functional imaging, lesional, and behavioral studies suggest that widespread and coordinated networks are required for complex cognitive function.[89] These distributed networks are linked by projection, association, and commissural white matter fiber tracts that connect cortical-subcortical, cortical-cortical, and interhemispheric regions.[90]

In macaque monkeys, interrupting major afferent pathways from the basal forebrain to the temporal lobe, without removal of the medial temporal structures, produces severe amnesia.[91] In addition, simply disconnecting the parietal lobe from the frontal lobe functionally, as can be done by white matter stimulation during surgery, leads to profound neglect in humans.[92] In certain cases, loss or disruption of cerebral connections can produce a greater magnitude of deficits than localized lesions, suggesting the importance of an integrated structural network in normal cognitive functions. This concept has led to a unifying hypothesis that disconnection between important cortical and subcortical regions impairs information transfer and contributes to cognitive impairments.[93] Indeed, such disconnection models can now be tested, using quantitative imaging techniques, such as diffusion tensor imaging (DTI), to interrogate the integrity of white matter tracts.[94]

In DTI, the primary measure of white matter integrity is fractional anisotropy (FA), which is determined by the directional magnitude of water diffusion in three-dimensional space.[95] Tightly packed white matter fascicles provide structural coherence, which results in water diffusion in a preferred direction (high FA). In contrast, white matter fascicles that have poor structural organizations allow water to diffuse more randomly (low FA). Other measures of white matter integrity include mean diffusivity (MD) or apparent diffusion coefficient, which calculates bulk water diffusion characteristic in the intracellular and extracellular water compartments.[96] Using these water diffusion parameters, studies have evaluated the coherence of specific white matter tracts and whole-brain white matter connectivity.

Initial DTI studies used a region of interest approach to investigate specific white matter tracts in the limbic network. One of the first DTI tractography studies evaluated the integrity of fornix and cingulum in patients with mTLE. In these fiber tracts, Concha and colleagues[97] observed diffusion abnormalities ipsilateral and contralateral to the side of seizure onset. Postulating a more diffuse epileptogenic network in TLE, other investigations have extended this initial finding to frontal-temporal (uncinate fasciculus and arcuate fasciculus),[98–100] temporal-occipital (inferior longitudinal fasciculus),[101] frontal-occipital (inferior frontal occipital fasciculus),[101] and interhemispheric (corpus callosum) connections.[102–104] Parallel to the gray matter region of interest studies, these DTI studies have also shown extensive bilateral abnormalities in cortical-cortical, cortical-subcortical, and interhemispheric connections, despite unilateral seizure onset.

More recently, whole-brain voxelwise analysis techniques of DTI data have been developed. These analyses allow mapping of white matter profiles and delineate systemic differences between TLE patients and healthy individuals, without a priori bias for specific tracts or brain regions. DTI data have poor anatomic resolution, which makes spatial matching across multiple subjects particularly challenging. Two methods have been developed to overcome these technical difficulties: VBM and tract-based spatial statistics. In patients with mTLE, both methods revealed extensive bilateral white matter diffusion abnormalities, particularly in the temporal and frontal lobes ipsilateral to the side of seizure onset.[105–107] Tract-based spatial statistics seemed to be more a sensitive method by detecting more extensive white matter changes when compared with traditional VBM methods in the same patient population.[106]

TLE: A LOCALIZATION-RELATED DISORDER?

The essential theme is that although the primary epileptic zone may be contained within the confines of the hippocampus and temporal lobe, considerable anatomic abnormality exists outside this region affecting a myriad of cortical, subcortical, and cerebellar regions and their direct and indirect connectivity. Importantly, the sum of these distributed structural abnormalities, not to mention associated abnormalities in other aspects of brain integrity, such as metabolism and blood flow, may result in a cumulative cognitive and behavioral burden that may be substantial on average, but with a mosaic that may be highly individualized depending on the underlying architecture of a given patient's structural and functional pathology.

LINKING DISTRIBUTED COGNITIVE IMPAIRMENTS WITH DISTRIBUTED NEUROIMAGING ABNORMALITIES: THE MOSAIC OF STRUCTURE-FUNCTION RELATIONSHIPS IN CHRONIC TLE

A developing literature has begun to characterize the links between cognition and the diverse regions of anatomic abnormality in TLE. This section touches on representative examples of these links. Although the focus is on associations between cognition and structural abnormalities, additional investigations albeit smaller in number have examined associations between cognition and behavior with other measures of brain integrity (eg, metabolism, functional MRI [fMRI] activation), and a few representative examples of those studies are included.

Hippocampus

Early studies demonstrated the expected relationship between memory performance and hippocampal pathology characterized by neuronal loss and sclerosis.[108] Subsequent studies demonstrated a link between hippocampal volumes and memory performance before epilepsy surgery, and preoperative left hippocampal volumes were also predictive of the risk of preoperative to postoperative memory change.[58,109,110] Abnormalities in left hippocampal volume have also been shown to be associated with some language-based abilities including confrontation naming[111] and fluency.[112]

Thalamus

The degree to which the thalamus is affected in chronic mTLE is increasingly recognized and there is now a demonstrated link between atrophy of the thalamus and performance on measures of memory and intelligence in TLE.[113,114] In addition, prior fluorodeoxyglucose positron emission tomography research demonstrated that verbal memory was affected in the context of ipsilateral thalamic hypometabolism in patients with left TLE.[115]

Basal Ganglia

Negative symptoms including affective flattening, alogia and avolition, anergia, apathy, anhedonia, and loss of social drive have been reported in patients with TLE.[116,117] These patients also exhibit cognitive and psychosocial correlates that are not seen in patients with TLE without negative symptoms, but neuroimaging correlations with cortical regions were nonspecific and limited only to increased total CSF.[116,117] Geary and coworkers[118] hypothesized that basal ganglia and anterior cingulate regions of interest play a role in the expression of negative symptoms in epilepsy and compared a matched group of TLE patients with and without negative symptoms with healthy controls (N = 22 per group). They found that TLE patients with negative symptoms exhibited significantly reduced volumes in the putamen and globus pallidus, that these volumetric abnormalities were independent of self-reported depression, and that there were specific significant relationships between alogia with volumes of the putamen and globus pallidus, and affective flattening with volume of the putamen.[118]

Frontal Lobe

There has been considerable interest in the neural basis of reported impairments in executive function among patients with TLE and their relevance to "secondary" frontal lobe or frontostriatal pathology. Keller and colleagues[119] examined prefrontal and hippocampal volume using sterology and VBM in 30 controls and 26 left and 17 right TLE patients. Assessment of executive functions included evaluation of response inhibition, working memory, and lexical fluency. They found volume reduction of the ipsilateral hippocampus as expected, but also volume reduction in regions of the prefrontal cortex. In addition, there were significant associations between prefrontal cortex and executive function including working memory with all prefrontal regions examined except right dorsal prefrontal cortex; lexical fluency with left dorsal prefrontal cortex, whole left prefrontal cortex, and left hippocampus; and response inhibition with left ventral prefrontal cortex). Along related lines, an earlier positron emission tomography investigation of patients with TLE showed that extension of hypometabolism into the ipsilateral frontal lobe was associated with cognitive consequences.[120]

Examining 36 patients with unilateral mTLE using VBM, Bonilha and colleagues[121] addressed the extrahippocampal correlates of memory performance. In addition to the contributions of hippocampus, entorhinal, and perirhinal cortices to general and verbal memory, they found that atrophy of the cingulate and orbitofrontal cortex was also associated with disrupted memory performance.

Temporal Lobe

In addition to the investigations of memory and the integrity of the hippocampus reviewed previously, there have been several investigations of temporal lobe structure and memory for unfamiliar and familiar faces.[122,123] These studies include bilateral investigation of T2 relaxation time in hippocampus, amygdala, and fusiform gyrus, showing that worse immediate but not delayed memory was correlated with greater differences in T2 values between left and right fusiform gyrus and hippocampus. Griffith and colleagues[124] examined the relationship between [18F] fluorodeoxyglucose positron emission tomography and performance on a task of famous face recognition, naming, and generation of semantic information in 12 patients with TLE. Strong relationships between all aspects of the Famous Faces Task and the left temporal pole were revealed, whereas Famous Faces Task correlations with the right temporal pole were not significant. These findings indicated that the left temporal pole was associated with lexical and semantic retrieval of knowledge of famous persons in patients with TLE.

Cerebellum

The traditional view of cerebellar function is that it contributes primarily to movement and motor control; however, converging animal and human studies indicate that the cerebellum contributes to a variety of higher cognitive abilities, including specific types of memory.[125,126] Human memory is composed of multiple systems, each mediating specific forms of learning and each dependent on different neuronal networks for efficient operation.[127,128] A clear behavioral and anatomic distinction exists between the conscious recollection of facts and events (explicit or declarative memory) versus memories that are inaccessible to conscious recollection but that are expressed through changes in skills, habits, and other forms of simple associative learning (implicit or procedural memory).[127,128] Classical conditioning, a fundamental form of implicit associative learning, is one type of procedural memory, and conditioning of the eyeblink response is the most commonly investigated conditioning paradigm. The neural circuitry underlying this associative learning has been well characterized and shown to be dependent on the cerebellum.[129] There is now evidence that cerebellar atrophy in TLE is associated with compromised classical eyeblink conditioning.[130]

Cortical Surface Features

Several studies have demonstrated distributed abnormalities in the cortical mantle of patients with unilateral TLE. Only one investigation has examined the association of cognition with cortical surface features (gyral and sulcal curvature, cortical area, and thickness).[56] Among TLE patients, measures of cortical curvature (gyral and sulcal) were significantly associated with performance IQ, verbal and visual memory, simple and complex psychomotor processing, and speeded fine motor dexterity. Total surface area was associated only with verbal IQ.

Amygdala

Abnormalities of the amygdala have been shown to have a relationship with psychopathology both in children[131] and adults with epilepsy.[132] In addition, early onset right mTLE has been shown to be associated with poor facial recognition[133] or for facial emotional processing to be affected following right anterior temporal lobectomy.[134]

CSF

Links between measures of CSF and cognition are uncommon but robust. Indices of total CSF have been associated with measures of cognition including total impairment index.[135,136] Total CSF has also been found to be related to measures of negative symptoms (eg, apathy, anhedonia) but not positive symptoms (eg, hallucinations) or depression in TLE.[117]

Cerebrum Volume

Investigating 28 adult patients with lateralized TLE, Baxendale and coworkers[137] found 15 to exhibit extrahippocampal abnormalities on quantitative MRI analysis. Thirteen of the patient group overall had global or bilateral memory impairment. Bilateral memory deficits were significantly associated with both the presence of cerebral abnormalities and poor postoperative seizure control ($P<.05$). They concluded that disproportions in the regional distribution of gray and white matter in patients with hippocampal sclerosis may form the structural basis of global memory disturbance in patients with TLE.

White Matter Volumes: Cerebrum

Traditional volumetric measures of cerebral white matter volume have been found to have significant associations with multiple cognitive domains including nonverbal intelligence, memory, executive function, and psychomotor processing speed.[138] In addition, total cerebral white matter volumes have been shown to be associated with reaction time and mental scanning efficiency.[139]

White Matter Volume: Corpus Callosum

Volume of the corpus callosum has been found to be reduced in TLE, particularly those with childhood onset.[77,140] Volume of the corpus callosum was found to be significantly related to measures of nonverbal problem solving, immediate memory, complex psychomotor processing, and speeded fine motor dexterity.[140]

White Matter Microstructure: DTI

Recent studies have examined relationships between specific white matter regions or tracts and aspects of cognition and behavior. Flugel and colleagues[141] evaluated diffusion characteristics of TLE patients with (N = 18) and without (N = 20) interictal psychosis and correlated diffusion measures with neuropsychological test scores. The investigators sampled frontal and temporal white matter regions and found that TLE patients with interictal psychosis had greater white matter compromise, as measured by FA, in these brain regions. Further, FA reductions were correlated with cognitive dysfunction and increased negative symptoms. Diehl and colleagues[142] compared the integrity of the uncinate fasciculus, an important frontotemporal white matter tract, between healthy controls (N = 10) and patients with lateralized TLE (N = 28). They demonstrated that TLE patients have bilateral uncinate fasciculus diffusion abnormalities. In patients with left TLE, the integrity of the left uncinate fasciculus was related to verbal memory performances, whereas the integrity of the right uncinate fasciculus was associated with visual memory scores. McDonald and colleagues[143] examined the relationship between cognitive performances and the integrity of several white matter tracts including the uncinate fasciculus, arcuate fasciculus, fornix, parahippocampal cingulum, inferior frontooccipital fasciculus, and corticospinal tract in 17 patients with TLE and 17 healthy controls. Verbal memory and language performances were correlated with MD and FA values of multiple cortical-to-cortical association tracts and limbic projection tracts, particularly in the left hemisphere. Further, cognitive performance was related to anatomic derangements in connections that were germane to the specific cognitive task, such as the relationship between arcuate fasciculus and language scores. These studies demonstrated a clear association between abnormal white matter connections and adverse cognitive outcomes and supported the disconnection model of cognitive dysfunction in patients with TLE.

Multimodality Imaging

Several studies have used fMRI to examine language reorganization in TLE and found that patients with left TLE have a greater propensity for bilateral language representation.[144,145] It was unclear, however, whether such functional reorganization was associated with structural asymmetry in the language network. Recent investigations have combined fMRI and DTI tractography to answer this question.[146] In these studies, patients underwent fMRI tasks, such as reading comprehension and verb generation, to activate language areas in the inferior frontal and superior temporal lobes. DTI tractography was then used to delineate the structural connections between fMRI-defined language areas. Using this combined imaging technique, Powell and colleagues[147] found that left TLE patients had reduced left hemisphere and increased right hemisphere white matter connections, when compared with controls and right TLE patients. Further, a greater degree of lateralization to the left hemisphere was correlated with greater decline in naming function after a dominant hemisphere temporal lobe surgery.[148] The abnormal structural lateralization found in DTI was congruent with fMRI activation patterns and established the important relationship between structure and function in brain regions salient for language processing.

There is no question that anatomic abnormalities in TLE are distributed in nature throughout the brain and have clinical relevance through their association with cognition or behavior. The unique and nonoverlapping associations between specific cognitive abilities and anatomic areas remain to be further determined.

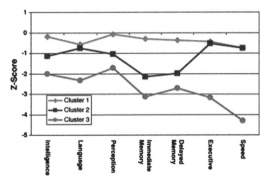

Fig. 5. Cognitive Phenotypes in TLE. (*From* Hermann B, Seidenberg M, Lee EJ, et al. Cognitive phenotypes in temporal lobe epilepsy. J Int Neuropsychol Soc 2007;13:12–20.)

THE LIMITATIONS OF MODAL COGNITIVE PROFILES

Modal or average cognitive profiles clearly help to convey a sense of the overall cognitive burden associated with TLE, an average burden that seems surprisingly onerous. Similarly, modal or average neuroimaging profiles convey a similar impression regarding the neuroanatomic burden. The symmetry between these modal cognitive and neuroimaging profiles helps to make the cognitive pathology understandable. Although helpful, these average profiles are just that, averages, and may not be

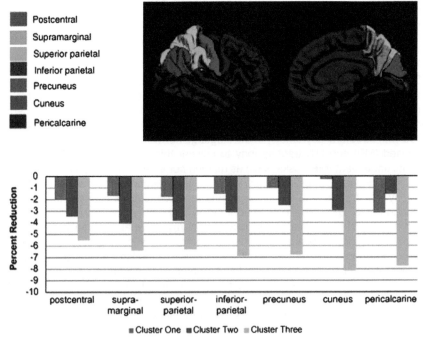

Fig. 6. Bilateral reductions in cortical thickness across cognitive phenotypes. (*From* Dabbs K, Jones J, Seidenberg M, et al. Neuroanatomical correlates of cognitive phenotypes in temporal lobe epilepsy. Epilepsy Behav 2009;15(4):445–51.)

particularly representative of individual patients. There is considerable variability across patients in their patterns of both cognitive and structural abnormalities and the authors have argued that one way to understand this variability is through the study of so-called "cognitive phenotypes."[149–151]

Using cluster analysis and analyzing age- and education-adjusted cognitive domain scores, the authors identified three neuropsychological profile types in adult TLE (**Fig. 5**). One group was characterized by relatively preserved mentation (47% of sample); a second group demonstrated more generally affected mentation but with particular memory impairment (24% of sample); and a third group exhibited diffuse cognitive impairment with especially impaired memory, executive function, and motor-psychomotor processing speed (29% of sample).[149]

Within the context of an average profile of generally affected mentation (see **Fig. 1**), discrete underlying cognitive profile types could be identified. In addition, these groups exhibited varying cognitive prognoses over a subsequent 4-year interval.

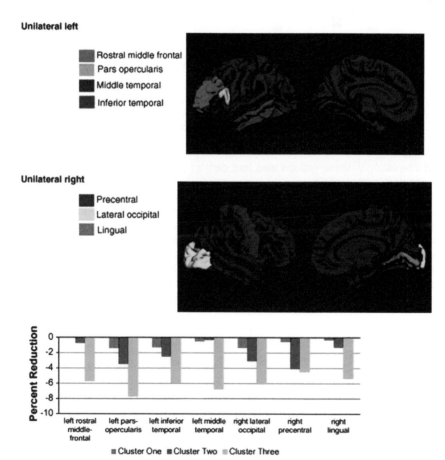

Fig. 7. Unilateral reductions in cortical thickness across cognitive phenotypes. (*From* Dabbs K, Jones J, Seidenberg M, et al. Neuroanatomical correlates of cognitive phenotypes in temporal lobe epilepsy. Epilepsy Behav 2009;15(4):445–51.)

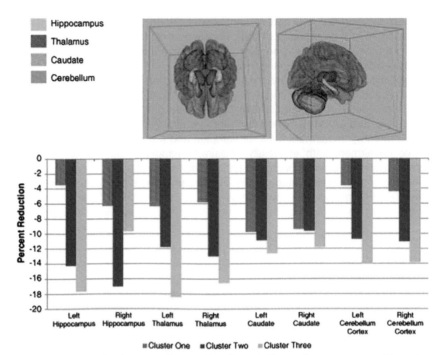

Fig. 8. Volumetric reductions in subcortical and cerebellar regions across cognitive pheno-types. (*From* Dabbs K, Jones J, Seidenberg M, et al. Neuroanatomical correlates of cognitive phenotypes in temporal lobe epilepsy. Epilepsy Behav 2009;15(4):445–51.)

Most interestingly, these groups also had distinct patterns of associated underlying neuroanatomic abnormality.

Specifically, depicted in the accompanying figures and bar graphs are patterns of anatomic abnormality associated with these cognitive phenotypes. Abnormalities in cortical thickness are evident across the cognitive phenotypes detected bilaterally in several areas (**Fig. 6**), unilaterally in others (**Fig. 7**), along with volumetric abnormal-ities in subcortical structures and cerebellum (**Fig. 8**), and targeted white matter tracts (corpus callosum) (**Fig. 9**). The link between cognitive profile and corresponding neuroanatomic abnormality is telling and speaks to the anatomic reality of identified neuropsychological profiles in TLE.[150] Buried within modal profiles of both cognition

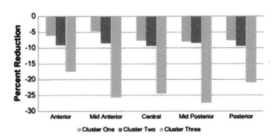

Fig. 9. Volumetric reductions of the corpus callosum across cognitive phenotypes. (*From* Dabbs K, Jones J, Seidenberg M, et al. Neuroanatomical correlates of cognitive phenotypes in temporal lobe epilepsy. Epilepsy Behav 2009;15(4):445–51.)

and anatomic abnormality are groups that vary substantially in their cognitive and associated anatomic status.

IS TLE UNIQUE?

The evidence presented indicates that patients with chronic TLE often exhibit cognitive and quantitative neuroimaging abnormalities that extend beyond the primary zone of seizure onset with significant associations between specific "extratemporal" structural abnormalities and cognitive impairments. These patterns may have their origin in considerable part from the effects of epilepsy and its causes on neurodevelopment as well as progressive abnormalities in a subset of patients. There is suggestive evidence that similar patterns may be evident in other epilepsy syndromes (eg, juvenile myoclonic epilepsy). Early neuropsychological investigations reported impairments in higher level executive functions consistent with the primary thalamofrontal pathophysiology of juvenile myoclonic epilepsy.[152–154] Some recent reports suggest more

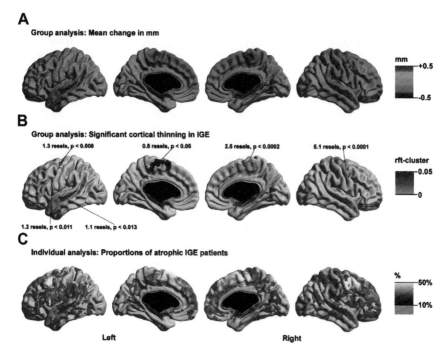

Fig. 10. Group and individual analyses of cortical thickness. (*A*) Absolute differences in cortical thickness (in millimeters) between idiopathic generalized epilepsy (IGE) patients and controls. (*B*) Areas of significant cortical thinning in IGE compared with controls. Peak positions and resolution elements (ie, resels) of significant clusters after random field theory (rft) correction are shown (cluster threshold $t \leq -3.2$, cluster extent threshold 0.8 resels). (*C*) Individual analysis. At each vertex, the corresponding proportion of atrophic patients with a thickness z-score of ≤ -2 SD with respect to healthy controls is shown. Only fractions above 10% are displayed. In controls, no vertex displayed a prevalence of atrophy above 10%. Individual analysis showed widespread atrophy in more than 10% of patients; up to 40% of them had atrophy localized in the same areas detected by the group analysis. (*From* Bernhardt BC, Rozen DA, Worsley KJ, et al. Thalamo-cortical network pathology in idiopathic generalized epilepsy: insights from MRI-based morphometric correlation analysis. Neuroimage 2009;46:373–81.)

distributed neuropsychologic impairment,[155] findings that become understandable in the context of recently reported widely distributed cortical thinning in juvenile myoclonic epilepsy (**Fig. 10**).[156] The degree to which extrathalamofrontal abnormalities are linked to distributed neuropsychologic impairments and the presence and characteristics of phenotypes of structure-function abnormalities remain to be investigated in this and other epilepsy syndromes.

It is hypothesized that within most if not all epilepsy syndromes there exists a distribution of cognitive phenotypes that are linked to structural, metabolic, and other neuroimaging features. These structural abnormalities will lend shape to the patients' neuropsychologic profile. In addition to these structural abnormalities with associated neurobehavioral consequences will be the added the perhaps more variable influence of factors such as antiseizure medications and their particular adverse cognitive profiles,[21] variations in epileptiform and other waveform abnormalities,[157–160] complications of the disorder,[25] and postictal effects. In addition, familial susceptibilities and other factors will influence cognitive status.[161,162]

EPILEPSY AND COGNITION: BRIDGING THE OLD AND NEW LITERATURES

This article describes a developing architecture of cognitive impairment in the epilepsies, moving from the long established traditional focus on the relationship between neuropsychological status and clinical epilepsy characteristics (eg, seizure frequency, seizure severity, duration of epilepsy, age of onset, etiology, medications), to one focusing on interrelationships between underlying anatomic, metabolic, and other neurobiologic correlates of the epilepsies with critical cognitive and behavioral functions. This is a paradigm shift that has a strong influence on the understanding of the neuropsychology of epilepsy. The older literature, however, is reliable, well understood, and clinically meaningful. Is there some way to understand the intersection of the cognition and clinical seizure feature and the cognition and neuroanatomy literatures (**Fig. 11**), and are there methods that might help inform the understanding of

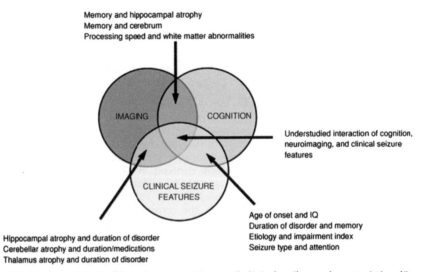

Fig. 11. The intersection of imaging, cognition, and clinical epilepsy characteristics. (*From* Oyegbile TO, Bhattacharya A, Seidenberg M, et al. Quantitative MRI biomarkers of cognitive morbidity in temporal lobe epilepsy. Epilepsia 2006;47:143–52.)

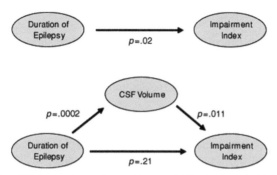

Fig. 12. Quantitative MRI biomarkers of cognitive morbidity in temporal lobe epilepsy. (From Oyegbile TO, Bhattacharya A, Seidenberg M, et al. Epilepsia 2006;47(1):143–52.)

the neuroanatomic pathways through which clinical seizure features exert their impact on cognition in epilepsy?

In a first step to address this issue, the authors tested a mediator-moderator model to determine how overall cognitive impairment, total CSF, and duration of epilepsy were associated and whether duration of epilepsy affected cognition directly or through a structural neuroimaging marker (brain atrophy reflected in total CSF) (**Fig. 12**). It was found that total CSF mediated the relationship between duration of epilepsy and cognitive impairment.[136] That is, the longer the duration of epilepsy, the more abnormal the total CSF, with resulting greater cognitive impairment. The impact of duration of epilepsy on cognition was mediated by the degree of overall brain atrophy reflected in total CSF. This represents a crude initial approach to a complex problem, but this statistical approach may have some use in understanding these complex relationships and the move toward a more unified understanding of the neuropsychologic consequences of the epilepsies.

CONCLUSION

The landscape of cognitive impairment is clearly in transition from a long-standing focus on the relationship between cognitive function and clinical epilepsy features to one linking cognitive impairment to a multitude of neuroimaging parameters. Whether it will be possible to derive a broad understanding of cognition, clinical epilepsy features and neuroimaging markers remains to be determined. This represents an interesting research challenge for the future.

REFERENCES

1. Folsom A. Psychological testing in epilepsy. Epilepsia 1952;1:15–22.
2. Keating LE. A review of the literature on the relationship of epilepsy and intelligence in school children. J Ment Sci 1960;106:1042–59.
3. Tarter RE. Intellectual and adaptive functioning in epilepsy: a review of 50 years of research. Dis Nerv Syst 1972;33:763–70.
4. Trimble MR, Thompson PJ. Neuropsychological and behavioral sequelae of spontaneous seizures. Ann N Y Acad Sci 1986;462:284–92.
5. Novelly RA. The debt of neuropsychology to the epilepsies. Am Psychol 1992; 47:1126–9.

6. Elger CE, Helmstaedter C, Kurthen M. Chronic epilepsy and cognition. Lancet Neurol 2004;3:663–72.

7. Boake C. From the Binet-Simon to the Wechsler-Bellevue: tracing the history of intelligence testing. J Clin Exp Neuropsychol 2002;24:383–405.

8. Wallin JEW. Eight months of psycho-clinical research at the New Jersey state village for epileptics, with some results from the Binet-Simon testing. Epilepsia 1912;A3:366–80.

9. Angers WP. Intelligence quotients of institutionalized and non-institutionalized epileptics. J Psychol Studies 1962;13:152–6.

10. Lennox WG. Epilepsy and related disorders. Boston: Little, Brown and Co; 1960.

11. Berg AT, Langfitt JT, Testa FM, et al. Global cognitive function in children with epilepsy: a community-based study. Epilepsia 2008;49:608–14.

12. Hackett R, Hackett L, Bhakta P. Psychiatric disorder and cognitive function in children with epilepsy in Kerala, South India. Seizure 1998;7:321–4.

13. Hoie B, Mykletun A, Sommerfelt K, et al. Seizure-related factors and non-verbal intelligence in children with epilepsy: a population-based study from Western Norway. Seizure 2005;14:223–31.

14. Hoie B, Sommerfelt K, Waaler PE, et al. The combined burden of cognitive, executive function, and psychosocial problems in children with epilepsy: a population-based study. Dev Med Child Neurol 2008;50:530–6.

15. Tuxhorn I, Kotagal P. Classification. Semin Neurol 2008;28:277–88.

16. Seino M. Classification criteria of epileptic seizures and syndromes. Epilepsy Res 2006;70(Suppl 1):S27–33.

17. Nolan MA, Redoblado MA, Lah S, et al. Intelligence in childhood epilepsy syndromes. Epilepsy Res 2003;53:139–50.

18. Nolan MA, Redoblado MA, Lah S, et al. Memory function in childhood epilepsy syndromes. J Paediatr Child Health 2004;40:20–7.

19. Macallister WS, Schaffer SG. Neuropsychological deficits in childhood epilepsy syndromes. Neuropsychol Rev 2007;17:427–44.

20. Hommet C, Sauerwein HC, De Toffol B, et al. Idiopathic epileptic syndromes and cognition. Neurosci Biobehav Rev 2006;30:85–96.

21. Loring DW, Marino S, Meador KJ. Neuropsychological and behavioral effects of antiepilepsy drugs. Neuropsychol Rev 2007;17:413–25.

22. Klove H, Matthews CG. Psychometric and adaptive abilities in epilepsy with differential etiology. Epilepsia 1966;7:330–8.

23. Matthews CG, Klove H. MMPI performances in major motor, psychomotor and mixed seizure classifications of known and unknown etiology. Epilepsia 1968;9:43–53.

24. Dodrill CB. Neuropsychological aspects of epilepsy. Psychiatr Clin North Am 1992;15:383–94.

25. Dodrill CB. Neuropsychological effects of seizures. Epilepsy Behav 2004; 5(Suppl 1):S21–4.

26. Aldenkamp AP, Bodde N. Behaviour, cognition and epilepsy. Acta Neurol Scand Suppl 2005;182:19–25.

27. Gibbs FA, Gibbs EL, Lennox WG. Epilepsy: a paroxysmal cerebral dysrhythmia. Brain 1937;60:377–88.

28. Dejong RN. Psychomotor or temporal lobe epilepsy: a review of the development of our present concepts. Neurology 1957;7:1–14.

29. Gibbs FA, Gibbs EL, Lennox WG. Cerebral dysrhythmias of epilepsy: measures for their control. Arch Neurol Psychiatr 1938;39:298–314.

30. Jasper H, Kershman J. Electroencephalographic classification of the epilepsies. Arch Neurol Psychiatr 1941;45:903.

31. Gibbs EL, Gibbs FA, Fuster B. Psychomotor epilepsy. Arch Neurol Psychiatr 1948;60:331–9.
32. Hermann BP, Stone JL. A historical review of the epilepsy surgery program at the University of Illinois Medical Center: the contributions of Bailey, Gibbs, and collaborators to the refinement of anterior temporal lobectomy. J Epilepsy 1989;2:155–63.
33. Feindel W, Leblanc R, de Almeida AN. Epilepsy surgery: historical highlights 1909–2009. Epilepsia 2009;50(Suppl 3):131–51.
34. Hebb DO, Penfield W. Human behavior after extensive bilateral removal from the frontal lobes. Not Found In Database 1940;44:421–38.
35. Milner B. Intellectual function of the temporal lobes. Psychol Bull 1954;51: 42–62.
36. Milner B, Penfield W. The effect of hippocampal lesions on recent memory. Trans Am Neurol Assoc 1955;80:42–8.
37. Halsted WC. Some behavioral aspects of partial temporal lobectomy in man. In: Proceedings of the association for research in nervous and mental disease. Baltimore (MD): Williams & Wilkins; 1958. p. 478–89.
38. Meyer V, Yates AJ. Intellectual changes following temporal lobectomy for psychomotor epilepsy: preliminary communication. J Neurol Neurosurg Psychiatr 1955;18:44–52.
39. Bladin PF. Murray Alexander Falconer and the Guy's-Maudsley hospital seizure surgery program. J Clin Neurosci 2004;11:577–83.
40. Engel J. Surgical treatment of the epilepsies. 2nd edition. New York: Raven Press; 1993.
41. Engel J Jr. Update on surgical treatment of the epilepsies. Summary of the Second International Palm Desert Conference on the Surgical Treatment of the Epilepsies (1992). Neurology 1993;43:1612–7.
42. French JA, Williamson PD, Thadani VM, et al. Characteristics of medial temporal lobe epilepsy: I. Results of history and physical examination. Ann Neurol 1993; 34:774–80.
43. Sass KJ, Spencer DD, Kim JH, et al. Verbal memory impairment correlates with hippocampal pyramidal cell density. Neurology 1990;40:1694–7.
44. Williamson PD, French JA, Thadani VM, et al. Characteristics of medial temporal lobe epilepsy: II. Interictal and ictal scalp electroencephalography, neuropsychological testing, neuroimaging, surgical results, and pathology. Ann Neurol 1993;34:781–7.
45. Janszky J, Janszky I, Ebner A. Age at onset in mesial temporal lobe epilepsy with a history of febrile seizures. Neurology 2004;63:1296–8.
46. Fox JT. The response of epileptic children to mental and educational tests. Br J Med Psychol 1924;4:235–48.
47. Dikmen S, Matthews CG, Harley JP. The effect of early versus late onset of major motor epilepsy upon cognitive-intellectual performance. Epilepsia 1975;16: 73–81.
48. Dikmen S, Matthews CG, Harley JP. Effect of early versus late onset of major motor epilepsy on cognitive-intellectual performance: further considerations. Epilepsia 1977;18:31–6.
49. Dodrill CB, Matthews CG. The role of neuropsychology in the assessment and treatment of persons with epilepsy. Am Psychol 1992;47:1139–42.
50. Glosser G, Cole LC, French JA, et al. Predictors of intellectual performance in adults with intractable temporal lobe epilepsy. J Int Neuropsychol Soc 1997;3: 252–9.

51. O'Leary DS, Seidenberg M, Berent S, et al. Effects of age of onset of tonic-clonic seizures on neuropsychological performance in children. Epilepsia 1981;22: 197–204.

52. O'Leary DS, Lovell MR, Sackellares JC, et al. Effects of age of onset of partial and generalized seizures on neuropsychological performance in children. J Nerv Ment Dis 1983;171:624–9.

53. Schoenfeld J, Seidenberg M, Woodard A, et al. Neuropsychological and behavioral status of children with complex partial seizures. Dev Med Child Neurol 1999;41:724–31.

54. Hermann BP, Seidenberg M, Schoenfeld J, et al. Neuropsychological characteristics of the syndrome of mesial temporal lobe epilepsy. Arch Neurol 1997;54: 369–76.

55. Oyegbile TO, Dow C, Jones J, et al. The nature and course of neuropsychological morbidity in chronic temporal lobe epilepsy. Neurology 2004;62: 1736–42.

56. Oyegbile T, Hansen R, Magnotta V, et al. Quantitative measurement of cortical surface features in localization-related temporal lobe epilepsy. Neuropsychology 2004;18:729–37.

57. Marques CM, Caboclo LO, da Silva TI, et al. Cognitive decline in temporal lobe epilepsy due to unilateral hippocampal sclerosis. Epilepsy Behav 2007;10: 477–85.

58. Lencz T, McCarthy G, Bronen RA, et al. Quantitative magnetic resonance imaging in temporal lobe epilepsy: relationship to neuropathology and neuropsychological function. Ann Neurol 1992;31:629–37.

59. Cendes F, Andermann F, Gloor P, et al. MRI volumetric measurement of amygdala and hippocampus in temporal lobe epilepsy. Neurology 1993;43: 719–25.

60. Salmenpera T, Kalviainen R, Partanen K, et al. Hippocampal and amygdaloid damage in partial epilepsy: a cross-sectional MRI study of 241 patients. Epilepsy Res 2001;46:69–82.

61. Bernasconi N, Bernasconi A, Caramanos Z, et al. Mesial temporal damage in temporal lobe epilepsy: a volumetric MRI study of the hippocampus, amygdala and parahippocampal region. Brain 2003;126:462–9.

62. Bernasconi N, Bernasconi A, Andermann F, et al. Entorhinal cortex in temporal lobe epilepsy: a quantitative MRI study. Neurology 1999;52:1870–6.

63. Bonilha L, Rorden C, Halford JJ, et al. Asymmetrical extra-hippocampal grey matter loss related to hippocampal atrophy in patients with medial temporal lobe epilepsy. J Neurol Neurosurg Psychiatr 2007;78:286–94.

64. Kuzniecky R, Bilir E, Gilliam F, et al. Quantitative MRI in temporal lobe epilepsy: evidence for fornix atrophy. Neurology 1999;53:496–501.

65. DeCarli C, Hatta J, Fazilat S, et al. Extratemporal atrophy in patients with complex partial seizures of left temporal origin. Ann Neurol 1998;43:41–5.

66. Dreifuss S, Vingerhoets FJ, Lazeyras F, et al. Volumetric measurements of subcortical nuclei in patients with temporal lobe epilepsy. Neurology 2001;57: 1636–41.

67. Natsume J, Bernasconi N, Andermann F, et al. MRI volumetry of the thalamus in temporal, extratemporal, and idiopathic generalized epilepsy. Neurology 2003; 60:1296–300.

68. Szabo CA, Lancaster JL, Lee S, et al. MR imaging volumetry of subcortical structures and cerebellar hemispheres in temporal lobe epilepsy. AJNR Am J Neuroradiol 2006;27:2155–60.

69. Marsh L, Morrell MJ, Shear PK, et al. Cortical and hippocampal volume deficits in temporal lobe epilepsy. Epilepsia 1997;38:576–87.
70. Lee JW, Andermann F, Dubeau F, et al. Morphometric analysis of the temporal lobe in temporal lobe epilepsy. Epilepsia 1998;39:727–36.
71. Jutila L, Ylinen A, Partanen K, et al. MR volumetry of the entorhinal, perirhinal, and temporopolar cortices in drug-refractory temporal lobe epilepsy. AJNR Am J Neuroradiol 2001;22:1490–501.
72. Moran NF, Lemieux L, Kitchen ND, et al. Extrahippocampal temporal lobe atrophy in temporal lobe epilepsy and mesial temporal sclerosis. Brain 2001; 124:167–75.
73. Hermann B, Seidenberg M, Bell B, et al. The neurodevelopmental impact of childhood-onset temporal lobe epilepsy on brain structure and function. Epilepsia 2002;43:1062–71.
74. Sandok EK, O'Brien TJ, Jack CR, et al. Significance of cerebellar atrophy in intractable temporal lobe epilepsy: a quantitative MRI study. Epilepsia 2000; 41:1315–20.
75. Sisodiya SM, Moran N, Free SL, et al. Correlation of widespread preoperative magnetic resonance imaging changes with unsuccessful surgery for hippocampal sclerosis. Ann Neurol 1997;41:490–6.
76. Theodore WH, DeCarli C, Gaillard WD. Total cerebral volume is reduced in patients with localization-related epilepsy and a history of complex febrile seizures. Arch Neurol 2003;60:250–2.
77. Weber B, Luders E, Faber J, et al. Distinct regional atrophy in the corpus callosum of patients with temporal lobe epilepsy. Brain 2007;130:3149–54.
78. Ronan L, Murphy K, Delanty N, et al. Cerebral cortical gyrification: a preliminary investigation in temporal lobe epilepsy. Epilepsia 2007;48:211–9.
79. Pulsipher DT, Seidenberg M, Morton JJ, et al. MRI volume loss of subcortical structures in unilateral temporal lobe epilepsy. Epilepsy Behav 2007;11:442–9.
80. Keller SS, Roberts N. Voxel-based morphometry of temporal lobe epilepsy: an introduction and review of the literature. Epilepsia 2008;49:741–57.
81. Lin JJ, Salamon N, Lee AD, et al. Reduced neocortical thickness and complexity mapped in mesial temporal lobe epilepsy with hippocampal sclerosis. Cereb Cortex 2007;17:2007–18.
82. McDonald CR, Hagler DJ Jr, Ahmadi ME, et al. Regional neocortical thinning in mesial temporal lobe epilepsy. Epilepsia 2008;49:794–803.
83. Bernhardt BC, Worsley KJ, Besson P, et al. Mapping limbic network organization in temporal lobe epilepsy using morphometric correlations: insights on the relation between mesiotemporal connectivity and cortical atrophy. Neuroimage 2008;42:515–24.
84. Mueller SG, Laxer KD, Barakos J, et al. Widespread neocortical abnormalities in temporal lobe epilepsy with and without mesial sclerosis. Neuroimage 2009; 46(2):353–9.
85. Lin JJ, Salamon N, Lee AD, et al. Reduced neocortical thickness and complexity mapped in mesial temporal lobe epilepsy with hippocampal sclerosis. Cereb Cortex 2007;17(9):2007–18.
86. Seidenberg M, Kelly KG, Parrish J, et al. Ipsilateral and contralateral MRI volumetric abnormalities in chronic unilateral temporal lobe epilepsy and their clinical correlates. Epilepsia 2005;46:420–30.
87. McMillan AB, Hermann BP, Johnson SC, et al. Voxel-based morphometry of unilateral temporal lobe epilepsy reveals abnormalities in cerebral white matter. Neuroimage 2004;23:167–74.

88. Bernasconi N, Duchesne S, Janke A, et al. Whole-brain voxel-based statistical analysis of gray matter and white matter in temporal lobe epilepsy. Neuroimage 2004;23:717–23.
89. Gaffan D. Against memory systems. Philos Trans R Soc Lond B Biol Sci 2002; 357:1111–21.
90. Filley C. The behavioral neurology of white matter. New York: Oxford University Press; 2001.
91. Gaffan D, Parker A, Easton A. Dense amnesia in the monkey after transection of fornix, amygdala and anterior temporal stem. Neuropsychologia 2001;39: 51–70.
92. Thiebaut de Schotten M, Urbanski M, Duffau H, et al. Direct evidence for a parietal-frontal pathway subserving spatial awareness in humans. Science 2005;309:2226–8.
93. Catani M, ffytche DH. The rises and falls of disconnection syndromes. Brain 2005;128:2224–39.
94. Catani M, Howard RJ, Pajevic S, et al. Virtual in vivo interactive dissection of white matter fasciculi in the human brain. Neuroimage 2002;17:77–94.
95. Pierpaoli C, Barnett A, Pajevic S, et al. Water diffusion changes in wallerian degeneration and their dependence on white matter architecture. Neuroimage 2001;13:1174–85.
96. Gass A, Niendorf T, Hirsch JG. Acute and chronic changes of the apparent diffusion coefficient in neurological disorders: biophysical mechanisms and possible underlying histopathology. J Neurol Sci 2001;186(Suppl 1):S15–23.
97. Concha L, Beaulieu C, Gross DW. Bilateral limbic diffusion abnormalities in unilateral temporal lobe epilepsy. Ann Neurol 2005;57:188–96.
98. Rodrigo S, Oppenheim C, Chassoux F, et al. Uncinate fasciculus fiber tracking in mesial temporal lobe epilepsy: initial findings. Eur Radiol 2007;17:1663–8.
99. Lin JJ, Riley JD, Juranek J, et al. Vulnerability of the frontal-temporal connections in temporal lobe epilepsy. Epilepsy Res 2008;82:162–70.
100. Matsumoto R, Okada T, Mikuni N, et al. Hemispheric asymmetry of the arcuate fasciculus: a preliminary diffusion tensor tractography study in patients with unilateral language dominance defined by Wada test. J Neurol 2008;255:1703–11.
101. Ahmadi ME, Hagler DJ Jr, McDonald CR, et al. Side matters: diffusion tensor imaging tractography in left and right temporal lobe epilepsy. AJNR Am J Neuroradiol 2009. June 9, 2009 [epub ahead of print].
102. Arfanakis K, Hermann BP, Rogers BP, et al. Diffusion tensor MRI in temporal lobe epilepsy. Magn Reson Imaging 2002;20:511–9.
103. Concha L, Gross DW, Wheatley BM, et al. Diffusion tensor imaging of time-dependent axonal and myelin degradation after corpus callosotomy in epilepsy patients. Neuroimage 2006;32:1090–9.
104. Concha L, Beaulieu C, Collins DL, et al. White-matter diffusion abnormalities in temporal-lobe epilepsy with and without mesial temporal sclerosis. J Neurol Neurosurg Psychiatr 2009;80:312–9.
105. Thivard L, Lehericy S, Krainik A, et al. Diffusion tensor imaging in medial temporal lobe epilepsy with hippocampal sclerosis. Neuroimage 2005;28: 682–90.
106. Focke NK, Yogarajah M, Bonelli SB, et al. Voxel-based diffusion tensor imaging in patients with mesial temporal lobe epilepsy and hippocampal sclerosis. Neuroimage 2008;40:728–37.
107. Schoene-Bake JC, Faber J, Trautner P, et al. Widespread affections of large fiber tracts in postoperative temporal lobe epilepsy. Neuroimage 2009;46:569–76.

108. Sass KJ, Sass A, Westerveld M, et al. Specificity in the correlation of verbal memory and hippocampal neuron loss: dissociation of memory, language, and verbal intellectual ability. J Clin Exp Neuropsychol 1992;14:662–72.
109. Trenerry MR, Jack CR Jr, Ivnik RJ, et al. MRI hippocampal volumes and memory function before and after temporal lobectomy. Neurology 1993;43:1800–5.
110. Trenerry MR, Jack CR Jr, Cascino GD, et al. Gender differences in post-temporal lobectomy verbal memory and relationships between MRI hippocampal volumes and preoperative verbal memory. Epilepsy Res 1995;20:69–76.
111. Seidenberg M, Geary E, Hermann B. Investigating temporal lobe contribution to confrontation naming using MRI quantitative volumetrics. J Int Neuropsychol Soc 2005;11:358–66.
112. Alessio A, Bonilha L, Rorden C, et al. Memory and language impairments and their relationships to hippocampal and perirhinal cortex damage in patients with medial temporal lobe epilepsy. Epilepsy Behav 2006;8:593–600.
113. Seidenberg M, Hermann B, Pulsipher D, et al. Thalamic atrophy and cognition in unilateral temporal lobe epilepsy. J Int Neuropsychol Soc 2008;14:384–93.
114. Stewart CC, Griffith HR, Okonkwo OC, et al. Contributions of volumetrics of the hippocampus and thalamus to verbal memory in temporal lobe epilepsy patients. Brain Cogn 2009;69:65–72.
115. Rausch R, Henry TR, Ary CM, et al. Asymmetric interictal glucose hypometabolism and cognitive performance in epileptic patients. Arch Neurol 1994;51:139–44.
116. Getz K, Hermann B, Seidenberg M, et al. Negative symptoms and psychosocial status in temporal lobe epilepsy. Epilepsy Res 2003;53:240–4.
117. Getz K, Hermann B, Seidenberg M, et al. Negative symptoms in temporal lobe epilepsy. Am J Psychiatry 2002;159:644–51.
118. Geary B, Hermann B, Seidenberg M, et al. Anatomic correlates of negative symptoms in temporal lobe epilepsy. J Neuropsychiatry Clin Neurosci 2009;21(2):152–9.
119. Keller SS, Baker G, Downes JJ, et al. Quantitative MRI of the prefrontal cortex and executive function in patients with temporal lobe epilepsy. Epilepsy Behav 2008;49(5):741–57.
120. Jokeit H, Seitz RJ, Markowitsch HJ, et al. Prefrontal asymmetric interictal glucose hypometabolism and cognitive impairment in patients with temporal lobe epilepsy. Brain 1997;120(Pt 12):2283–94.
121. Bonilha L, Alessio A, Rorden C, et al. Extrahippocampal gray matter atrophy and memory impairment in patients with medial temporal lobe epilepsy. Hum Brain Mapp 2007;28(12):1376–90.
122. Bengner T, Malina T, Lindenau M, et al. Face memory in MRI-positive and MRI-negative temporal lobe epilepsy. Epilepsia 2006;47:1904–14.
123. Bengner T, Siemonsen S, Stodieck S, et al. T2 relaxation time correlates of face recognition deficits in temporal lobe epilepsy. Epilepsy Behav 2008;13:670–7.
124. Griffith HR, Richardson E, Pyzalski RW, et al. Memory for famous faces and the temporal pole: functional imaging findings in temporal lobe epilepsy. Epilepsy Behav 2006;9(1):173–80.
125. Botez MI, Botez T, Elie R, et al. Role of the cerebellum in complex human behavior. Ital J Neurol Sci 1989;10:291–300.
126. Schmahmann JD. The cerebellum and cognition. New York: Academic Press; 1997.
127. Eichenbaum H, Chhen N. From conditioning to conscious recollection: memory systems of the brain. New York: Oxford University Press; 2001.

128. Squire LR, Zola-Morgan S. The medial temporal lobe memory system. Science 1991;253:1380–6.
129. Wooduff-Pak D, Steinmetz J. Eyeblink classical conditioning: applications in humans. New York: Plenum Press; 2000.
130. Hermann B, Seidenberg M, Sears L, et al. Cerebellar atrophy in temporal lobe epilepsy affects procedural memory. Neurology 2004;63:2129–31.
131. Daley M, Siddarth P, Levitt J, et al. Amygdala volume and psychopathology in childhood complex partial seizures. Epilepsy Behav 2008;13:212–7.
132. Tebartz Van Elst L, Baeumer D, Lemieux L, et al. Amygdala pathology in psychosis of epilepsy: a magnetic resonance imaging study in patients with temporal lobe epilepsy. Brain 2002;125:140–9.
133. Meletti S, Benuzzi F, Rubboli G, et al. Impaired facial emotion recognition in early-onset right mesial temporal lobe epilepsy. Neurology 2003;60: 426–31.
134. McClelland S, Garcia RE, Peraza DM, et al. Facial emotion recognition after curative nondominant temporal lobectomy in patients with mesial temporal sclerosis. Epilepsia 2006;47:1337–42.
135. Focke NK, Thompson PJ, Duncan JS. Correlation of cognitive functions with voxel-based morphometry in patients with hippocampal sclerosis. Epilepsy Behav 2008;12:472–6.
136. Oyegbile TO, Bhattacharya A, Seidenberg M, et al. Quantitative MRI biomarkers of cognitive morbidity in temporal lobe epilepsy. Epilepsia 2006;47:143–52.
137. Baxendale SA, Sisodiya SM, Thompson PJ, et al. Disproportion in the distribution of gray and white matter: neuropsychological correlates. Neurology 1999; 52:248–52.
138. Hermann BP, Seidenberg M, Bell B, et al. Extratemporal quantitative MRI volumetrics and neuropsychological function in temporal lobe epilepsy. J Int Neuropsychol Soc 2003;9:353–62.
139. Dow C, Seidenberg M, Hermann B. Relationship between information processing speed in temporal lobe epilepsy and white matter volume. Epilepsy Behav 2004;5:919–25.
140. Hermann B, Hansen R, Seidenberg M, et al. Neurodevelopmental vulnerability of the corpus callosum to childhood onset localization-related epilepsy. Neuroimage 2003;18:284–92.
141. Flugel D, Cercignani M, Symms MR, et al. Diffusion tensor imaging findings and their correlation with neuropsychological deficits in patients with temporal lobe epilepsy and interictal psychosis. Epilepsia 2006;47:941–4.
142. Diehl B, Busch RM, Duncan JS, et al. Abnormalities in diffusion tensor imaging of the uncinate fasciculus relate to reduced memory in temporal lobe epilepsy. Epilepsia 2008;49:1409–18.
143. McDonald CR, Ahmadi ME, Hagler DJ, et al. Diffusion tensor imaging correlates of memory and language impairments in temporal lobe epilepsy. Neurology 2008;71:1869–76.
144. Waites AB, Briellmann RS, Saling MM, et al. Functional connectivity networks are disrupted in left temporal lobe epilepsy. Ann Neurol 2006;59:335–43.
145. Janszky J, Mertens M, Janszky I, et al. Left-sided interictal epileptic activity induces shift of language lateralization in temporal lobe epilepsy: an fMRI study. Epilepsia 2006;47:921–7.
146. Powell HW, Parker GJ, Alexander DC, et al. Hemispheric asymmetries in language-related pathways: a combined functional MRI and tractography study. Neuroimage 2006;32:388–99.

147. Powell HW, Parker GJ, Alexander DC, et al. Abnormalities of language networks in temporal lobe epilepsy. Neuroimage 2007;36:209–21.
148. Powell HW, Parker GJ, Alexander DC, et al. Imaging language pathways predicts postoperative naming deficits. J Neurol Neurosurg Psychiatr 2008;79: 327–30.
149. Hermann B, Seidenberg M, Lee EJ, et al. Cognitive phenotypes in temporal lobe epilepsy. J Int Neuropsychol Soc 2007;13:12–20.
150. Dabbs K, Jones J, Seidenberg M, et al. Neuroanatomical correlates of cognitive phenotypes in temporal lobe epilepsy. Epilepsy Behav 2009;15(4):445–51.
151. Paradiso S, Hermann BP, Somes G. Patterns of academic competence in adults with epilepsy: a cluster analytic study. Epilepsy Res 1994;19:253–61.
152. Devinsky O, Gershengorn J, Brown E, et al. Frontal functions in juvenile myoclonic epilepsy. Neuropsychiatry Neuropsychol Behav Neurol 1997;10: 243–6.
153. Piazzini A, Turner K, Vignoli A, et al. Frontal cognitive dysfunction in juvenile myoclonic epilepsy. Epilepsia 2008;49:657–62.
154. Sonmez F, Atakli D, Sari H, et al. Cognitive function in juvenile myoclonic epilepsy. Epilepsy Behav 2004;5:329–36.
155. Pascalicchio TF, de Araujo Filho GM, da Silva Noffs MH, et al. Neuropsychological profile of patients with juvenile myoclonic epilepsy: a controlled study of 50 patients. Epilepsy Behav 2007;10:263–7.
156. Bernhardt BC, Rozen DA, Worsley KJ, et al. Thalamo-cortical network pathology in idiopathic generalized epilepsy: insights from MRI-based morphometric correlation analysis. Neuroimage 2009;46:373–81.
157. Dodrill CB, Wilkus RJ. Relationships between intelligence and electroencephalographic epileptiform activity in adult epileptics. Neurology 1976;26:525–31.
158. Wilkus RJ, Dodrill CB. Neuropsychological correlates of the electroencephalogram in epileptics: I. Topographic distribution and average rate of epileptiform activity. Epilepsia 1976;17:89–100.
159. Koop JI, Fastenau PS, Dunn DW, et al. Neuropsychological correlates of electroencephalograms in children with epilepsy. Epilepsy Res 2005;64:49–62.
160. Binnie CD. Cognitive impairment during epileptiform discharges: is it ever justifiable to treat the EEG? Lancet Neurol 2003;2:725–30.
161. Iqbal N, Caswell HL, Hare DJ, et al. Neuropsychological profiles of patients with juvenile myoclonic epilepsy and their siblings: a preliminary controlled experimental video-EEG case series. Epilepsy Behav 2009;14:516–21.
162. Clarke T, Strug LJ, Murphy PL, et al. High risk of reading disability and speech sound disorder in rolandic epilepsy families: case-control study. Epilepsia 2007; 48:2258–65.

The Etiology of Psychogenic Non-Epileptic Seizures: Toward a Biopsychosocial Model

Markus Reuber, MD, PhD, FRCP

KEYWORDS

- Psychogenic non-epileptic seizures • Conversion
- Dissociation • Epilepsy • Pseudoseizures • Etiology

Many paroxysmal neurologic disorders cause impairment of consciousness, but most patients are diagnosed with one of three: epilepsy, syncope, or psychogenic nonepileptic seizures (PNES). In one study, a neurologist was able to establish a diagnosis in 87% of 158 consecutive patients newly referred to her clinic, with 43% having epilepsy, 25% syncope, 12% PNES, and 7% other disorders.[1] The authors of another study, which reportedly captured all patients experiencing a blackout who first presented to a neurologist, emergency room, or primary care physician, believed that 57.4% had epilepsy, 22.3% syncope, and 18.0% PNES.[2]

Although PNES are therefore among the most important differential diagnoses of epilepsy, they are not well understood, and are therefore often not well treated.[3–5] Diagnostic delay, the mistreatment of PNES as epilepsy (or less commonly of epilepsy as PNES), and poor communication between patients and doctors remain commonplace. Neurologists have a crucial role in explaining the disorder to patients.

PNES are episodes of altered movement, sensation, or experience resembling epileptic seizures, but not associated with ictal electrical discharges in the brain. They are a behavioral response to mental, physical, or social distress characterized by a temporary loss of control. The most common semiology involves excessive movement of limbs, trunk, and head resembling tonic–clonic seizures. PNES with stiffening and tremor, or atonia and unresponsiveness also occur.[6]

Most experts assume that PNES are an unintentional manifestation of emotional distress. They are called "dissociative convulsions" (F44.5) in the International Classification of Diseases (ICD-10) and "conversion disorder with seizures or convulsions"

Funding support: The author did not receive any funding for this review. There is no conflict of interest to declare.

Academic Neurology Unit, University of Sheffield, Royal Hallamshire Hospital, Glossop Road, Sheffield, S10 2JF, UK

E-mail address: mreuber@doctors.org.uk

(300.11) in the Diagnostic and Statistical Manual of Mental Disorders (DSM-IV-TR). However, experts recognize that PNES are occasionally simulated (in malingering and factitious disorders).[7]

PNES have been the subject of many recent review articles, which have focused on the differential diagnosis,[8] the process of making the diagnosis,[9,10] the relationship with neurologic pathology,[11] the management by neurologists,[12] and further treatment by psychotherapists.[13–16] This article focuses on developing an explanatory model for PNES that integrates the results of a wide range of studies. It is aimed at general neurologists, psychiatrists, and clinical psychologists who would like to gain a better understanding of a complex disorder. Reflecting the author's expertise in the area, it focuses on adults.

ETIOLOGIC FRAMEWORK

PNES occur in a heterogeneous patient population. No single mechanism or even contributing factor has been identified that is necessary and sufficient to explain PNES in all patients. PNES are best understood based on the biopsychosocial, multifactorial etiologic model outlined in **Fig. 1**.

In most patients several interacting causes can be identified. *Predisposing factors* increase vulnerability to the development of PNES in later life. *Precipitating factors* occur over the days to months before the onset of seizures and seem to cause PNES to start. *Perpetuating factors* make it harder for patients to regain control of seizures or aggravate the problem once seizures have started. *Triggering factors* seem to start recurrent seizures within seconds or minutes. Even if one factor seems to play a predominant role in a particular patient, other factors are likely to have contributed and should not be ignored.

PREDISPOSING FACTORS
Genetic factors

The relationship between inherited factors or childhood antecedents of a particular disorder such as PNES and its later development is typically indirect or probabilistic. Many other factors codetermine whether PNES will develop in an individual. Little is currently known about specific genetic factors conferring vulnerability or resilience

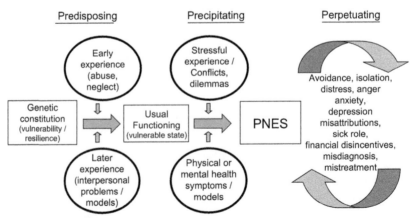

Fig. 1. Etiology of psychogenic nonepileptic seizures: a multifactorial model.

to adverse life events or the development of mental disorders.[17] However, large studies show that these factors exist, and that they are not always active from birth but may exert their effects during later periods of development.[18,19]

The most obvious genetically determined risk factor for the development of PNES is female gender. Lesser[20] examined the sex distribution in 21 studies and found descriptions of 734 women and 250 men who had PNES. Similar to the sex distribution in other somatoform disorders,[21] women are therefore three times more likely to develop PNES than men. This gender difference is not fully explained by readily recognizable experiential differences between men and women, such as the higher rates of sexual abuse experienced by women.[22] Similar to other forms of somatization, PNES may be an acquired and culturally determined predominantly female expression of helplessness or anger.[23,24] However, more direct biologic reasons may exist as to why women are more likely than men to develop PNES.

Childhood Abuse and Neglect

The relationship between childhood sexual abuse (CSA) and PNES has received particular attention since Freud[25] highlighted a possible link. Although CSA is only reported by a minority of patients who have PNES, it is a good example of the complex relationship between a distant antecedent and an adult manifestation of psychopathology (see Case A). The largest study comparing CSA in groups of patients who had PNES (n = 71) and those who had epilepsy (n = 140) found significantly higher rates of both sexual (24.0% versus 7.1%) and physical (15.5% versus 2.9%) childhood abuse in those who had PNES.[26] Although the etiologic relevance of CSA for PNES is not undisputed, these results have been replicated in most other studies of this issue.[27,28]

As with other psychiatric conditions linked to CSA, the adverse childhood experience probably must combine with other factors to lead to PNES in later life. Although the effects of CSA can also be reduced by optimal support from at least one parent,[29] several recent studies have identified a range of different mechanisms that may link CSA or physical abuse and neglect in early life with PNES in adulthood. Holman and colleagues[30] showed that (unlike controls affected by epilepsy) patients who have PNES often have a fearful attachment style, making secure interpersonal relationships harder for them to develop and maintain in adulthood. The presence of a fearful attachment style was correlated with a history of adverse experience in early life.

Salmon and colleagues[31] showed that CSA is often associated with childhood physical abuse, neglect, and a dysfunctional family environment. Patients who had PNES and reported CSA were also more likely to report adult sexual abuse, suggesting that a history of CSA can be a marker of more extensive and pervasive adverse experience. Bewley and colleagues[32] found that more than 90% of patients who had PNES scored in the abnormal range on a standardized measure of alexithymia, meaning that they had difficulties feeling or perceiving emotions. Others have shown that etiologic links exist between trauma and deprivation in early life and alexithymia in later life.[33]

Alexithymia is not the only form of abnormal emotional reactivity related to CSA. Individuals who have a history of CSA may also experience sudden and extreme emotional fluctuations in adulthood.[34] In two studies using personality inventories, the largest subgroups of patients who had PNES reported experiencing this form of emotional dysregulation,[35,36] with borderline personality disorder (which is characterized by emotional dysregulation) overrepresented.[37,38]

Furthermore, Bakvis and colleagues[39] showed that patients who have PNES and a history of sexual abuse have a heart rate variability than healthy controls. In a masked emotional Stroop test, comparing color-naming latencies for backwardly masked angry, neutral, and happy faces, patients who had PNES showed a positive attentional bias for angry faces, suggesting that their previous adverse experience had produced measurable changes in (preconscious) information processing. These findings suggest that patients with PNES who have experienced sexual abuse remain in a persistently hypervigilant state.

The fact that sexual abuse (including CSA) is likely to be relevant to PNES is also supported by the finding that this history shapes the way in which PNES present. Those who experienced previous sexual abuse developed their seizures earlier, had more anxiety prodromes or ictal flashbacks, more severe seizures (with more frequent injuries, incontinence, and "pseudostatus"), and more seizures from apparent sleep than other patients who have PNES.[22]

Physical Factors

The author's understanding about the mechanisms through which apparently physical or biologic factors such as epilepsy or learning disabilities predispose to the development of PNES is limited.[11] Structural or functional brain abnormalities are found more commonly in patients who have PNES than in the general population.[40–42] The percentage of patients found to have concurrent epilepsy has varied from 3.6% to 58% in different PNES series,[43] but the risk for developing PNES is increased in patients who have epilepsy.

In the author's own series, the clinical history suggested additional epilepsy in 119 of 329 patients who had PNES (36.2%).[43] Similar to other large case series, the development of epileptic seizures almost always preceded the manifestation of PNES.[44] However, the mechanisms through which epilepsy predisposes to PNES remain uncertain. In a study comparing patients affected by epilepsy (n = 90) and those affected by epilepsy and PNES (E+P, n = 90), no particular epileptologic features that made the development of comorbid PNES more likely could be identified. Patients in the E+P group were more likely to have neuropsychological impairment and low IQ (see Case B).[43]

Epilepsy may contribute to the risk for developing PNES not only through biologic mechanisms but also because the experience (or observation) of epileptic seizures may provide an opportunity for model learning (see Case C).[45] Studies showing that patients who have PNES are more likely to report a family history than those with epilepsy and are more likely to have witnessed someone else have a seizure before developing their own seizure disorder offer some support for this idea.[46,47]

PRECIPITATING FACTORS
Adult Life Events

Although patients will often state initially that their seizures started "out of the blue" and without any identifiable cause, significant precipitants for the development of PNES can often be identified. One small study comparing patients who had recent-onset PNES (n = 20) with those who had recent-onset epilepsy (n = 20) found that the PNES group reported more (typically adverse or traumatic) life events over the 12 months before the onset of the seizures than the epilepsy group.[48] The authors of one descriptive study found precipitating traumatic life events in all but 9% of patients.[49]

Factors that have been described as precipitating PNES include rape,[50–52] injury,[50,53] "symbolic" traumatic experience in adulthood after childhood abuse,[50,51,54] death of or separation from family members or friends,[50,55] job loss,[49,50] road traffic and other accidents,[49,50] giving birth,[56] minor surgical procedures,[57] earthquakes,[58] relationship difficulties,[49,50] and legal action.[59] In women, precipitating events are most commonly linked to sexual abuse (see Case A). In men, loss of employment or enforced role changes are more important (see Case D).[49,50,60] In older people, physical illness is the most common identifiable precipitant.[61]

Although approximately 75% to 90% of patients who have PNES report a history of significant trauma,[27,50] and some evidence shows that a history of trauma or adverse life events is more closely associated with the development of PNES than of other unexplained neurologic symptoms,[50,62] these potential precipitants are clearly not specific for the development of PNES.

One study showed that in 76% of patients the precipitating event was only significant in the context of a history of other trauma or previous or ongoing conflict (see Case D).[49] Another study based on a detailed analysis of 14 video-recorded patient interviews showed that in 13 of 14 cases, any precipitating events seemed less relevant to the cause of the seizures than the forced choices or unspeakable dilemmas forced on patients by family or social circumstances.[54]

Two studies comparing patients who had PNES with those who had epilepsy found that PNES were not so much explained by stressful life events (which were reported equally as often by patients who had epilepsy) as by the use of less-effective coping mechanisms.[63,64]

Psychopathology

Clinical experience suggests that PNES commonly start in association with or during a period of exacerbation of another mental disorder. A lifetime history of other somatoform or dissociative disorders is found in more than 50% of patients who have PNES. Anxiety or psychotic and bipolar disorders are less common but are found more frequently in patients who have PNES than in the general population.[38,53] Many patients who have PNES have features of posttraumatic stress disorder (PTSD) and, according to a range of (small) studies, 22% to 100% of patients who have PNES fulfill the DSM-IV criteria for PTSD.[65]

Physical Factors

In some patients (at least potentially), physical precipitating factors can be identified. PNES have been observed after epilepsy surgery and other neurosurgical procedures. Although some studies suggest that patients who have right-sided brain abnormalities were at particular risk,[42,66] this was not confirmed by other studies.[40,67–69] A history of head injuries is given by 24% to 65% of patients.[70–72] In most cases, investigations fail to show any physical sequelae of injury, although PNES have also been reported more after traumatic brain injury.[73] PNES may also be facilitated by antiepileptic drugs (AEDs) or AED intoxication (see Case C).[74]

TRIGGERS

Clinical experience suggests that PNES often also have more immediate triggers.[75] PNES have been observed in patients emerging from general anesthesia.[57,67,76–78] Video-EEG studies with intracranial electrodes have shown that PNES can develop from focal epileptic seizures[79] or even EEG-documented sleep.[80]

Much more commonly, however, an episode of apparent loss of consciousness is directly preceded by physical symptoms of arousal (eg, dry mouth, racing heart, increased sweating, hand tremor, shortness of breath), suggesting panic as a trigger (even if the patient was unaware that the symptoms were associated with anxiety) (see Case D).[81] Some patients describe PNES when exposed to a sudden sensory stimulus, or during sensory overload when many things seemed to occur simultaneously.

Not uncommonly, an increasing number of different sensations (eg, flashing lights, stepping into dark rooms, sudden noises) seem to trigger seizures as the disorder becomes more chronic (see Case A). Many patients seem to become so weary of triggering their seizures that they begin to make great efforts to avoid all emotional fluctuations, perhaps best described as *emotion phobia*. In keeping with this observation, a study comparing patients who had PNES, those who had epilepsy, and healthy controls found evidence of increased fear sensitivity in the PNES group.[82]

Patients may also become highly sensitized to (and avoidant of) physical sensations, such as mild presyncopal symptoms, perhaps as a consequence of an initial blackout fully explained by syncope. Unfortunately, whether an initial blackout may have been truly syncopal is difficult to determine because the semiology of PNES can be hard to distinguish from that of syncope.[83,84] The phenomenon of PNES directly arising from simple partial (epileptic) seizures observed with video-EEG could be explained by a similar phobic/dissociative mechanism (although different explanations have also been proposed).[85] This mechanism could also explain why some PNES are triggered by manifestations of psychopathology, such as visual flashbacks in PTSD or hallucinations in psychotic disorders.

PERPETUATING FACTORS
Avoidance

Once PNES have developed, it is usually possible to identify perpetuating factors that inhibit ability to gain control over seizures. Perhaps the most important of these is anxiety/avoidance. In a study describing etiologic factors in patients who had PNES and other functional symptoms, the authors identified anxiety (including health anxiety or hypochondriasis) as a relevant perpetuating factor in more than 50% of patients in both groups.[50]

Comparative studies have shown that patients who have PNES feel more strongly than healthy controls or those affected by epilepsy that their health is determined by factors beyond their own control, and that they have a stronger tendency to escape or avoid dealing with problems (see Cases B and D).[86,87] Perhaps persistent avoidance causes patients who have PNES to be less likely to consider negative life events relevant to the cause of their seizures than patients affected by epilepsy,[86] although they report these adverse experiences more commonly.[48] Avoidant behavior and the failure to consider life events as relevant may also explain why nearly 50% of patients who have PNES (or other functional neurologic disorders) fail to engage in psychotherapy.[88]

Avoidant behavior may even be apparent in the communication between doctors and patients. Several studies have shown that if the doctor adopts a receptive stance, avoids early interruption, and opens the encounter with an open question (eg, "how can I help you today?" or "what was your expectation when you came to see me?"), patients who have epilepsy will focus on their subjective seizure experiences without any further prompting.[89–91] In contrast, patients who have PNES and who are approached in this way avoid talking about seizure symptoms and focus on the situations in which their seizures occur or the consequences.[92]

Isolation and "sick role"

Perhaps the increasing avoidance of potential seizure triggers and normal social interaction causes patients to become isolated and their social contact group to contract.[93] Some become angry,[94] and a substantial number (22% in the author's study) become depressed.[50] Many develop additional physical symptoms, such as fatigue or pain (see Cases A and D),[95,96] with the number of additional symptoms correlating to the degree of emotional distress and severity of PNES disorder.[97]

Many patients become disabled and dependent on others. One study showed that 69% of 84 patients were employed at the start of their seizure disorder, and only 20% were still working by the time they were referred for video-EEG.[98] Four years after diagnosis, 56.4% were receiving health benefits.[99] In fact, two studies suggest that patients who have PNES are more likely than those who have similarly disabling epileptic seizures to be receiving health-related benefits, providing them with a financial disincentive to getting better.[100,101] For some patients the "sick role" becomes an important part of their identity (see Cases A, B, and D).[24]

The fact that patients and doctors commonly misattribute PNES to physical causes (especially epilepsy) means that the psychodynamic causes are not addressed. Misdiagnosis rates between 5% and 50% have been reported in different settings.[102–105] Patients' misplaced belief that there must be something physically wrong may be strengthened by repeated cycles of investigation and the prescription of more and more drugs (see Case D).[106,107]

In a study describing more than 300 patients, the authors found that the diagnosis of PNES was delayed by a mean of more than 7 years after the manifestation of seizures and that three quarters of the patients had been treated inappropriately with AEDs by the time the correct diagnosis was made.[108] More than 20% of these patients had at least one hospital admission with prolonged PNES ("pseudostatus"). Repeated admissions with prolonged PNES can lead to significant iatrogenic harm, including death.[109,110] Even patients who have been formally diagnosed with PNES commonly report being confused by their physicians' explanations of their diagnosis.[93,111]

SUMMARY

This account shows how a wide range of nonspecific factors collude to cause PNES, which is a very particular manifestation of psychopathology. The case reports show in what complex ways a predisposing traumatic experience, such as CSA, can be intimately linked to precipitating and perpetuating experiences in later life, or how one factor, such as comorbid epilepsy, can predispose to, precipitate, and perpetuate PNES. Although considering the cause of PNES in terms of the etiologic framework described in this article can help clinicians understand their patients,[75] and perhaps to communicate the diagnosis more credibly,[112] the identification of particular etiologic factors is not directly linked to specific interventions. Often the interaction of different factors is more readily addressed with psychotherapy than the specific factors themselves.

The fact that current understanding of the cause of PNES is limited to such a complex model of interacting etiologic factors, and that no specific pathogen has been identified, does not mean that the cause of the disorder remains unknown. In clinical practice, psychodynamic factors explain the presence of PNES to the satisfaction of experienced psychologists or psychotherapists in 95% of cases,[50,113] which means that individually adapted variants of psychotherapy are the preferred treatment.[75,114,115] However, other forms of intervention may also prove useful in the future. The biologic underpinning of an increased vulnerability to PNES is just beginning to be understood.[39] This work may enable better targeted medical interventions to be developed in the future.

APPENDIX: CASES
Case A

History

Mrs. A was referred to a specialist epilepsy clinic by a general neurologist at 55 years of age. Her seizures did not respond to several antiepileptic drugs (AEDs). She described blank spells for which she had no memory (duration: seconds to minutes; onset: 36 years of age; frequency: daily) and episodes involving loss of consciousness, shaking, incontinence, and tongue biting (duration: 5 to 20 minutes; onset: 36 years of age; frequency: two per week).

She had a history of medically unexplained fatigue, which caused her to use a wheelchair for 2 years (19 years of age); depression and a deliberate medication overdose (31 years of age); asthma (33 years of age); and a hysterectomy for dysfunctional bleeding (35 years of age). Her first blackout occurred during an episode of shortness of breath and anxiety triggered by an argument with her partner. An interictal EEG showed a "very considerable amount of sharp wave activity" with a "possible left-sided sharp wave focus" amounting to "strong support for the diagnosis of epilepsy." AED treatment was started, but her family doctor never observed any relationship between changes in her drug treatment and seizure frequency, although he noticed that seizures got worse during times of "social difficulty."

When she was 36 years old, she was admitted to the hospital after a seizure left her with a weak and stiff left arm and walking difficulties. The neurologic symptoms were considered functional and resolved without treatment after 3 months. The timing of these symptoms coincided with child custody proceedings.

Further emergency admissions occurred with prolonged seizures. When she was 46 year old, she had another admission with left-sided weakness. An MRI scan of the head showed no abnormalities. Emergency admissions continued as a result of seizures.

When she was 54 years of age, a typical convulsive seizure (without epileptic EEG changes) was captured during an admission for video-EEG. The interictal EEG showed nonspecific changes in the left temporal leads. After the diagnosis of psychogenic nonepileptic seizures was discussed with the patient, she stopped having seizures completely for 1 year, although her AEDs were withdrawn.

Her blank spells later returned (frequency: fewer than one per week), but did not cause much anxiety or disability, and 3 years later she remains disabled by medically unexplained facial and joint pains. A state-funded caregiver takes her out once a week. Twenty sessions of psychotherapy have revealed sexual abuse by several family members starting in childhood, and followed by sexually and physically abusive relationships in adulthood with a range of partners. Seizure exacerbations often seemed to be triggered by close contact with her son (who looked like one of her abusers) or her daughter (who was abused by a neighbor when the patient was too unwell to look after her).

Formulation

Predisposing factors: Childhood sexual abuse and neglect; somatization disorder with inappropriate medical and no psychological interventions; attachment problems with exploitative and abusive relationships in adulthood.

Precipitating factors: Ongoing sexual abuse and emotional exploitation; court proceedings.

Perpetuating factors: Inappropriate AED treatment; establishment of codependent relationship with new ("nice") partner; constant reminders of previous abuse through ongoing contact with children; other functional symptoms; perceives self as chronically disabled; receives long-term disability benefits.

Triggers: Flashing lights; sudden noises; seeing son or daughter; flashbacks of abuse.

Case B

History

Mr. B presented to a specialist epilepsy clinic at 56 years of age. He was a nursing home resident with a lifelong history of epilepsy and severe learning disability. He was able to feed himself with a spoon but unable to communicate verbally, was doubly incontinent, and had recently become unable to walk unaided. Mr. B had stopped undergoing regular neurologic follow-up 5 years previously. His antiepileptic drugs (AEDs) (phenytoin, 500 mg/d; carbamazepine, 1000 mg/d; phenobarbitone 180 mg/d) had not been altered since.

He experienced three different seizure types:

(1) Blank spells with head flopping to one side and drooling. The patient could slap himself on head or face when disturbed (duration: 5–10 minutes; onset: uncertain; frequency: several per week).

(2) Attack during which the patient would throw himself on floor, banging his head repetitively until it bled (duration: 5–10 minutes; onset: recent; frequency: several per week).

(3) Sudden collapse, rigidity, violent shaking followed by limp unresponsive state with recovery over 10 minutes (duration: 5–10 minutes; onset: always; frequency: 2 per year).

Examination showed the facial appearance of fragile-X (later confirmed with genetic testing), downbeat nystagmus, refusal to walk, normal tone, tendon reflexes, and plantar responses.

Diagnosis: Severe learning disability and epilepsy (seizure type 3) secondary to fragile-X. Additional psychogenic nonepileptic seizures (PNES) facilitated by antiepileptic drug toxicity.

Treatment: Withdrawal of phenytoin followed by withdrawal of phenobarbitone and introduction of levetiracetam. Encouragement of care staff to ignore PNES and reward appropriate interpersonal behavior.

Outcome: Type 1 and 2 seizures stopped when phenytoin was discontinued, walking unaided. At 2 years later, he experienced three type 3 seizures per year.

Formulation

Predisposing factors: Epilepsy, AED treatment, communication difficulties caused by learning disabilities.

Precipitating factors: AED toxicity.

Perpetuating factors: Failure to recognize PNES, inappropriate response to seizures by caregivers.

Triggers: "Not getting his own way," frustrations.

Case C

History

Mrs. C was referred to a specialist epilepsy clinic at 41 years of age for consideration of epilepsy surgery. From 3 years of age, she experienced seizures that occurred with a warning, allowing her to sit down (but which the patient was unable to recall);

unresponsiveness; drooling of saliva; chewing and fumbling movements; shuddering of arms and legs; and gradual recovery after 5 minutes, followed by confusion for 30 minutes. Seizures continued at a rate of two to three per month despite treatment with different AEDs.

At 40 years of age, the seizure frequency suddenly rose to ten per month. The patient ensured that she was with her mother 24 hours a day. An MRI scan of the head showed left mesial temporal sclerosis. Further history in the epilepsy clinic suggested that eight of ten attacks had a different semiology (slumping to the ground with closed eyes, unresponsiveness, appearing asleep for 10 to 20 minutes followed by immediate recovery). The new seizure type had started 1 year after she found her husband had died in bed beside her, and days after her son married and moved out.

Video-EEG captured one nocturnal complex partial seizure with left temporal seizure onset and one PNES manifesting as a limp, unresponsive state. PNES stopped after two sessions with a clinical psychologist. The patient underwent a left selective amygdalohippocampectomy 2 years later. All seizures have been controlled for more than 1 year.

Formulation

Predisposing factors: Epilepsy since childhood; fostering a codependent relationship with the patient's mother; chronic anxiety disorder.

Precipitating factors: Traumatic discovery of husband's death; loss of husband's support; conflict between perceived abandonment by son and unwillingness to stand in the way of son's happiness.

Perpetuating factors: Ongoing epilepsy; failure to recognize PNES; reestablishment of codependent relationship with mother.

Triggers: Being left alone; panic attacks; flashbacks.

Case D

History

Mr. D presented to a specialist epilepsy clinic at 46 years of age. His symptoms had started 5 years previously. Before his first blackout, he had come under increasing pressure as an information technology project manager. His memory seemed poor and he was taking increasingly more notes. His first blackout occurred at a business meeting. He struggled to get his words out although he knew what he wanted to say. He could not recall the names of the people around him and felt hot and tired. He developed blurred and double vision and collapsed after these symptoms had been present for 4 to 5 hours. He looked like he was asleep but lost control of his bladder. No shaking or injury was present. He recovered after 1 minute. He returned to his hotel room on his own but had no recollection of doing so. The next day he felt confused and experienced chest pain. He went to the hospital for a checkup, where a doctor noticed a droopy left eyelid.

He was unable to return to work for 6 months because of persisting fatigue. His attempt to return to work on a part-time basis failed because of fatigue, double vision, and further collapses (3–4 per year). Treatment for myasthenia was started after an equivocal edrophonium test. Further investigations for myasthenia failed to confirm this diagnosis. Other tests for muscle diseases were unremarkable. In 20 sessions of psychotherapy, the patient was able to link his driven work habits and tendency to avoid emotional experiences with his symptoms. He learned to pace himself and recognize his limits. He stopped having blackouts. Pyridostigmine treatment was stopped without a significant worsening of symptoms, but withdrawal of steroid treatment (prednisolone) below 5 mg/d caused a marked increase in lethargy.

Formulation

Predisposing factors: Strict and competitive but emotionally deprived upbringing with awards only for achievements; tendency to avoid emotional challenge in his own family through excessive commitment to work.

Precipitating factors: Exhaustion; inability to manage work demands to own satisfaction; inability to recruit support; panic attacks.

Perpetuating factors: Other functional symptoms (with chronic fatigue offering the opportunity to avoid emotional challenges); unhelpful medical tests and treatments; delayed psychological intervention.

Triggers: Fatigue; overactivity; demanding social situations.

REFERENCES

1. Angus-Leppan H. Diagnosing epilepsy in neurology clinics: a prospective study. Seizure 2008;17(5):431–6.
2. Kotsopoulos IA, de Krom MC, Kessels FG, et al. The diagnosis of epileptic and non-epileptic seizures. Epilepsy Res 2003;57(1):59–67.
3. LaFrance WC Jr, Rusch MD, Machan JT. What is "treatment as usual" for non-epileptic seizures? Epilepsy Behav 2008;12(3):388–94.
4. Reuber M. Psychogenic nonepileptic seizures: answers and questions. Epilepsy Behav 2008;12:622–35.
5. LaFrance WC Jr, Alper K, Babcock D, et al. Nonepileptic seizures treatment workshop summary. Epilepsy Behav 2006;8(3):451–61.
6. Groppel G, Kapitany T, Baumgartner C. Cluster analysis of clinical seizure semiology of psychogenic nonepileptic seizures. Epilepsia 2000;41(5):610–4.
7. Reuber M, Zeidler M, Chataway J, et al. Münchausen syndrome by phone. Lancet 2000;365:1358.
8. Benbadis S. The differential diagnosis of epilepsy: a critical review. Epilepsy Behav 2009;15(1):15–21.
9. Reuber M, Elger CE. Psychogenic nonepileptic seizures: review and update. Epilepsy Behav 2003;4(3):205–16.
10. Cragar DE, Berry DTR, Fakhoury TA, et al. A review of diagnostic techniques in the differential diagnosis of epileptic and nonepileptic seizures. Neuropsychol Rev 2002;12(1):31–64.
11. Reuber M. Are non-epileptic seizures a manifestation of neurologic pathology? In: Kanner AM, Schachter S, editors. Controversies in epilepsy and behavior. New York: Elsevier; 2008. p.151–75.
12. Reuber M, House AO. Treating patients with psychogenic non-epileptic seizures. Curr Opin Neurol 2002;15(2):207–11.
13. Baker GA, Brooks JL, Goodfellow L, et al. Treatments for non-epileptic attack disorder. Cochrane Database Syst Rev 2007;(1):CD006370.
14. Reuber M, Howlett S, Kemp S. Psychologic treatment for patients with psychogenic nonepileptic seizures. Expert Rev Neurother 2005;5:737–52.
15. LaFrance WC, Barry JJ. Update on treatments of psychological nonepileptic seizures. Epilepsy Behav 2005;7:364–74.
16. LaFrance WC, Devinsky O. Treatment of nonepileptic seizures. Epilepsy Behav 2002;3:S19–23.
17. Jaffee SR, Caspi A, Moffitt TE, et al. Individual, family, and neighborhood factors distinguish resilient from non-resilient maltreated children: a cumulative stressors model. Child Abuse Negl 2007;31(3):231–53.

18. Kendler KS, Aggen SH, Czajkowski N, et al. The structure of genetic and environmental risk factors for DSM-IV personality disorders: a multivariate twin study. Arch Gen Psychiatry 2008;65(12):1438–46.
19. Kendler KS, Gardner CO, Lichtenstein P. A developmental twin study of symptoms of anxiety and depression: evidence for genetic innovation and attenuation. Psychol Med 2008;38(11):1567–75.
20. Lesser RP. Psychogenic seizures. Neurology 1996;46(6):1499–507.
21. Chodoff P. Hysteria and women. Am J Psychiatry 1982;139(5):545–51.
22. Selkirk M, Duncan R, Oto M, et al. Clinical differences between patients with nonepileptic seizures who report antecedent sexual abuse and those who do not. Epilepsia 2008;49(8):1446–50.
23. Rosenbaum M. Psychogenic seizures—why women? Psychosomatics 2000; 41(2):147–9.
24. Ford C. Somatization and non-epileptic seizures. In: Gates JR, Rowan AJ, editors. Non-epileptic seizures. 1st edition. Boston: Butterworth-Heinemann; 1993. p.153–64.
25. Freud S, Breuer J. Studien über Hysterie. Leipzig and Vienna: Deuticke 1895 [in German].
26. Alper K, Devinsky O, Perrine K, et al. Nonepileptic seizures and childhood sexual and physical abuse. Neurology 1993;43(10):1950–3.
27. Duncan R, Oto M. Predictors of antecedent factors in psychogenic nonepileptic attacks: multivariate analysis. Neurology 2008;71(13):1000–5.
28. Sharpe D, Faye C. Non-epileptic seizures and child sexual abuse: a critical review of the literature. Clin Psychol Rev 2006;26:1020–40.
29. Kooiman CG, van Rees Vellinga S, Spinhoven P, et al. Childhood adversities as risk factors for alexithymia and other aspects of affect dysregulation in adulthood. Psychother Psychosom 2004;73(2):107–16.
30. Holman N, Kirby A, Duncan S, et al. Adult attachment style and childhood interpersonal trauma in non-epileptic attack disorder. Epilepsy Res 2008; 79(1):84–9.
31. Salmon P, Al-Marzooqi SM, Baker G, et al. Childhood family dysfunction and associated abuse in patients with nonepileptic seizures: towards a causal model. Psychosom Med 2003;65:695–700.
32. Bewley J, Murphy PN, Mallows J, et al. Does alexithymia differentiate between patients with nonepileptic seizures, patients with epilepsy and nonpatient controls? Epilepsy Behav 2005;7(3):1165–73.
33. Joukamaa M, Luutonen S, von RH, et al. Alexithymia and childhood abuse among patients attending primary and psychiatric care: results of the RADEP Study. Psychosomatics 2008;49(4):317–25.
34. Briere J, Rickards S. Self-awareness, affect regulation, and relatedness: differential sequels of childhood versus adult victimization experiences. J Nerv Ment Dis 2007;195(6):497–503.
35. Cragar DE, Berry DTR, Schmitt FA, et al. Cluster analysis of normal personality traits in patients with psychogenic nonepileptic seizures. Epilepsy Behav 2005; 6:593–600.
36. Reuber M, Pukrop R, Derfuss R, et al. Multidimensional assessment of personality in patients with psychogenic nonepileptic seizures. J Neurology Neurosurg Psychiatry 2003;75:743–8.
37. Lacey C, Cook M, Salzberg M. The neurologist, psychogenic nonepileptic seizures, and borderline personality disorder. Epilepsy Behav 2007;11(4): 492–8.

38. Galimberti CA, Ratti MT, Murelli R, et al. Patients with psychogenic nonepileptic seizures, alone or epilepsy associated, share a psychological profile distinct of epilepsy patients. J Neurology 2003;250(3):338–46.
39. Bakvis P, Roelofs K, Kuyk J, et al. Trauma, stress and preconscious threat processing in patients with psychogenic non-epileptic seizures. Epilepsia 2009; 50(5):1001–11.
40. Reuber M, Fernández G, Helmstaedter C, et al. Evidence of brain abnormality in patients with psychogenic nonepileptic seizures. Epilepsy Behav 2002;3:246–8.
41. Reuber M, Fernández G, Bauer J, et al. Interictal EEG abnormalities in patients with psychogenic non-epileptic seizures. Epilepsia 2002;43:1013–20.
42. Devinsky O, Mesad S, Alper K. Nondominant hemisphere lesions and conversion nonepileptic seizures. J Neuropsychiatry Clin Neurosci 2001;13(3): 367–73.
43. Reuber M, Fernández G, Helmstaedter C, et al. Are there physical risk factors for psychogenic nonepileptic seizures in patients with epilepsy? Seizure 2003;12: 561–7.
44. Rabe F. Die Kombination hysterischer und epileptischer Anfälle—das Problem der 'Hysteroepilepsy' in neuer Sicht. Berlin: Springer; 1970 [in German].
45. Sirven JI, Glosser DS. Psychogenic nonepileptic seizures. Neuropsychiatry Neuropsychol Behav Neurol 1998;11(4):225–35.
46. Bautista RE, Gonzales-Salazar W, Ochoa JG. Expanding the theory of symptom modeling in patents with psychogenic nonepileptic seizures. Epilepsy Behav 2008;13(2):407–9.
47. Stewart RS, Lovitt R, Stewart RM. Are hysterical seizures more than hysteria? A research diagnostic criteria, DMS-III, and psychometric analysis. Am J Psychiatry 1982;139(7):926–9.
48. Binzer M, Stone J, Sharpe M. Recent onset pseudoseizures—clues to aetiology. Seizure 2004;13(3):146–55.
49. Bowman ES, Markand ON. The contribution of life events to pseudoseizure occurrence in adults. Bull Menninger Clin 1999;63(1):70–88.
50. Reuber M, Howlett S, Khan A, et al. Non-epileptic seizures and other functional neurological symptoms: predisposing, precipitating and perpetuating factors. Psychosomatics 2007;48:230–8.
51. Bowman ES. Etiology and clinical course of pseudoseizures. Relationship to trauma, depression, and dissociation. Psychosomatics 1993;34(4):333–42.
52. Cartmill A, Betts T. Seizure behaviour in a patient with post-traumatic stress disorder following rape. Notes on the aetiology of "pseudoseizures". Seizure 1992;1:33–6.
53. Bowman ES, Markand ON. Psychodynamics and psychiatric diagnoses of pseudoseizure subjects. Am J Psychiatry 1996;153(1):57–63.
54. Griffith JL, Polles A, Griffith ME. Pseudoseizures, families, and unspeakable dilemmas. Psychosomatics 1998;39(2):144–53.
55. Gardner DL, Goldberg RL. Psychogenic seizures and loss. Int J Psychiatry Med 1982;12(2):121–8.
56. Miller HR. Psychogenic seizures treated by hypnosis. Am J Clin Hypn 1983; 25(4):248–52.
57. Ward PE, McCarthy DJ, Nyman GW. Podiatric implications of psychogenic seizures. J Foot Surg 1988;27:222–5.
58. Watson NF, Doherty MJ, Dodrill CB, et al. The experience of earthquakes by patients with epileptic and psychogenic nonepileptic seizures. Epilepsia 2002; 43:317–20.

59. Guberman A. Psychogenic pseudoseizures in non-epileptic patients. Can J Psychiatry 1982;27(5):401–4.
60. Oto M, Conway P, McGonigal A, et al. Gender differences in psychogenic non-epileptic seizures. Seizure 2005;14:33–9.
61. Duncan R, Oto M, Martin E, et al. Late onset psychogenic nonepileptic attacks. Neurology 2006;66(11):1644–7.
62. Stone J, Sharpe M, Binzer M. Motor conversion symptoms and pseudoseizures: a comparison of clinical characteristics. Psychosomatics 2004;45(6):492–9.
63. Tojek TM, Lumley M, Barkley G, et al. Stress and other psychosocial characteristics of patients with psychogenic nonepileptic seizures. Psychosomatics 2000;41(3):221–6.
64. Frances PL, Baker GA, Appleton PL. Stress and avoidance in pseudoseizures: testing the assumptions. Epilepsy Res 1999;34(2–3):241–9.
65. Fiszman A, Alves-Leon SV, Nunes RG, et al. Traumatic events and posttraumatic stress disorder in patients with psychogenic nonepileptic seizures: a critical review. Epilepsy Behav 2004;5:818–25.
66. Glosser G, Roberts D, Glosser DS. Nonepileptic seizures after resective epilepsy surgery. Epilepsia 1999;40(12):1750–4.
67. Reuber M, Kurthen M, Kral T, et al. New-onset psychogenic seizures after intracranial neurosurgery. Acta Neurochir 2002;144:901–8.
68. Davies KG, Blumer DP, Lobo S, et al. De novo nonepileptic seizures after intracranial surgery for epilepsy: incidence and risk factors. Epilepsy Behav 2000;1:436–43.
69. Ney GC, Barr WB, Napolitano C, et al. New-onset psychogenic seizures after surgery for epilepsy. Arch Neurol 1998;55(5):726–30.
70. Kalogjera-Sackellares D, Sackellares JC. Impaired motor function in patients with psychogenic pseudoseizures. Epilepsia 2001;42(12):1600–6.
71. Westbrook LE, Devinsky O, Geocadin R. Nonepileptic seizures after head injury. Epilepsia 1998;39(9):978–82.
72. Barry E, Krumholz A, Bergey GK, et al. Nonepileptic posttraumatic seizures. Epilepsia 1998;39(4):427–31.
73. Hudak AM, Trivedi K, Harper CR, et al. Evaluation of seizure-like episodes in survivors of moderate and severe traumatic brain injury. J Head Trauma Rehabil 2004;19(4):290–5.
74. Niedermeyer E, Blumer D, Holscher E, et al. Classical hysterical seizures facilitated by anticonvulsant toxicity. Psychiatr Clin (Basel) 1970;3(2):71–84.
75. Howlett S, Reuber M. An augmented model of brief psychodynamic interpersonal therapy for patients with nonepileptic seizures. Psychother Theory Res Pract Train 2009;46(1):125–38.
76. Lichter I, Goldstein LH, Toone BK, et al. Nonepileptic seizures following general anaesthetics: a report of five cases. Epilepsy Behav 2004;5(6):1005–13.
77. Reuber M, Enright SM, Goulding PJ. Postoperative pseudostatus: not everything that shakes is epilepsy. Anaesthesia 2000;55(1):74–8.
78. Parry T, Hirsch N. Psychogenic seizures after general anaesthesia. Anaesthesia 1992;47(6):534.
79. Devinsky O, Gordon E. Epileptic seizures progressing into nonepileptic conversion seizures. Neurology 1998;51(5):1293–6.
80. Orbach D, Ritaccio A, Devinsky O. Psychogenic nonepileptic seizures associated with video-EEG confirmed sleep. Epilepsia 2003;44:64–8.

81. Goldstein LH, Mellers JD. Ictal symptoms of anxiety, avoidance behaviour, and dissociation in patients with dissociative seizures. J Neurol Neurosurg Psychiatry 2006;77(5):616–21.

82. Hixson JD, Balcer LJ, Glosser G, et al. Fear sensitivity and the psychological profile of patients with psychogenic nonepileptic seizures. Epilepsy Behav 2006;9(4):587–92.

83. Benbadis SR, Chichkova R. Psychogenic pseudosyncope: an underestimated and provable diagnosis. Epilepsy Behav 2006;9(1):106–10.

84. Zaidi A, Crampton S, Clough P, et al. Head-up tilting is a useful test for psychogenic nonepileptic seizures. Seizure 1999;8:353–5.

85. Blumer D, Adamolekun B. Treatment of patients with coexisting epileptic and nonepileptic seizures. Epilepsy Behav 2006;9(3):498–502.

86. Stone J, Binzer M, Sharpe M. Illness beliefs and locus of control: a comparison of patients with pseudoseizures and epilepsy. J Psychosom Res 2004;57(6):541–7.

87. Goldstein LH, Drew C, Mellers J, et al. Dissociation, hypnotizability, coping styles and health locus of control: characteristics of pseudoseizure patients. Seizure 2000;9(5):314–22.

88. Howlett S, Grünewald R, Khan A, et al. Engagement in psychological treatment for functional neurological symptoms - barriers and solutions. Psychother Theory Res Pract Train 2007;44(3):354–60.

89. Plug L, Reuber M. Making the diagnosis in patients with blackouts: it's all in the history. Pract Neurol 2009;9(1):4–15.

90. Schwabe M, Reuber M, Schöndienst M, et al. Listening to people with seizures: how can conversation analysis help in the differential diagnosis of seizure disorders? Commun Med 2008;5(1):59–72.

91. Plug L, Reuber M. Conversation analysis can help in the differential diagnosis of patients with seizures: a case comparison. Seizure 2009;18:43–50.

92. Schwabe M, Howell SJ, Reuber M. Differential diagnosis of seizure disorders: a conversation analytic approach. Soc Sci Med 2007;65(4):712–24.

93. Thompson R, Isaac CL, Rowse G, et al. What is it like to receive the diagnosis of non-epileptic seizures? Epilepsy Behav 2009;14(3):508–15.

94. Mokleby K, Blomhoff S, Malt UF, et al. Psychiatric comorbidity and hostility in patients with psychogenic nonepileptic seizures compared with somatoform disorders and healthy controls. Epilepsia 2002;43(2):193–8.

95. Ettinger AB, Devinsky O, Weisbrot DM, et al. Headaches and other pain symptoms among patients with psychogenic non-epileptic seizures. Seizure 1999; 8(7):424–6.

96. Benbadis SR. A spell in the epilepsy clinic and a history of "chronic pain" or "fibromyalgia" independently predict a diagnosis of psychogenic seizures. Epilepsy Behav 2005;6(2):264–5.

97. Reuber M, House AO, Pukrop R, et al. Somatization, dissociation and psychopathology in patients with psychogenic nonepileptic seizures. Epilepsy Res 2003; 57:159–67.

98. Martin R, Bell B, Hermann B, et al. Nonepileptic seizures and their costs: the role of neuropsychology. In: Prigatano GP, Pliskin NH, editors. Clinical neuropsychology and cost outcome research: a beginning. 1st edition. New York: Psychology Press; 2003. p.235–58.

99. Reuber M, Pukrop R, Bauer J, et al. Outcome in psychogenic nonepileptic seizures: 1 to 10 year follow-up in 164 patients. Ann Neurol 2003;53:305–11.

100. Kristensen O, Alving J. Pseudoseizures–risk factors and prognosis. A case-control study. Acta Neurol Scand 1992;85(3):177–80.

101. Binder LM, Salinsky MC, Smith SP. Psychological correlates of psychogenic seizures. J Clin Exp Neuropsychol 1994;16(4):524–30.
102. Benbadis SR, O'Neill E, Tatum WO, et al. Outcome of prolonged video-EEG monitoring at a typical referral epilepsy center. Epilepsia 2004;45(9):1150–3.
103. Smith D, Defalla BA, Chadwick DW. The misdiagnosis of epilepsy and the management of refractory epilepsy in a specialist clinic. QJM 1999;92(1):15–23.
104. Scheepers B, Clough P, Pickles C. The misdiagnosis of epilepsy: findings of a population study. Seizure 1998;7(5):403–6.
105. Howell SJ, Owen L, Chadwick DW. Pseudostatus epilepticus. QJM 1989;71(266):507–19.
106. Hantke NC, Doherty MJ, Haltiner AM. Medication use profiles in patients with psychogenic nonepileptic seizures. Epilepsy Behav 2007;10(2):333–5.
107. Page LA, Wessely S. Medically unexplained symptoms: exacerbating factors in the doctor-patient encounter. J R Soc Med 2003;96:223–7.
108. Reuber M, Fernández G, Bauer J, et al. Diagnostic delay in psychogenic non-epileptic seizures. Neurology 2002;58(3):493–5.
109. Reuber M, Baker GA, Gill R, et al. Failure to recognize psychogenic nonepileptic seizures may cause death. Neurology 2004;62(5):834–5.
110. Gunatilake SB, De Silva HJ, Ranasinghe G. Twenty-seven venous cutdowns to treat pseudostatus epilepticus. Seizure 1997;6(1):71–2.
111. Carton S, Thompson PJ, Duncan JS. Non-epileptic seizures: patients' understanding and reaction to the diagnosis and impact on outcome. Seizure 2003;12:287–94.
112. Hall-Patch L, Brown R, House A, et al. Acceptability and effectiveness of a communication strategy for the diagnosis of non-epileptic attacks. Epilepsy Behav, in press.
113. Frances PL, Baker GA. Non-epileptic attack disorder (NEAD): a comprehensive review. Seizure 1999;8:53–61.
114. LaFrance WC Jr, Miller IW, Ryan CE, et al. Cognitive behavioral therapy for psychogenic nonepileptic seizures. Epilepsy Behav 2009;14(4):591–6.
115. Goldstein LH, Deale A, Mitchell-O'Malley S, et al. An evaluation of cognitive behavioral therapy as a treatment for dissociative seizures. Cogn Behav Neurol 2004;17:41–9.

Predicting Seizures: A Behavioral Approach

Sheryl R. Haut, MD[a],*, Richard B. Lipton, MD[a,b]

KEYWORDS

- Seizure prediction • Premonitory features
- Seizure precipitants • Trigger factors • Pre-ictal state

Epilepsy is the prototype for chronic neurologic disorders with episodic attacks (CDEA).[1] Like other CDEAs, the episodic attack (the seizure itself) is the most prominent manifestation of epilepsy. Nonetheless, between attacks, persons with epilepsy have alterations in brain structure and function that result in an enduring predisposition to seizures. Under certain circumstances, persons with epilepsy undergo a physiologic transition from the interictal state to the ictal state. This transition is generally regarded as a random, unpredictable event. Much of epilepsy treatment has been directed toward stabilizing the interictal brain state in hopes of preventing the transition to the ictal state, largely through the daily use of antiepilepsy drugs.

Despite optimal therapy, up to 40% of persons with epilepsy have refractory seizures.[2] Whereas much of the burden of epilepsy is related to the seizures themselves, the disorder also has a major impact on seizure-free days. Part of this interictal burden arises from the unpredictability of attacks.[3] Persons with attacks just 1 day a month may worry every day about having a seizure, potentially decreasing health-related quality of life.[4] More than 80% of persons with epilepsy are afraid of seizures; many regard the unpredictability of seizures as the single most problematic aspect of epilepsy,[3] and this unpredictability likely contributes to the reduced internal health locus of control exhibited in patients with epilepsy.[5] Clinical experience suggests that if patients recognize that attacks are predictable, that will, in itself, reduce the burden of unpredictability and improve quality of life.

Seizure prediction has arisen from the hope of making seizures predictable and perhaps preventable. The most widespread approaches to seizure prediction rely

Conflict of Interest Statement: Dr. S.R. Haut serves on the Speaker's Bureau and Advisory Board of UCB Pharma. She has served as a paid consultant for Jazz and King Pharma, and has received grant support from Endo. Dr. R.B. Lipton has served as a consultant for, and received grant support from Pfizer and Endo.

[a] Department of Neurology, Montefiore Medical Center, Albert Einstein College of Medicine, 111 East 210th Street, Bronx, New York, NY 10467, USA
[b] Department of Epidemiology and Population Health, Albert Einstein College of Medicine, Bronx, New York, NY 10461, USA
* Corresponding author.
E-mail address: haut@aecom.yu.edu (S.R. Haut).

on examination of electroencephalographic (EEG) changes, often recorded from intracranial electrodes.[6,7] These approaches could lead to direct intervention during the preictal period, using brain stimulation or pharmacologic agents, to abort or preempt an impending attack.[8] Thus far these approaches have not yet translated into significant clinical interventions, though at least one clinical trial is in progress.[9] More recently, clinical and behavioral strategies for seizure prediction in localization-related epilepsy have emerged.

This approach began with 2 simple clinical observations. First, some patients report that they can predict an impending seizure and second, individuals vary in the predictors they rely on and in the accuracy of predictions. Patients use different strategies to predict seizures. Some rely on premonitory features, changes in mood, behavior, or clinical experience that are harbingers of an impending attack, such as impaired concentration, increased anxiety, malaise, nausea, headache, and sleep disturbance.[10–13] Others identify specific trigger factors or precipitants, events associated with an increased probability of seizure over a circumscribed period of time. Candidate trigger factors may include stressful life events, missed medications, and altered sleep, among others.[14–17] Still others simply describe a feeling of impending seizure, and report that they can make accurate predictions.[18] Firm causal connections between putative trigger factors or premonitory features and the occurrence of seizures cannot be established based on patient self-report alone. Methods for establishing these connections are discussed later in this article.

Identifying reliable trigger factors and premonitory features would be of considerable clinical importance. For example, patients might learn to take precautionary measures during times of increased vulnerability to seizures. Insight into the factors that drive the transition from the interictal to the ictal state might provide a window into the mechanisms of epilepsy initiation. Finally, the ability to successfully predict seizures clinically could lead to a new paradigm of treatment in epilepsy, namely preemptive therapy, during periods of elevated seizure risk. These approaches depend on expanding our knowledge about the premonitory phase of a seizure, identifying reliable trigger factors, educating patients to become more aware of an impending attack, and developing interventions that decrease the probability of seizures over clinically relevant time frames.

In this article, the authors begin by considering fundamental underpinnings of seizure prediction, the epilepsy cycle, and the nonrandom distribution of seizures in time. Four categories of candidate predictor variables are then considered: EEG, premonitory features, trigger factors, and self-prediction. The methodological issues and approaches to studying seizure prediction are discussed, and the authors recommend that e-diaries offer considerable advantages. Results for the association of candidate predictors examined one at a time are presented, and the development of multivariate models to estimate the probability of seizures over clinically meaningful time periods is discussed. The article closes with a discussion of potential preemptive treatments and the steps necessary to make preemptive treatment of epilepsy a reality.

ISSUES IN SEIZURE PREDICTION

Emerging evidence suggests that seizures may be predictable in a subset of persons with epilepsy and that patients differ in their ability to make predictions. This section first describes the epilepsy cycle, which provides a conceptual context for viewing seizure prediction. The evidence reviewed shows that the temporal distribution of seizures is not random, again setting the stage for seizure prediction.

The Epileptic Cycle and Seizure Prediction

The "epileptic cycle" comprises the interictal phase, a preictal phase, an ictal phase, and a postictal phase (**Fig. 1**). The preictal phase represents a transition between the "usual" interictal state and the clinical seizure. Detecting this preictal phase is an area of great promise in seizure prediction. In the preictal phase, preemptive therapy intended to prevent the transition to the ictal phase may be possible. Once the transition from preictal to ictal state has occurred, preemption is no longer an option. Thus successful seizure prediction depends on the assumption that the preictal state differs from the interictal state in ways that can be identified and measured. These differences may be detected clinically, neurophysiologically, or functionally.

There is objective and subjective evidence that a preictal phase exists and that it can be identified. Some changes may be detected hours before a clinical seizure,

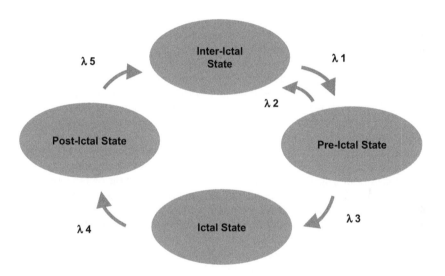

Transition	Goal	Treatment strategies
λ1 Transition to pre-ictal state	↓	Standard preventive therapy Trigger avoidance
λ2 Transition from pre-ictal to interictal state	↑	Potential role of pre-emptive therapy
λ3 Transition from pre-ictal to ictal state	↓	Potential role of pre-emptive therapy
λ4 Transition from ictal to post-ictal state	↑	Abortive antiepileptic therapies Possible role of VNS magnet
Transition from post-ictal to interictal period	↑	Unknown

Fig. 1. Transition phases in epilepsy and potential interventions.

such as quantitative EEG changes[19] and changes in cortical excitability as measured by transcranial magnetic stimulation threshold.[20,21] Measurable changes in affect or cognition in the preictal phase have also been reported,[22,23] and an increasing number of investigations are focusing on patient-reported features of the preictal state,[24] including premonitory symptoms and, for some patients, a feeling of impending seizure, referred to here as "self prediction."[18] It is likely that a maximally successful seizure prediction algorithm will incorporate multimodal features of objective and subjective predictive variables. To date, the investigations remain preliminary, and seizure prediction and preemption in the preictal period remain elusive. However, as evidenced by the studies discussed, the field continues to evolve with promise.

Seizures are Not Randomly Distributed in Time

The temporal distribution of seizures has been assessed using Markov models and by searching for deviations from a Poisson distribution. The available evidence indicates that the temporal profile of seizures is not random.[25–31]

Using Markov models, the probability of seizure on a particular day can be assessed based on the probability of seizures on the previous day or days. These approaches show that seizure occurrence is a nonrandom event. Using these methods, probability estimates for the expected incidence of subsequent seizure days can be calculated.[30] Tauboll and colleagues[25] computed transitional probabilities between seizures and no seizures and demonstrated this dependence in half of their subjects. Negative dependence, or a lower probability of seizure events following a day of high seizure activity, has also been noted.[27]

An alternative approach tests the hypothesis that seizures are randomly distributed in time by looking for deviation from a Poisson process. A Poisson model describes a stochastic (random) system whereby the number of events in disjointed (nonoverlapping) time intervals are independent random variables, and the number of events within each time variable occurs as random variables with a Poisson distribution. For a Poisson process the probability of an event is not influenced by the temporal distribution of recent events. Seizure patterns do not follow a Poisson distribution. Deviations from a Poisson process may reflect clustering, periodic patterns, or other types of regularity. Seizure clustering has been reviewed elsewhere[32] and seizure clusters have been shown to significantly deviate from a Poisson process.[25,27,29,30] Clinical examples of seizures as periodic events are well recognized, and seizure regularity is seen largely in patients who experience daily seizures.

CANDIDATE PREDICTORS OF SEIZURES

Given that seizures are not randomly distributed in time, they may have several predictors. In this section EEG-based approaches are briefly mentioned and 3 sorts of behavioral predictors considered: premonitory features, trigger factors, and self-prediction based on a subjective state.

Electroencephalographic-based Approaches

The electrophysiology of the preictal state has been under investigation since the 1970s, but the advent of computerized methods of linear and nonlinear EEG analysis significantly enhanced the progress in this area.[8] Neurophysiologic seizure prediction techniques attempt to identify characteristic changes in EEG that precede a seizure by days, hours, or seconds, typically by examining EEG changes obtained during intracranial monitoring.[33] The ultimate goals of this line of research are to reliably identify preictal changes leading to successful seizure prediction, particularly toward the development of closed-loop devices that actively record EEG signals, process these signals, and trigger an intervention. To date, one closed-loop device, the responsive neurostimulator, is under evaluation in a randomized double-blind clinical trial.[9] These investigations have been recently well reviewed[8,34] and are outside the scope of this article.

Premonitory Features and the Prodrome

Clinical seizure prediction paradigms must consider the presence of subjective feelings preceding the seizure. These premonitory features occur during a period called the prodrome. Although the presence of a prodrome is less common in epilepsy than in other CDEAs such as migraine, many reports have documented specific signs or symptoms endorsed by patients to occur up to 24 hours preceding a clinical seizure.[10–13,24] It is important to distinguish between a prodrome, which implies a pre-ictal state, and an aura, which occurs as the first part of the seizure. The presence of premonitory features and duration of the prodrome figure prominently in identification of, and treatment during, a high-risk seizure state.

Premonitory features during the preictal state may include functional changes such as behavioral disturbance or cognitive slowing.[22,35] The frequency of epileptiform discharges has been shown to increase as early as 7 hours before a seizure,[19] and studies have indicated that paroxysmal epileptiform activity can contribute to cognitive impairment in the absence of clinical seizure activity.[36,37] Efforts to elucidate the characteristics of the preictal state will have to focus on examination of function during this phase, although this area has received little attention to date.

The Role of Trigger Factors/Seizure Precipitants

Triggers, or precipitants, are factors that increase the probability of an attack over a brief, defined time period in people who have a disease. Understanding trigger factors is crucial, as persons with epilepsy are eager to understand what initiates their attacks, and trigger management can potentially reduce attack frequency and enhance self-efficacy.[38] Identifying trigger factors may also provide clues to the neurobiological mechanisms that lead to the transition from the preictal to the ictal state. On the other hand, misidentification of triggers can lead to unhelpful and unnecessary changes in lifestyle. Therefore, robust methods to identify triggers are necessary for both clinical practice and research. As it is likely that seizure self-prediction is based in part on the recognition of specific trigger factors in the time period before the prediction, any clinical seizure prediction algorithms should include data on precipitants.

Patient Self-Prediction

Many patients with CDEA report that they can predict whether an attack is imminent. Whereas the ability to successfully predict an attack has been previously demonstrated in persons with migraine,[39] this direction has not been widely pursued in the epilepsy literature to date. One study has specifically addressed the patient's ability to self-predict seizures.[18] Using a prospective paper diary design, seizure self-prediction was assessed by the following question, completed on a daily basis: "Do you think you will have a seizure in the next 24 hours?" Response options included extremely likely (1), somewhat likely (2), somewhat unlikely (3), and extremely unlikely (4). The results of this study, discussed later, indicated that a significant subset of the cohort were able to successfully predict up to 40% of their seizures.

METHODOLOGIC ISSUES IN STUDYING SEIZURE PREDICTION

The goal is to link the candidate predictors of seizures to the actual occurrence of seizures by measuring each and assessing their relationship. In efforts to accomplish this seemingly simple goal, the authors have encountered several methodological issues and challenges. In general, the authors capture data on candidate risk factors for attacks and the occurrence of attacks at least once a day; they then study the relation of the exposures to the attacks within an individual or within a population taking the individual into account. In these designs, each patient provides data regarding exposures followed by seizures and exposures not followed by seizures. There are opportunities to develop models for individuals, models for specified populations, or models that take both the individual and the population into account.

Selecting Patients for Seizure Prediction Studies

Seizure prediction is not plausible for a patient with one seizure per year. The probability of an event on any given day is very low and it is not possible to collect enough data over a reasonable period to develop robust statistical models. Nor is seizure prediction appropriate for persons with daily or near daily seizures, as the probability of an event on any given day approaches 1. Rather, seizure prediction is most relevant for individuals with an intermediate frequency of seizures, which occur at a frequency of 1 to 20 days per month. In this group, events are frequent enough to gather meaningful data over realistic time periods but not so frequent that there is no variability to explain.

Distinguishing Within-person and Population Level Prediction

It is useful to distinguish individual (within-person) models and population models. An individual model is developed only using data from a particular person and answers questions about factors that predict seizures in that individual. The strength of this approach is that only factors germane to a particular patient are identified. The great weakness is that it takes many seizures (at least 10) to fit a reliable within-person model. As a consequence, it may take a year to get sufficient data from a single individual to fit a robust prediction model.

Population level models are informative about factors that predict seizures in the group of patients under study. The great strength of this model is that large amounts of data (a large number of attacks) can be captured quickly. The great weakness is that a factor that is very important in a single person, but only in that person, may not be detected.

An optimal modeling strategy, discussed in a recent study,[40] takes advantage of the known phenomenon that borrowing strength from cohort models can be used to develop individual models.[41] In this study, diary-based population data were used to predict the occurrence of future seizures using individual-level models.

Diary Formats and Data Sampling Approaches

The traditional paper diary format is being replaced by electronic platforms in many diary studies.[42] Paper diaries allow for frequent data capture and allow patients to report putative risk factors before seizures occur. Electronic diaries provide significant advantages over paper diaries for seizure prediction. Electronic diaries can be used to examine within-day temporal dynamics with precise timing, and provide a time stamp to ensure the prospective nature of the data. As data entry portals they are small and portable, allowing for multiple entries throughout the day. The Internet is also emerging as a potential diary data collection tool.

Diary investigations in behavioral science have increasingly relied on intensive repeated within-person designs to capture affective states and physical symptoms in real time or close to real time.[43] Published literature suggests that whereas people can recall concrete behavioral events and stressful encounters across short time intervals (ie, several days to a week),[44,45] emotional experiences[46] and coping efforts[47,48] recalled even just a few days after their occurrence bear only modest concordance with their close to real time assessment. This fact was recently demonstrated in a study of affect during epilepsy monitoring,[23] discussed later, which used an experience-based sampling method (ESM), also called ecological momentary assessment, to assess affect in relation to seizure occurrence. The ESM methodology is useful in capturing affective states in real time or close to real time.[49] Robust clinical seizure prediction models will likely require a combination of interval contingent, or fixed, data sampling, and ESM sampling.

Adequately Sampling the Preictal State

Sampling intervals also need to consider the duration of the preictal state. If the preictal state is relatively brief, a long sampling interval may miss the relevant preictal features required for prediction. With frequent sampling, one can examine the time lag between the predictor and the seizure. For example, losing sleep the night before last may influence seizure probability today.

Defining the duration of the preictal state is also critical for clinically relevant therapeutic interventions. A relatively brief time window may preclude intervention; in contrast, defining a preictal state as the 24 hours preceding a seizure may be too long a window for a behavioral or pharmacologic intervention. Very little data are yet available on this issue. The duration of prodromes from a recent article[13] ranged from 30 minutes to several hours, whereas other studies suggest a preictal state of up to 24 hours.[24]

RESULTS OF DIARY STUDIES
Premonitory Features and the Prodrome

Premonitory symptoms have been reported in 6% to 47% of the epilepsy population.[10–13,24] Many premonitory features reported in epilepsy lie in the neuropsychiatric domain, including behavioral, cognitive, and mood changes[13] such as impaired concentration, and increased anxiety. Other frequently reported symptoms include malaise, nausea, headache, and sleep disturbance. The premonitory symptoms most frequently reported in cross-sectional studies are summarized in **Table 1**.

Of the reported prodromal symptoms, mood changes have been the most widely investigated. In 2 prospective studies, seizure occurrence followed low mood reported the previous day[50] or increased stress and anxiety ratings reported the previous day.[51] These studies were limited by once daily sampling, thus the exact time frame between mood change and seizure occurrence is unknown.

In an inpatient study of patients undergoing epilepsy monitoring,[52] retrospective report of affect was compared with ESM-based affective state ratings collected during interictal, preictal, and postictal periods in a small number of subjects. The prodromal, or preictal phase was characterized by a statistically significant elevation of unactivated negative affect and decrease in activated positive affect. Of note, subjects retrospectively reported more positive feeling during the monitoring than they actually reported in real time by the ESM data collection, demonstrating the increased reliability of momentary assessment.

Table 1
Premonitory features reported in epilepsy studies

	Scaramelli et al, 2009[13]	Schultze-Bonhage et al, 2006[12]	Rajna et al, 1997[11]	Hughes et al, 1993[10]
Most common	Behavioral changes	Restlessness	Poorly described funny feeling	Irritability
	Cognitive disturbance	Headache	Epigastric sensation	Anxiety/mood changes
	Anxiety/mood changes	Malaise	Headache	Cognitive disturbance
	Fatigue/malaise	Nausea	–	Headache
	Sleep disturbance	Impaired concentration	–	Funny feeling
	Speech disturbance	Dizziness	–	Speech disturbance
	Gastrointestinal symptoms	Tiredness	–	Polyuria
	Headache	–	–	Elation
Less common	Appetite/thirst changes	–	–	–

At least one study has examined measurable changes of clinical behavior during the preictal period. Administering a methodology previously used in schizophrenia, Bruzzo and colleagues[22] examined the performance of a mental stimulation task during various phases of the epileptic cycle in a small sample of patients with epilepsy. In 2 patients with right temporal lobe epilepsy, timing precision of nonbiological movement simulation demonstrated patterns that differed based on the temporal vicinity to a forthcoming seizure. Although preliminary, these findings suggest that behavioral tasks may be used for clinical seizure prediction. These findings are consistent with the high incidence of cognitive changes reported as premonitory features.[13]

Trigger Factors or Precipitants

In the general epilepsy population, up to 90% of persons with epilepsy identify at least one seizure precipitant.[14–17,52,53] Patients with poorly controlled epilepsy are more likely to report precipitants than those with infrequent seizures,[15,17] as are patients with higher anxiety levels and lower health locus of control.[17] Emotional stress and stressful life events, sleep deprivation, depression, anxiety, menstruation, and alcohol use are among the most commonly reported seizure precipitants.[14–17,52–55]

Most studies rely on patient self-report to identify precipitants. As can be seen in **Table 2** and **Fig. 2**, patients may report seizure triggers that have not been documented in prospective studies, such as drinking coffee. However, emotional stress and sleep deprivation are the 2 most commonly reported precipitants in most studies; the associations between these factors and seizure occurrence have been confirmed prospectively.

An intriguing hypothesis reported recently by Rajna and colleagues[56] supposes that true unprovoked seizures are rare and that most seizures are in fact related to seizure-precipitating factors. These investigators suggest that the occurrence of seizures in epilepsy relies on both an epileptic susceptibility of a tonic nature and an acute occasional seizure-precipitating factor of a phasic nature. When the tonic dysfunction is predominant, a seizure may occur from a subtle precipitant not easily observable, and the patient will conclude that this was an unprovoked seizure. If the tonic

Table 2
Most frequently reported seizure-precipitating factors across populations ($n = 1677$)

	United States	Denmark	Norway	Total
1. Emotional stress	106 (18.2%)	73 (24.3%)	171 (21.5%)	350 (20.9%)
2. Sleep deprivation	32 (5.5%)	54 (17.9%)	108 (13.6%)	194 (11.6%)
3. Tiredness	51 (8.8%)	35 (11.6%)	74 (9.3%)	160 (9.5%)
4. Alcohol	21 (3.6%)	28 (9.3%)	46 (5.8%)	95 (5.7%)
5. Fever	37 (6.4%)	22 (7.3%)	27 (3.4%)	86 (5.1%)
6. Flickering light	10 (1.7%)	28 (9.3%)	35 (4.4%)	73 (4.4%)
7. Noncompliance	27 (4.6%)	21 (7.0%)	14 (1.8%)	62 (3.7%)
8. Menstruation	4 (1.3%)	5 (3.2%)	20 (4.8%)	29 (3.3%)
9. Physical exercise	4 (0.7%)	1 (0,3%)	47 (5.9%)	52 (3.1%)
10. Health	10 (1.7%)	7 (2.3%)	10 (1.3%)	27 (1.6%)
11. Other	26 (4.5%)	10 (3.3%)	38 (4.8%)	74 (4.4%)

From Nakken KO, Solaas MH, Kjeldsen MJ, et al. Which seizure-precipitating factors do patients with epilepsy most frequently report? *Data from* Epilepsy Behav 2005;6(1):85–9.

dysfunction is not strong, a more dramatic precipitant is required. This hypothesis, if true, lends support to the concept that seizures may be predictable if precipitants for an individual patient, both subtle and dramatic, can be identified.

Patient Self-Prediction During the Preictal State

One study has specifically addressed the patient's ability to self-predict seizures.[18] Using a prospective paper diary design, seizure self-prediction was assessed by the following question, completed on a daily basis: "Do you think you will have a seizure in the next 24 hours?" Response options included extremely likely (1), somewhat likely (2), somewhat unlikely (3), and extremely unlikely (4). The 71 subjects had 1488 seizure days, of which 475 had an antecedent prediction of "extremely likely" or "somewhat likely," yielding a population sensitivity of 31.9%. For the 13,691 seizure-free days for which there was a prediction, 11,388 had been rated "somewhat unlikely" or "extremely unlikely" (83.2% specificity). Adjusting for heterogeneity across subjects, an overall specificity of 87% and sensitivity of 21% were obtained. The Cochran-Mantel-Haenzel odds ratio (OR) for positive prediction was 2.25 (95% confidence interval [CI] 1.91–2.65), indicating that seizures were twice as likely in the 24-hour epoch following a prediction.

While the overall group demonstrated significant seizure self-prediction, 12 subjects demonstrated significant individual predictability and were termed "predictors." The Mantel-Haenzel estimate of the OR for the predictor group was 3.14 (95% CI 2.53–3.89), indicating that following a positive prediction, the subject was more than 3 times more likely to experience a seizure. In this subgroup, the unadjusted mean specificity of prediction was 88% and the sensitivity was 57%; adjusting for heterogeneity across subjects resulted in specificity of 90% and sensitivity of 37%. Accuracy of seizure prediction for the subjects with significant predictive ability, adjusted for individual contribution, is presented in **Fig. 3**. The investigators subsequently demonstrated[51] that subjects appeared to be drawing on stress and anxiety ratings to derive this sense of impending seizure (see later discussion).

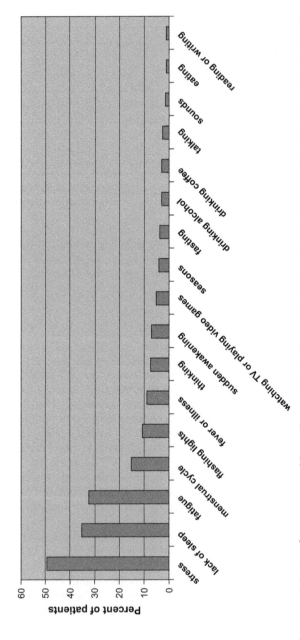

Fig. 2. Seizure precipitating factors reported by epilepsy patients. (*Reproduced from* Sperling MR, Schilling CA, Glosser D, et al. Self-perception of seizure precipitants and their relation to anxiety level, depression, and health locus of control in epilepsy. Seizure 2008;17(4):302–7; with permission.)

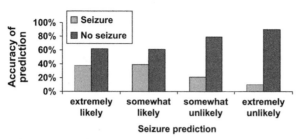

Fig. 3. Accuracy of seizure predictors. positive predictive values and negative predictive values for the subgroup (n = 12) of subjects demonstrating significant seizure prediction. Values are adjusted for within-person correlation.

The major limitation of this initial study was the use of paper diaries, which potentially allowed for back-filling. A current electronic diary study is in process; preliminary analysis supports the findings of the paper diary study (Haut et al, 2009, unpublished data).

BUILDING A PREDICTIVE MODEL

The next step in clinical seizure prediction is the development of robust prediction modeling using several predictors. In the paper diary study described above,[51] precipitants were entered into predictive models. Self-reported levels of stress, anxiety, and hours of sleep for the night before the seizure remained significant in the model. When patient self seizure prediction was included, variables that remained in the model included self-prediction (OR 3.7; 95% CI 1.8–7.2), and hours of sleep for the night before the seizure (OR 0.90; 95% CI 0.82–0.99). Self-reported stress and anxiety levels did not remain significant; the implication being that subjects felt most likely to experience a seizure when they were reporting greater stress and anxiety.

Based on these data, several hypothetical scenarios (**Table 3**) were calculated for a 40-year-old female subject. Although this study was preliminary and based on paper diary data, the demonstrated potential for developing predictive models is exciting.

PROSPECTS FOR PREEMPTIVE THERAPY

The treatment of epilepsy is traditionally divided into acute and preventive treatments. Acute treatments have only limited use, and are generally taken during prolonged

Table 3
Building predictive models: Hypothetical scenarios. Seizure self-prediction replaces stress and anxiety in the model; the implication being that subjects felt most likely to experience a seizure when they were reporting greater stress and anxiety

Stress		Anxiety	Hours of Sleep	Risk of Seizure %
Low		Low	High	4.1
Moderate		Moderate	Moderate	5.9
High		High	Low	8.5

Stress	Anxiety	Hours of Sleep	Self-prediction	Risk of Seizure %
Any	Any	High	Low	2.9
Any	Any	Moderate	Moderate	6.7
Any	Any	Low	High	13.1

seizures, seizure clusters, or episodes of status epilepticus. Preventive treatments are nearly standard in epilepsy, consisting of medication that is taken on a regular basis to reduce the probability of an attack. Preemptive therapy is the next logical step in the treatment of CDEAs such as epilepsy. The strategy involves treating in anticipation of the next attack before it begins. As a treatment strategy, preemptive treatment is inter-mediate between acute and preventive treatment. Preemptive therapy may be highly advantageous, in part because treatment is given only when it is most likely to be useful, reducing patient exposure to medications and cost. Successful preemption of attacks would greatly reduce the health and economic burden of episodic disease.

Potential Pharmacologic Preemptive Treatments

The mainstay of acute pharmacologic therapy in epilepsy is benzodiazepine therapy; there is ample evidence that these agents successfully abort seizure clusters, or termi-nate prolonged seizures/status epilepticus.[57,58] It is likely that the use of benzodiaze-pines will figure prominently in preemptive epilepsy therapy. For example, a patient might take a long-acting benzodiazepine when an attack is likely. Alternative pharmacotherapies might include an increased dose of a preventive antiepileptic drug, although this presents a significant risk of toxicity. With the exception of preemp-tive treatment during periods of fever for patients with febrile seizures[59] and preemptive treatment with acetozolamide for catamenial seizures,[60] no studies of preemptive therapy in epilepsy have been reported to date; presumably this investiga-tion will expand when seizure prediction improves.

Nonpharmacologic Preemptive Therapies

Nonpharmacologic preemptive approaches include taking precautionary measures to reduce the consequences of a seizure, trigger avoidance, and other behavioral methods.

Precautionary Measures

If at-risk seizure states can be identified, patients may be able to institute precau-tionary measures to increase their safety on "high-risk" days. Examples might include such measures as avoiding travel by public transportation, or alerting family members or friends to "check in" periodically. For this approach to be effective without need-lessly increasing anxiety and limiting the patient's quality of life, a high specificity for a high-risk day would be necessary.

Trigger Avoidance

Trigger avoidance is a technique that is already practiced by many patients.[15,24,52] Patients may try to avoid precipitants that they associate with their own seizure occur-rence, or those reported in the literature.[38] There are several limitations to trigger avoidance. Not surprisingly, patients are anxious to identify triggers to improve their sense of seizure self-control in an otherwise unpredictable disorder. Recollection bias will ascribe associations of seizures and triggers that do not show significant associations when studied prospectively. Furthermore, for many triggers there is a high level of variation from person to person; even within persons, susceptibility to a particular trigger may depend on the overall level of seizure risk. Therefore, nonper-sonalized trigger avoidance may lead to needless restrictions of lifestyle. Finally, whereas certain triggers may be avoided (ie, sleep deprivation), others remain out of the patient's control (ie, stressful life events).

Other Behavioral Techniques

The measures that patients report of being able to "prevent a seizure from happening" can be considered a form of behavioral preemptive therapy. Several studies have discussed this reported ability, called by various terms including "seizure countermeasures" and seizure self-control.[11,15,52,61,62] The ability to self-terminate a focal seizure before it spreads, termed "seizure arrest," has also been discussed.[38] These techniques, often self-developed by patients, range from relaxation to concentration. Reported relaxation strategies include deep breathing, progressive muscle relaxation, biofeedback, or yoga.[38,62,63] In contrast, some patients report that focusing on a thought, performing mental calculations, or concentrating on a task may be effective in aborting an impending seizure. Specific seizure arrest by activation of an adjacent cortical area has been described; for example, a patient whose seizures began with sensory paresthesias found that clenching his fist at the onset of the symptoms could prevent secondary generalization.[38] Although intriguing, to date no large study has examined patients' ability to preempt seizures with behavioral methodologies.

SUMMARY

This article reviews the epilepsy cycle, distinguishing the interictal, preictal, ictal, and postictal phases. Evidence suggesting that the preictal phase can sometimes be identified based on neurophysiologic signals, premonitory features, the presence of trigger factors, or self-report is also reviewed. Diary studies have shown that seizures are not randomly distributed in time and that a subgroup of persons with epilepsy can predict an impending seizure. Paper diary data and preliminary analysis of electronic diary data suggest that seizure prediction is feasible.

Whereas all of this evidence sets the stage for seizure prediction and preemptive therapy, several questions remain unanswered. First, what proportion of persons with epilepsy can predict their seizures? Second, within and among individuals, how accurate is prediction? Third, can prediction be improved through education about group level or individual predictors? And finally, in a group that can make robust predictions what are the most effective interventions for reducing seizure probability at times of high risk?

The answers to these questions could reduce the burden of epilepsy by making seizures predictable and setting the stage for preemptive therapy. This work could improve the understanding of epilepsy by providing a context for studying the transitions from the interictal to preictal and ictal states. More prospective studies are needed; challenges certainly exist, but as the studies discussed here demonstrate, the field is rich with promise for improving the lives of patients with epilepsy.

ACKNOWLEDGMENTS

The authors gratefully acknowledge their collaboration with Dr. Charles B. Hall and Dr. Howard Tennen.

REFERENCES

1. Haut SR, Bigal M, Lipton RB. Chronic disorders with episodic manifestations: Focus on epilepsy and migraine. Lancet Neurol 2006;5:148–57.
2. Kwan P, Brodie MJ. Early identification of refractory epilepsy. N Engl J Med 2000; 342(5):314–9.
3. Fisher RS, Vickrey BG, Gibson P, et al. The impact of epilepsy from the patient's perspective I. Descriptions and subjective perceptions. Epilepsy Res 2000;41:39–51.

4. Fisher RS. Epilepsy from the patient's perspective: review of results of a community-based survey. Epilepsy Behav 2000;1(4):S9–14.

5. Asadi-Pooya AA, Schilling CA, Glosser D, et al. Health locus of control in patients with epilepsy and its relationship to anxiety, depression, and seizure control. Epilepsy Behav 2007;11(3):347–50.

6. Mormann F, Kreuz T, Rieke C, et al. On the predictability of epileptic seizures. J Clin Neurophysiol 2005;116(3):569–87.

7. Litt B, Echauz J. Prediction of epileptic seizures. Lancet Neurol 2002;1(1):22–30.

8. Sackellares JC. Seizure prediction. Epilepsy Curr 2008;8(3):55–9.

9. Skarpaas TL, Morrell MJ. Intracranial stimulation therapy for epilepsy. Neurotherapeutics 2009;6(2):238–43.

10. Hughes J, Devinsky O, Feldmann E, et al. Premonitory symptoms in epilepsy. Seizure 1993;2:201–3.

11. Rajna P, Clemens B, Csibri E, et al. Hungarian multicenter epidemiologic study of the warning and initial symptoms (prodrome, aura) of epileptic seizures. Seizure 1997;6:361–8.

12. Schulze-Bonhage A, Kurth C, Carius A, et al. Seizure anticipation by patients with focal and generalized epilepsy: a multicentre assessment of premonitory symptoms. Epilepsy Res 2006;70:83–8.

13. Scaramelli A, Braga P, Avellanal A, et al. Prodromal symptoms in epileptic patients: Clinical characterization of the pre-ictal phase. Seizure 2009;18(4):246–50.

14. Nakken KO, Solaas MH, Kjeldsen MJ, et al. Which seizure-precipitating factors do patients with epilepsy most frequently report? Epilepsy Behav 2005;6(1):85–9.

15. Spector S, Cull C, Goldstein LH. Seizure precipitants and perceived self-control of seizures in adults with poorly controlled epilepsy. Epilepsy Res 2000;38(2–3):207–16.

16. Neugebauer R, Paik M, Hauser WA, et al. Stressful life events and seizure frequency in patients with epilepsy. Epilepsia 1994;35(2):336–43.

17. Sperling MR, Schilling CA, Glosser D, et al. Self-perception of seizure precipitants and their relation to anxiety level, depression, and health locus of control in epilepsy. Seizure 2008;17(4):302–7.

18. Haut SR, Hall CB, LeValley AJ, et al. Can patients with epilepsy predict their seizures? Neurology 2007;68:262–6.

19. Litt B, Esteller R, Echauz J, et al. Epileptic seizures may begin hours in advance of clinical onset: a report of five patients. Neuron 2001;30(1):51–64.

20. Wright MA, Orth M, Patsalos PN, et al. Cortical excitability predicts seizures in acutely drug-reduced temporal lobe epilepsy patients. Neurology 2006;67(9):1646–51.

21. Badawy R, Macdonell R, Jackson G, et al. The peri-ictal state: cortical excitability changes within 24 h of a seizure. Brain 2009;132(Pt 4):1013–21.

22. Bruzzo AA, Gesierich B, Rubboli G, et al. Predicting epileptic seizures with a mental simulation task: a prospective study. Epilepsy Behav 2008;13(1):256–9.

23. Willard KS, Licht BG, Gilmore RL, et al. Affect in patients with epilepsy undergoing video/EEG monitoring: retrospective versus momentary assessment and temporal relationship to seizures. Epilepsy Behav 2006;8(3):625–34.

24. Petitmengin C, Baulac M, Navarro V. Seizure anticipation: are neurophenomenological approaches able to detect preictal symptoms? Epilepsy Behav 2006;9(2):298–306.

25. Tauboll R, Lundervold A, Gjerstad L. Temporal distribution of seizures in epilepsy. Epilepsy Res 1991;8:153–65.

26. Binnie CD, Aarts JHP, Houtkooper MA, et al. Temporal characteristics of seizures and epileptiform discharges. Electroencephalogr Clin Neurophysiol 1984;58: 498–505.
27. Balish M, Albert P, Theodore WH. Seizure frequency in intractable partial epilepsy: a statistical analysis. Epilepsia 1991;32(5):642–9.
28. Milton JG, Gotman J, Remillard GM, et al. Timing of seizure recurrence in adult epileptic patients: a statistical analysis. Epilepsia 1987;28(5):471–8.
29. Haut SR, Lipton RB, LeValley A, et al. Identifying seizure clusters in patients with epilepsy. Neurology 2005;65(8):1313–5.
30. Hopkins A, Davies P, Dobson C. Mathematical models of patterns of seizures: their use in the evaluation of drugs. Arch Neurol 1985;42:463–7.
31. Bauer J, Burr W. Course of chronic focal epilepsy resistant to anticonvulsant treatment. Seizure 2001;10:239–46.
32. Haut SR. Seizure clustering. Epilepsy Behav 2006;8(1):50–5.
33. Iasemidis LD, Shiau DS, Pardalos PM, et al. Long-term prospective on-line real-time seizure prediction. Clin Neurophysiol 2005;116(3):532–44.
34. Stacey WC, Litt B. Technology insight: neuroengineering and epilepsy—designing devices for seizure control. Nat Clin Pract Neurol 2008;4(4): 190–201.
35. Boylan LS. Peri-ictal behavioral and cognitive changes. Epilepsy Behav 2002; 3(1):16–26.
36. Binnie CD, Kasteleijn-Nolst Trenité DG, Smit AM, et al. Interactions of epileptiform EEG discharges and cognition. Epilepsy Res 1987;1(4):239–45.
37. Aarts JH, Binnie CD, Smit AM, et al. Selective cognitive impairment during focal and generalized epileptiform EEG activity. Brain 1984;107(Pt 1):293–308.
38. Wolf P. The role of nonpharmaceutic conservative interventions in the treatment and secondary prevention of epilepsy. Epilepsia 2002;43(Suppl 9):2–5.
39. Giffin NJ, Ruggiero L, Lipton RB, et al. Premonitory symptoms in migraine: an electronic diary study. Neurology 2003;60(2):935–40.
40. Hall CB, Lipton RB, Tennen H, et al. Early follow-up data from seizure diaries can be used to predict subsequent seizures in same cohort by borrowing strength across participants. Epilepsy Behav 2009;14(3):472–5.
41. Efron B, Morris C. Stein's paradox in statistics. Sci Am 1977;236:119–27.
42. Burton C, Weller D, Sharpe M. Are electronic diaries useful for symptoms research? A systematic review. J Psychosom Res 2007;62(5):553–61.
43. Tennen H, Affleck G, Armeli S. Personality and daily experience revisited. J Pers 2005;73(6):1465–83.
44. Zautra AJ, Affleck GG, Davis MC, et al. Assessing the ebb and flow of daily life with an accent on the positive. Handbook of methods in positive psychology. New York: Oxford University Press; 2007.
45. Ekholm O. Influence of the recall period on self-reported alcohol intake. Eur J Clin Nutr 2004;58(1):60–3.
46. Robinson MD, Clore GL. Episodic and semantic knowledge in emotional self-report: evidence for two judgment processes. J Pers Soc Psychol 2002;83(1): 198–215.
47. Todd M, Tennen H, Carney MA, et al. Do we know how we cope? Relating daily coping reports to global and time-limited retrospective assessments. J Pers Soc Psychol 2004;86:310–9.
48. Ptacek JT, Patterson DR, Montgomery BK, et al. Pain, coping, and adjustment in patients with burns: preliminary findings from a prospective study. J Pain Symptom Manage 1995;10(6):446–55.

49. Csikszentmihalyi M, Larson R. Validity and reliability of the Experience-Sampling Method. J Nerv Ment Dis 1987;175(9):526–36.
50. Blanchet P, Frommer GP. Mood change preceding epileptic seizures. J Nerv Ment Dis 1986;174(8):471–6.
51. Haut SR, Hall CB, Masur J, et al. Seizure occurrence: precipitants and prediction. Neurology 2007;69(20):1905–10.
52. Antebi D, Bird J. The facilitation and evocation of seizures. A questionnaire study of awareness and control. Br J Psychiatry 1993;162:759–64.
53. Frucht MM, Quigg M, Schwaner C, et al. Distribution of seizure precipitants among epilepsy syndromes. Epilepsia 2000;41:1534–9.
54. Temkin NR, Davis GR. Stress as a risk factor for seizures among adults with epilepsy. Epilepsia 1984;25(4):450–6.
55. Haut SR, Vouyiouklis M, Shinnar S. Stress and epilepsy: a patient perception survey. Epilepsy Behav 2003;4:511–4.
56. Rajna P, Sólyom A, Mezofi L, et al. Are there real unprovoked/unprecipitated seizures? Med Hypotheses 2008;71(6):851–7.
57. Treatment of convulsive status epilepticus. Recommendations of the Epilepsy Foundation of America's working group on status epilepticus. JAMA 1993;270:854–9.
58. Costello DJ, Cole AJ. Treatment of acute seizures and status epilepticus. J Intensive Care Med 2007;22(6):319–47.
59. Verrotti A, Latini G, di Corcia G, et al. Intermittent oral diazepam prophylaxis in febrile convulsions: its effectiveness for febrile seizure recurrence. Europ J Paediatr Neurol 2004;8(3):131–4.
60. Lim LL, Foldvary N, Mascha E, et al. Acetozolamide in women with catamenial epilepsy. Epilepsia 2001;42(6):746–9.
61. Cull CA, Fowler M, Brown SW. Perceived self-control of seizures in young people with epilepsy. Seizure 1996;5(2):131–8.
62. Fenwick P. The behavioral treatment of epilepsy generation and inhibition of seizures. Neurol Clin 1994;12(1):175–202.
63. Yardi N. Yoga for control of epilepsy. Seizure 2001;10(1):7–12.

Hormonal Aspects of Epilepsy

Page B. Pennell, MD

KEYWORDS

- Seizure • Epilepsy • Catamenial • Progesterone
- Estrogen • Hormone

Several alterations in different hormonal profiles have been described for patients with epilepsy. The brain directly regulates hormonal status through hypothalamus-pituitary-endocrine gland feedback loops. Epilepsy itself, with both interictal and ictal effects, and the medications used to treat epilepsy can have direct effects on the regulation of these hormone systems. Epilepsy and antiepileptic drugs (AEDs) can target a number of substrates to affect hormone levels, including the limbic system, hypothalamus, pituitary, peripheral endocrine glands, liver, and adipose tissue.[1] Abnormalities of the sex steroid hormones have been described most frequently, but have also been reported for thyroid hormone levels, prolactin, and vitamin D.

HORMONAL ABNORMALITIES IN PEOPLE WITH EPILEPSY AND ON AEDs
Sex Steroid Hormone Axis

The sex steroid hormones directly affect brain function and excitability. Release of these hormones is controlled by the hypothalamic-pituitary-gonadal axis. The major sex steroid hormones are testosterone from the testis and estrogen and progesterone (PROG) from the ovaries. The adrenal gland is another primary steroid endocrine gland with significant contribution to androgen synthesis. Peripheral conversion to other biologically active forms also occurs in skin or adipose tissue. The main estrogen in women during reproductive years is estradiol. A complex bidirectional feedback loop occurs with the hypothalamic-pituitary-ovarian axis (**Fig. 1**). Gonadotropin-releasing hormone (GnRH) is secreted by the hypothalamus and stimulates the release of follicle-stimulating hormone (FSH) by the pituitary. FSH stimulates formation of the ovarian follicles, which secrete estradiol as they develop. FSH is inhibited whereas GnRH is stimulated by estrogen. This combination then leads to a surge of luteinizing hormone (LH), which induces oocyte maturation, ovulation, and conversion of the follicle into the corpus luteum. This marks the end of the follicular phase and the beginning of the luteal phase (**Fig. 2**). Following ovulation, the corpus luteum secretes

Funding Support: Supported in part by NIH NINDS RO3NS063233.
Division of Epilepsy, Department of Neurology, Brigham and Women's Hospital, Harvard Medical School, 75 Francis Street, Boston, MA 02115, USA
E-mail address: ppennell@partners.org

Neurol Clin 27 (2009) 941–965
doi:10.1016/j.ncl.2009.08.005
0733-8619/09/$ – see front matter © 2009 Elsevier Inc. All rights reserved.

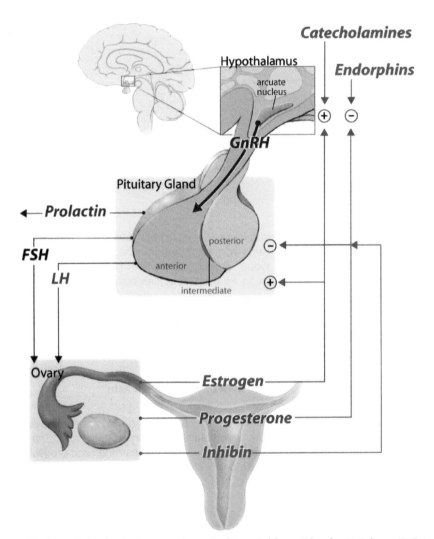

Fig. 1. The hypothalamic-pituitary-ovarian axis. (*From* Foldvary-Schaefer N, Falcone T. Catamenial epilepsy: Pathophysiology, diagnosis and management. Neurology 2003;61:2–15; with permission.)

PROG. The PROG inhibits secretion of GnRH, FSH, and LH. If there is no pregnancy, the corpus luteum regresses and production of PROG and estradiol declines. When PROG secretion tapers off and GnRH inhibition decreases, the cycle repeats. Because of the cyclic nature of hormone release and the direct neuronal effects of estrogen and PROG or metabolites, women are especially susceptible to the effects of these shifting hormones on seizure frequency and severity.

The interaction between the sex steroid hormonal axis, epilepsy, and the medications used to treat epilepsy is complex, with tridirectional interactions that affect both men and women in various ways. Both interictal and ictal discharges have been proposed as altering the sex steroid hormonal axis at the level of the hypothalamus and the pituitary.[2] Alterations in the reproductive hormone axis have been

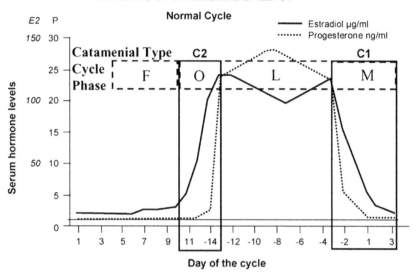

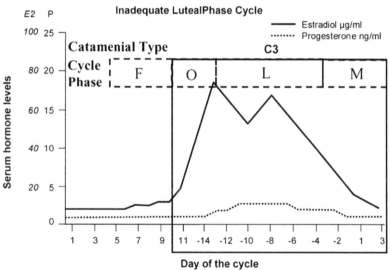

Fig. 2. Three patterns of catamenial epilepsy. During normal ovulatory cycles, both peri-menstrual (C1) and periovulatory (C2) patterns can occur in isolation or together. During inadequate luteral phase cycles, the (C3) pattern can occur with increased seizures during the entire second half of the cycle. Day 1 is the first day of menstrual flow and ovulation usually occurs at Day 14 in normal cycles. (*Adapted from* Herzog AG. Catamenial epilepsy: definition, prevalence pathophysiology and treatment. Seizure 2008;17:151; with permission.)

reported to occur commonly in both women and men with epilepsy. The most common reported manifestations in men are decreased sexual function with decreased libido and/or impotence. Women often have menstrual cycle irregularities and may have increased risk of infertility or signs of hyperandrogenism.[3] Both epilepsy and AEDs have been causally implicated.[1]

Hypogonadism

Among the abnormal patterns of reproductive function described in patients with epilepsy, hypogonadotropic hypogonadism is one of the more common ones. Hypothalamic amenorrhea is the most extreme form of this in women with epilepsy, characterized by amenorrhea (no menses) associated with low gonadotropin and estrogen levels and diminished LH response to GnRH, often tested with a GnRH challenge. Herzog and colleagues[3] studied 50 consecutive women with temporal lobe epilepsy. Fifty-six percent had amenorrhea, oligomenorrhea, or abnormally long or short menstrual cycle intervals, and 68% of these women had clearly identifiable reproductive endocrine disorders with polycystic ovarian syndrome (PCOS) in 20%, hypoandrogenism in 12%, severe premature menopause in 4%, and functional hyperprolactinemia in 2%. The estimated frequency for hypoandrogenism in the general population of women is 1.5%. Because there was no significant relationship between these menstrual disorders and the use of AEDs, the authors concluded that epilepsy itself may be a significant factor, which stimulated future investigations.

Hypogonadotopic hypogonadism has been found to be more common in women with right temporal lobe epilepsy compared with left temporal lobe epilepsy.[4,5] Herzog[4] studied 30 women with unilateral temporal lobe interictal epileptiform discharges and reproductive disorders. EEG laterality was significantly different for women with PCOS (left-sided discharges) and hypogonadotropic hypogonadism (right-sided discharges). Kalinin and Zheleznova[5] studied 80 women with temporal lobe epilepsy. They also reported that PCOS was more commonly associated with left temporal lobe epilepsy (TLE), and hypogonadotropic hypogonadism with right TLE. They also reported that a catamenial pattern was more common in the women with left TLE.

Other studies supporting the effect of epilepsy itself on reproductive dysfunction include the finding that women with idiopathic generalized epilepsy have higher pulse frequency GnRH secretion than control subjects.[6] Quigg and colleagues[7] studied LH secretion patterns in 10 men with TLE and in control men. They reported that the pulsatile secretion of LH was abnormal in the TLE group; interictal effects consisted mainly in loss of circadian fluctuations in LH burst amplitude, whereas postictal effects consist of altered burst timing.

In addition to the effects of the underlying disorder of epilepsy and seizures, several studies describe effects of the medications used to treat epilepsy on reproductive endocrine function. Lossius and colleagues[8] performed a prospective, randomized, and double-blinded study of the effects on reproductive endocrine function of AED withdrawal in 160 men and women with epilepsy, followed for 1 year. Patients were randomized to withdrawal or no withdrawal of AEDs. Blood samples were obtained before and 4 months after withdrawal or no withdrawal in 130 subjects. They reported that reversible endocrine changes in sex steroid hormone levels were observed in both sexes after withdrawal of AEDs. Carbamazepine (CBZ) was the most commonly used drug and withdrawal led to significant increases in serum testosterone concentrations and free androgen index (FAI) in both genders. Abnormalities in these parameters can lead to sexual dysfunction in both men and women with epilepsy.

Sexual Dysfunction (Related to Epilepsy and Antiepileptic Drug Effects)

AEDs can have a major impact on circulating sex steroid hormone levels, with effects on sexual function. Herzog and colleagues[9] studied men with localization-related epilepsy (LRE) on various AED regimens, on no AEDs, and control men without epilepsy. Sexual function scores (S-Scores) were obtained by a four-question self-administered questionnaire. Serum measurements included bioactive testosterone (BAT), bioactive estradiol (BAE), BAT/BAE, sex hormone binding globulin (SHBG), and LH. Gonadal efficiency was calculated as BAT/LH. Almost one-quarter of the men with epilepsy (MWE) had sexual dysfunction. S-scores were even lower in the men on enzyme-inducing AEDs (EIAEDs) compared with the MWE on lamotrigine (LTG) and compared with the control men. BAT levels correlated with S scores for men on EIAEDs, BAT levels, BAT/BAE and BAT/LH ratios were lower in this group, compared with control groups or the MWE on LTG.

A study of 40 men with refractory localization-related epilepsy by Kuba and colleagues[10] in the Czech Republic investigated sexual dysfunction and hormonal profiles. At least one type of sexual dysfunction was found in 55% of patients, with erectile dysfunction in 15%, orgasmic dysfunction in 15%, and loss of sexual desire in 40%. In the group of men with sexual dysfunction, there was an increase of FSH and SHBG, and a decrease of DHEAS and FAI in comparison with patients with normal sexual function. An increase in estrogen was also seen in men with erectile dysfunction. The observation was made that all patients with orgasmic dysfunction were being treated with CBZ, but when all patients with at least one type of sexual dysfunction were analyzed, a higher proportion were on valproic acid (VPA) than CBZ.

Testosterone supplementation can be an effective treatment for hypogonadal men with epilepsy and sexual dysfunction. It may improve not only sexual function, but mood and even seizure frequency.[1]

Morrell and colleagues[11] studied sexual function and hormones in women with epilepsy 18 to 40 years old with localization-related epilepsy, primary generalized epilepsy (PGE), and nonepilepsy controls. Questionnaires were administered examining sexual experience, arousability, anxiety, and depression (Beck Depression Inventory). Endocrine assessment was performed during the early follicular phase. Compared with the controls, women with LRE had significantly higher sexual dysfunction scores, lower mean arousal, and higher depression scores. Mean arousal scores were also lower in the PGE group. Women on EIAEDs, combined into one group, had statistically higher sexual dysfunction and lower sexual arousal compared with controls. Overall, estradiol negatively correlated with sexual anxiety, and dehydro-epiandrosterone (DHEAS) negatively correlated with sexual dysfunction and positively correlated with sexual arousal.

Another study reported similar adverse findings of altered hormone blood levels in association with lower sexual quality of life in men with epilepsy, but interestingly, not women with epilepsy.[12] Seventy-nine patients with different types of epilepsy or no epilepsy completed the Derogatis Interview for Sexual Function-Self-Report Inventory and had blood drawn for measurement of hormone studies. In men, increasing SHBG levels and duration of epilepsy were associated with decreased sexual quality of life. SHBG levels were related to EIAEDs and age. Women did not demonstrate an association between any hormone levels and sexual quality of life.

In summary, men and women with epilepsy are susceptible to sexual dysfunction. Questions about sexual function should be part of the routine evaluation in the outpatient clinic. The etiologies of sexual dysfunction in men and women with epilepsy are multifactorial, but AED type is one contributing factor that can be modified when indicated and available evidence suggests non-EIAEDs show more favorable profiles.

Fertility and Childbirth Rates

One study in North America compared fertility rates in 863 married adults with idiopathic/cryptogenic epilepsy and same-sex siblings without epilepsy. Reduced fertility rates occurred for both MWE and women with epilepsy (WWE) after but not before the onset of epilepsy. Factors reducing fertility rates further were localization-related epilepsy and early age at onset.[13]

Another study reported that the reduced rate of childbirths in married women with epilepsy (69% of expected number of live-born children) did not hold for married men with epilepsy.[14] A population- based cohort study in Finland from 1985 to 2001 of patients with newly diagnosed epilepsy (n = 14,077) reported that childbirth rates were lower than in a reference cohort among men (hazard ratio = 0.58, 95% confidence interval 0.54–0.62) and women (HR = 0.88, 0.83–0.93).[15] However, a comparable study from Iceland suggested no difference in childbearing rates for women with epilepsy.[16] Geographic and cultural differences are likely substantial factors and these will influence self-directed decisions. The "Ideal World" survey of Epilepsy Action UK women found that 33% of the women were not considering having children because of their epilepsy.[17]

For men with epilepsy, abnormalities on semen analysis have been reported, including decreased sperm count, abnormal morphology, or impaired motility, with some reports as high as 90% of men with epilepsy were affected.[1]

Premature Menopause

Premature menopause is characterized by amenorrhea, cessation of ovarian function, and elevated gonadotropin levels. This premature ovarian failure occurs more commonly in women with epilepsy. Klein and colleagues[18] evaluated the incidence of premature ovarian failure (POF) in 50 women with epilepsy, aged 38 to 64, compared with control women. Premature menopause was defined as amenorrhea for greater than 1 year with elevated Day 3 FSH levels in women younger than 42 years. Premature perimenopause was defined by the presence of perimenopausal symptoms. Of the women with epilepsy, 14% had premature perimenopause or menopause, compared with only 3.7% of the control women (P = .042). They did not find an association with epilepsy duration, seizure severity, or AEDs, although women with premature menopause were more likely to have had catamenial exacerbation of their seizures than were women without premature ovarian failure (POF) (P = .02).

Harden and colleagues[19] also found premature menopause in their multicenter cohort of women with epilepsy. The median age at menopause in the group of women with epilepsy was 47 years, compared with the median age of 51.4 years in the general US population.[20] When the investigators divided the patients into low, intermediate, and high seizure frequency groups, and there was an increasingly lower age at menopause with a negative correlation between the age at menopause and seizure group based on estimated lifetime seizures (P = .014). They also found no influence of enzyme-inducing AEDs. The authors concluded that the association of lifetime number of seizures with the timing of cessation of reproductive cycling may occur as a result of direct disruption of hypothalamic and pituitary function by the seizures.

Polycystic Ovarian Syndrome

PCOS is characterized by enlarged ovaries with multiple small cysts and a hypervascularized, androgen-secreting stroma leading to the associated signs of androgen excess (hirsutism, alopecia, acne), obesity, and menstrual-cycle disturbance (oligo- or amenorrhea).[21] This common endocrine disturbance occurs in approximately 4% to 7% of women of reproductive age in the general population, but in 10% to 25% of women with epilepsy.[1,22,23]

The definition of PCOS has been a source of debate and varies between Europe and North America, with stricter criteria adopted by North America. Minimal diagnostic criteria were defined by a 1990 National Institutes of Health (NIH) Consensus Panel: (1) menstrual irregularity, (2) biochemical or clinical evidence of hyperandrogenism, and (3) exclusion of other diseases that could cause female hyperandrogenism (such as congenital adrenal hyperplasia).[24] These North American minimal criteria do not include the need to identify the polycystic component of the ovaries by ultrasound. The signs and symptoms expressed by women with PCOS vary substantially (**Box 1**).[21] There is a familial tendency with some recent discoveries of potential underlying genetic contributions with genetic variants of LH, the pathway for androgen biosynthesis, and of regulation of expression of the insulin gene.[21] Women with PCOS are at long-term risk of developing diabetes and cardiovascular disease.

One of the most influential factors that affects the expression of PCOS is weight; weight gain causes a worsening of symptoms, and weight loss improves the endocrine and metabolic profile. Yet women with PCOS are prone to eating disorder, possibly because of a link with leptin. This is one of the reasons why the interplay between epilepsy, the use of VPA, weight gain, and PCOS has been so difficult to tease out. The underlying epilepsy itself likely contributes to

---

Box 1
Clinical manifestations of polycystic ovarian syndrome

Signs and symptoms (proportion of patients affected)

　　Obesity (38%)

　　Menstrual disturbance (66%)

　　　　Oligomenorrhea (47%)

　　　　Amenorrhea (19%)

　　　　[Regular cycle 30%]

　　Hyperandrogenism (48%)

　　Infertility (73% of anovulatory infertility)

　　Symptomless–20% of those with polycystic ovaries

Hormone systems that might be disturbed

　　Insulin ↑

　　Sex-hormone-binding globulin ↓

　　Androgens (testosterone and androstenedione) ↑

　　Luteinizing hormone ↑

　　Prolactin ↑

Possible late sequelae

　　Dyslipidemia

　　　　Low-density lipoprotein (LDL) ↑, High-density lipoprotein (HDL) ↓

　　　　Triglycerides ↑

　　Diabetes mellitus

　　Cardiovascular disease; hypertension

　　Endometrial carcinoma

Data from Balen A. Pathogenesis of polycystic ovary syndrome—the enigma unravels? Lancet 1999;354:966.

the expression of PCOS via effects on hypothalamic control of the menstrual cycle with the tendency toward more anovulatory cycles and oligomenorrhea. It is likely that both the underlying epilepsy and AED treatment play roles in the development of PCOS.[24]

Herzog and colleagues[3] were among the first to publish on the finding of PCOS in women with epilepsy. They reported that PCOS occurs significantly more often in women with TLE than in the general female population and is associated with predominantly left-sided lateralization of interictal epileptic discharges. These findings suggest that the underlying epilepsy contributes to the development of PCOS via the hypothalamic-pituitary-gonadal axis. Bilo and colleagues[25] also reported a higher incidence of reproductive endocrine disorders including PCOS, but in women with idiopathic generalized epilepsy syndromes. Neither group found an association with the type of AED being taken by the women.

Several studies by Isojarvi and colleagues[26] reported that the higher incidence of PCOS in women with epilepsy (WWE) was specifically associated with VPA use. One of the probable reasons for discrepancies in different studies is because of the differing definitions for PCOS. A study of 238 WWE in Finland on a variety of AEDs included vaginal ultrasonography and serum sex-hormone concentrations. Unlike the North American criteria for PCOS, they reported on findings of polycystic ovaries as an isolated finding as well as elevated testosterone concentrations. The VPA monotherapy group included findings of polycystic ovaries (43%) and elevated testosterone concentrations without polycystic ovaries (17%). Notably, 80% of the group that began VPA treatment before 20 years of age had polycystic ovaries or hyperandrogenism.

A later study by Isojarvi and colleagues[27] enrolled 16 women taking VPA for epilepsy who had polycystic ovaries or hyperandrogenism. They were converted to LTG monotherapy and followed for 1 year (n = 12 completers). The additional findings of weight gain, hyperinsulinemia, and lipid profiles were monitored. During the first year after drug conversion, the number of polycystic ovaries, body mass index (BMI), fasting serum insulin, and testosterone concentrations decreased, and the HDL/total cholesterol ratios increased.

A recent examination of 148 WWE by epilepsy type and AED use by Lofgren and colleagues[28] reported a higher prevalence of reproductive endocrine disorders in women with idiopathic generalized epilepsy than control subjects, but the specific findings of hyperandrogenism, polycystic ovaries, and polycystic ovary syndrome were more prevalent in WWE on VPA than in WWE taking other drugs or control women. The use of VPA and younger age predicted the development of hyperandrogenism.

Morrell and colleagues[29] studied 447 women prospectively with randomization to initiating 12 months of treatment with either VPA or LTG. More women in the VPA group than the LTG group developed ovulatory dysfunction (54% vs 38%; $P = .010$) and more women in the VPA group than the LTG group developed PCOS (9% vs 2%; $P = .007$). Development of hyperandrogenism was more frequent with VPA than LTG among those initiating treatment at age younger than 26 years (44% vs 23%; $P = .002$) but was similar if treatment was started at age 26 years or older (24% vs 22%).

In conclusion, WWE are a group at risk for reproductive health disorders regardless of AED use. Questions about reproductive health should be part of the evaluation of women with epilepsy, both during the initial evaluation and periodically during follow-up visits. History should include age at menarche, menstrual patterns and regularity, and fertility problems, as well as assessment of hirsutism, acne, and weight and height measurements.[24] When findings suggestive of a possible reproductive disorder are obtained, one should consider referral to a reproductive endocrinologist, gynecologist, or endocrinologist familiar with these issues. If women have signs of obesity, hyperandrogenism, or menstrual irregularities, then consideration should be given to avoidance of VPA use in women of reproductive age for these risks, in addition to the known increased risk for anatomic and neurodevelopmental teratogenicity.[30] Some experts suggest that women who are treated with VPA should not only be frequently monitored for weight gain, but also undergo laboratory investigation on a yearly basis for lipid and glucose metabolism, hyperandrogenism, and ultrasound for polycystic ovaries with more frequent monitoring if they develop menstrual pattern changes.[24] If PCOS develops, then the AED regimen should be reconsidered as to whether alternatives could still provide good seizure control, given the long-term health consequences and the potential to reverse the VPA-related risks by substituting VPA with another AED.[27]

Thyroid

Several studies evaluating thyroid function status in patients with epilepsy suggest that there are no alterations related directly to epilepsy, but that there can be some alterations in thyroid function tests associated with some of the AEDs. However, these laboratory abnormalities may not be clinically significant.[1] A study by Isojarvi and colleagues[31] of 90 men with epilepsy on either CBZ, VPA, or oxcarbazepine (OXC), and 25 control men demonstrated that serum thyroxine (T4) and free thyroxine (FT4) concentrations were low in men taking CBZ or OXC with 45% and 24% falling below the reference range, respectively, while serum triiodothyronine and thyrotropin (TSH) levels were normal. In men taking VPA, the concentrations of thyroid hormones and TSH were normal.

Another study in children with new-onset epilepsy[32] was performed prospectively with baseline thyroid testing before drug administration, followed by testing at 3, 6, and 12 months after initiation of CBZ or VPA; age-matched subjects served as controls. The epilepsy group included subjects with partial epilepsy and subjects with generalized epilepsy. Thyroid function tests were normal at baseline in all subjects. After 3 months and persisting until 12 months, CBZ-treated patients demonstrated significantly lower serum T4 and FT4 levels compared with baseline evaluation and control subjects, but normal serum T3 and TSH response to a thyrotropin-releasing hormone (TRH) test. Some of the CBZ-treated children were withdrawn from CBZ for other reasons, and reevaluation 6 months later revealed normalization of their values. All thyroid function test (TFT) values remained normal in the VPA group. Even with the alterations in the CBZ group, the authors concluded that the patients were euthyroid and therefore, that thyroid hormone alterations were not associated with clinical or subclinical hypothyroidism.

Gomez and colleagues[33] studied 96 patients on a variety of first-generation AEDs. They observed decreased T4 serum levels and free T4 index below the normal ranges (in 25 and 14 patients, respectively), decreased reverse triiodothronine (rT3), but normal levels of FT4, T3, and TSH. They concluded that TSH was the best measurement to indicate the euthyroid status of these patients.

Studies of other AEDs, especially the enzyme-inducing AEDs, have demonstrated somewhat similar findings of a tendency toward lower serum concentrations of T4, FT4, and thyroid-binding globulin while maintaining TSH at normal or slightly elevated levels.[1] TSH response to TRH is either unchanged or slightly increased as well.[34,35]

Another study of 35 patients on long-term phenytoin (PHT) or CBZ[35] reported that the mean concentrations of T4, FT4, FT3, and rT3, but not T3, of these patients were significantly lower than those of 19 controls of similar age and sex distribution. The mean serum TSH concentration was slightly but significantly higher in patients than in controls, but the serum TSH response to TRH was not significantly increased. Several other metabolic studies in these patients did not show other clinical signs of functional hypothyroidism. Response to thyroxine treatment was assessed in a smaller subset of subjects. Overall, the authors concluded that, on the basis of all data from the cross-sectional and thyroxine treatment studies, patients receiving AEDs chronically are eumetabolic and do not need thyroxine supplementation.

Because clinically significant thyroid disorders occur rarely with AED use, routine testing of thyroid function is generally not encouraged for patients on chronic AED therapy; exceptions would be when the patient exhibits potential signs of clinical hypo/hyperthyroidism or when the patient has a preexisting thyroid disorder. When thyroid function tests are obtained, any findings of lower concentrations of total or free thyroid hormones need to be considered in the context of the TSH, and other secondary metabolic effects.[35] Any benefit of thyroid supplementation needs to be weighed against the possible exacerbation of seizures in people with epilepsy.

Prolactin

Following seizures, a rise in prolactin levels following seizures has been reported.[36,37,38] In one study of measurements of more than 500 seizures, increased prolactin levels were documented after 88% of generalized tonic-clonic seizures, 78% of complex partial seizures, and 22% of simple partial seizures.[36] Absence seizures do not lead to a prolactin increase.[25] The mechanism is thought to be the propagation of the electrical activity (usually from the temporal lobe) to the hypothalamic-pituitary axis, causing the release of the hormone. The rise seen in approximately 60% of complex partial seizures may be related to the intensity and duration of the seizure; for example, generalized convulsive seizures are even more likely to be associated with a postictal rise in prolactin.[37] Because prolactin does not usually rise after psychogenic seizures, some authors propose that postictal prolactin levels can be used to differentiate between epileptic and psychogenic seizures. However, caution should be used, because a rise in prolactin is not detected after all epileptic seizures, and timing of the blood draw is critical and should be within 30 minutes after the seizure. Only in the case of a prolactin rise may one conclude that an epileptic seizure had occurred. Prolactin may not have a sustained increase following a flurry of seizures or in association with status epilepticus.

Bone Health

Bone disease occurs in both men and women with epilepsy and even in some children with epilepsy. Aging women can be at greater risk with estrogen loss that occurs in menopause. AED exposure is a cause of secondary osteoporosis with decreased bone mineral density (BMD) secondary to poor bone accrual in children or accelerated bone loss in adults. Fracture rates are higher in persons with epilepsy, owing to multifactorial causes including increased bone turnover with some AEDs, higher rates of osteopenia and osteoporosis, and falls as a result of seizures or medication side effects.

One differential risk factor is AED selection. Studies have cited decreased bone mineral density, increased markers for bone turnover, and/or fractures in patients on the enzyme-inducing AEDS and VPA, but the most consistent finding has been changes in bone metabolism and increased turnover and lower bone mineral density associated with phenytoin (PHT) use.[39,40] Pack and colleagues[40] studied premeno-pausal WWE on different monotherapy regimens. They reported that calcium concentrations were significantly lower in subjects on CBZ, PHT, or VPA monotherapy compared with women on LTG monotherapy ($P = .008$). Additionally, the PHT group demonstrated increases in markers of bone turnover.

All patients with epilepsy should be advised to receive at least the recommended daily allowance of calcium and vitamin D for their age, gender, and menopausal status. Recommendations vary for routine screening, and no consensus has been reached thus far. Some experts advise screening of 25-OH-vitamin D levels and bone mineral density screening for prolonged AED exposure, especially if other risk factors are present.[41] These screening measures should occur earlier if the woman is on PHT. If osteopenia is found, it is helpful to reinforce calcium and vitamin D daily requirements; if osteoporosis is found, then one should consider referral to an internist or endocrinologist for possible treatment interventions, such as with a bisphosphonate. If the patient is on PHT, then conversion to another AED should be considered.

ANTIEPILEPTIC DRUGS AND HORMONAL CONTRACEPTIVE INTERACTIONS
Reduced Efficacy of Contraceptive Hormones as a Result of Antiepileptic Drugs

Many of the AEDs induce the hepatic cytochrome P450 system, the primary metabolic pathway of the sex steroid hormones, and induce the production of sex hormone-binding globulin (SHBG). This leads to a lower concentration of free hormone to exert its targeted action and a more rapid clearance of the steroid hormones. This can allow ovulation in women taking oral contraceptive pills (OCPs) or other hormonal forms of birth control and contribute to the relatively high number of unplanned pregnancies in this patient population.[42] One recommended strategy is to prescribe an OCP containing 50 μg or more of ethinyl estradiol daily. However, more popular trends in the general population of women of childbearing age have been to prescribe especially low concentration hormonal contraceptives (through OCPs or other routes such as vaginal rings). Patients should be warned that midcycle bleeding indicates possible OCP failure but that the absence of such bleeding is not an indication of adequate contraceptive effectiveness.[42] The transdermal patch and vaginal ring formulations also have higher failure rates with these AEDs. Intramuscular medroxyprogesterone provides higher dosages of progestin but still may require dosing at 8- to 10-week intervals rather than 12-week intervals. Two types of intrauterine devices (IUDs) are available (hormone releasing and copper). The Mirena IUD is impregnated with PROG, but because its effect is at the local level of the endometrium, AEDs are unlikely to have an effect on its efficacy.

The 1998 guidelines by the American Academy of Neurology recommend use of an estradiol dose of 50 μg or its equivalent for 21 days of each cycle when using oral contraceptive agents with the enzyme-inducing AEDs,[43] but no studies have addressed whether this improves contraceptive efficacy. A higher progestin component may be as important as the estrogen component to prevent ovulation, but the combined oral contraceptive pills with a higher estradiol dose do usually also have a higher progestin content. Because this may still not be adequate protection against pregnancy, a backup barrier method is recommended. **Table 1** lists effects of the individual AEDs on hormonal contraceptive agents.[42,44]

The two newest AEDs approved in the United States have undergone interaction studies. Lacosamide studies of drug-drug interactions with a combination oral contraceptive pill containing ethinylestradiol and levonorgestrel demonstrated no pharmacokinetic interactions. Its primary route of elimination is renal excretion and

Table 1
Antiepileptic drug effects on hormonal contraceptive agents

Lowers Hormone Levels	No Significant Effects
Carbamazepine	Ethosuximide
Oxcarbazepine	Gabapentin
Phenobarbital	Lacosamide
Phenytoin	Lamotrigine
Primidone	Levetiracetam
Rufinamide	Tiagabine
Topiramate	Valproate
	Zonisamide

biotransformation. Rufinamide has been studied for hormonal contraceptive interaction. Coadministration with a common combination pill resulted in a mean decrease in the area under the curve (AUC) and the maximum concentration of the drug (C_{max}) for both ethinyl estradiol and norethindrone. Therefore, additional nonhormonal forms of contraception are recommended.

Davis and colleagues[45] administered a cross-sectional questionnaire to women with epilepsy (18–44 years) in an urban, academic medical center. They classified methods of contraception as highly effective ($\leq$10% experience pregnancy in the first year of typical use) or less effective (>10% will experience pregnancy in the first year of typical use). Half of the pregnancies in these women were unplanned, and among those who were sexually active in the preceding month, 74% used contraception but only 53% used highly effective methods of contraception (sterilization, intrauterine device, hormonal pill [any formulation], patch, and injection). Among the participants using hormonal contraception, 29% were on EIAEDs, with probable increased risk of unplanned pregnancy. One of the concerns these authors raised was that overall, highly effective methods of contraception were underprescribed, such as IUDs, intramuscular medroxyprogesterone, and even any form of OCPs. The effectiveness of OCPs in the setting of EIAEDs is still likely higher than that with condoms or withdrawal. This could be because of practitioner confusion about the interactions or worry about the possible effect of estrogen on seizure control. Despite the well-known effects of estrogen on lowering seizure threshold, observational studies have not shown that estrogen-containing oral contraceptives (OCs) worsen seizures in women with epilepsy.[42,46]

Influence of Exogenous Hormones on Antiepileptic Drug Concentrations

Studies in women with epilepsy have highlighted that during pregnancy clearances of AEDs increase.[47] Although serum concentrations of all AEDs are reduced during pregnancy, the magnitude of alterations in LTG concentrations exceeds that described for the older AEDs, which are primarily eliminated via the cytochrome P450 system.[48] Approximately 90% of LTG undergoes hepatic glucuronidation, catalyzed by UGT1A4, an isozyme of the UGT family of enzymes. This elimination pathway appears particularly susceptible to activation during pregnancy, possibly as a result of direct effects of rising sex steroid hormone levels[49] The effect of sex steroid hormones on LTG metabolism is not unique to pregnancy. Several recent studies have demonstrated increased clearance of LTG in women on hormonal contraceptives. In a study of 22 women on LTG in combination with OCs and 30 women on LTG without OC, the LTG plasma levels relative to dose and body weight were significantly reduced by more than 50% with coadministration of oral contraceptives.[50] A more recent prospective study separated the contraceptive group according to whether the women were on ethinyl estradiol (EE)-containing preparations or PROG-only containing compounds.[51] LTG serum concentration-to-dose ratio (CDR) was significantly lower in women using EE than in the control group; the CDR of the PROG group was not different from controls. Of the women who switched from the control to the EE group, considerable reductions in their CDRs occurred, and an increase in CDR occurred in the two women who changed from EE to PROG-containing compounds. It appears that it is the estrogen component of contraceptive preparations that induces the increase in LTG metabolism.

A double-blind placebo-controlled trial demonstrated that cessation of OCPs leads to an 84% increase in the concentration of LTG, and the change in LTG concentration occurs within 1 week of the shift in OCP status.[52] A study of hormone replacement therapy (HRT) in postmenopausal women with epilepsy also noted that subjects randomized to receive HRT had a decrease in LTG levels of 25% to 30% while taking conjugated equine estrogens/medroxyprogesterone acetate (CEE/MPA).[53] These findings should be considered when treating women during their reproductive and post-menopausal years. Initiation or discontinuation of estradiol-containing compounds may necessitate LTG serum concentration monitoring and dosage adjustment. Although none of these studies directly evaluated whether the alterations in LTG pharmacokinetics were clinically relevant with regard to seizure control or toxic side effects, it is unlikely that a controlled, randomized study would be performed to demonstrate seizure worsening with lowering of LTG serum concentrations by coadministration of exogenous EE. An observational study in women on LTG during pregnancy did demonstrate that lower LTG concentrations that occurred with the rising endogenous sex steroid hormone concentrations were predictive of worsening seizure frequency.[49]

The discovery that glucuronidation can be activated by hormonal shifts may apply to other AEDs. Metabolism of VPA is 30% to 50% by glucuronidation, and 50% to 60% of the clearance of OXC is via glucuronidation. Similar observations about increased clearance with possible worsening seizure control have been made about OXC during pregnancy, but reports about effects of concomitant OCP use are lacking.[47,54] Findings of a study of VPA with OCP use in women were that total and unbound VPA concentrations were higher during the OCP-free interval than during the OCP interval.[55] VPA clearance increased by 21.5% for total VPA and 45.0% for free VPA. The authors also commented the magnitude of the change varies across individuals, being potentially clinically relevant in some cases, and recommended monitoring of serum VPA concentrations when adding or discontinuing OCPs and possibly during the on-off intervals of an OCP cycle.

A recent study of VPA and LTG use with OCPs also demonstrated that total VPA and LTG levels were lower (23% and 33%, respectively) on active OCP than on inactive pill.[56] The authors also noted that with endogenous hormone fluctuations during normal menstrual cycles not on OCPs, serum LTG concentrations were lower during the mid-luteal phase, but the finding was not significant.

HORMONAL INFLUENCE ON SEIZURE SUSCEPTIBILITY

Both female patients with epilepsy and their treating physicians have observed a tendency for seizures to cluster in relationship to the menstrual cycle during the reproductive years. This phenomenon has been the source of much investigation in humans with epilepsy and in animal studies. It has been attributed to the neuroactive properties of sex steroid hormones and the cyclic variation of their serum levels. Results of animal studies of the effects of 17beta-estradiol (estradiol) and PROG are compelling. Estradiol has been shown to increase seizure activity, whereas PROG has been shown to have anticonvulsant properties.[57] Many cellular and molecular mechanisms have been identified contributing to the changes in brain excitability mediated by these hormones.

In animal studies, estrogen is generally proconvulsant.[58] Estradiol can create new cortical seizure foci when applied topically, activate preexisting cortical foci, increase the severity of pentylenetetrazol-induced seizures, lower the electroshock seizure threshold, and increase the number of dendritic spines and excitatory synapses on hippocampal CA1 pyramidal cells. Mechanisms are complex and likely include estrogen receptor-mediated effects, and action at glutamate and N-methyl-D-aspartate (NMDA) receptors. Progesterone, conversely, generally has an anticonvulsant effect.[58,59,60] Animal studies demonstrate that PROG elevates the seizure threshold, suppresses kindling, and decreases interictal spikes caused by cortically applied penicillin. Potential mechanisms include action at the progesterone receptor, but also through metabolism to γ-aminobutyric acid (GABA)$_A$ receptor modulating neuroactive steroids. Several studies suggest that allopregnanolone (ALLO) is the primary compound responsible for decreased seizure susceptibility when PROG is elevated and the anticonvulsant actions of PROG administration.[60] Putative steroid binding sites have been described on the GABA$_A$ receptor (see **Fig. 3**).[19]

Although many neuroactive steroids (NAS) can be synthesized in the brain from precursors such as PROG, experimental evidence demonstrates that blood levels correlate with seizure frequency and that administration of neuroactive steroids systemically can provoke or protect against seizures or the development of epilepsy.[3,59,61,62] Even natural fluctuations in sex steroid hormone levels during the menstrual cycle can affect not only epilepsy, but other neuropsychiatric symptoms including premenstrual syndrome, perimenstrual migraines, and dysphoria. Withdrawal from progesterone after chronic administration to rats via subcutaneous route results in increased seizure susceptibility.[63]

Androgens can also worsen seizures and some are felt to be proconvulsant in experimental models,[64] but given that major fluctuations do not occur except during puberty and gradually with aging, a regulatory role on seizure control is harder to demonstrate in men with epilepsy.

Catamenial Epilepsy During the Reproductive Years

In women with epilepsy during the reproductive years, a correlation has been observed between the cyclic monthly levels of estrogen and PROG and seizure frequency.[65,66] Catamenial epilepsy is the term applied when the pattern of seizure occurrence in a woman fluctuates with the menstrual cycle. The reported prevalence of a catamenial epilepsy among women varies because of differing definitions and few formal studies, with reports that it affects between 20% and 70% of women with epilepsy.[61,67,68,69] Work by Herzog[61] has led to a more uniform acceptance of the definition of catamenial epilepsy as a twofold increase in daily seizure frequency during specific phases of the menstrual cycle.

Herzog and colleagues[66] studied a cohort of 184 women with medically refractory localization-related epilepsy and were able to define three distinct patterns of catamenial epilepsy based on statistical evaluation of seizure frequency in women during their reproductive years. The definitions are based on Day 1 as the first day of menstrual flow and ovulation is presumed to occur 14 days before the subsequent onset of menses (Day 14). Seizures and menses were charted and midluteal serum progesterone levels were obtained on day 22. PROG concentrations greater than 5 ng/mL were considered ovulatory. Cycles were divided into four phases: menstrual (M) = −3 to +3, follicular

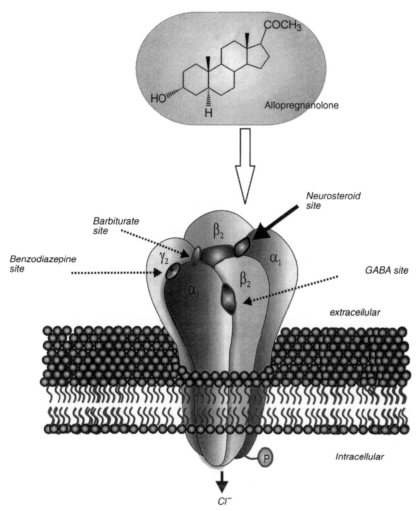

Fig. 3. Schematic diagram of allopregnanolone and its neuroactive steroid binding site on the GABA$_A$-BDZ receptor.

(F) = 4 to 9, ovulatory (O) = 10 to −13, and luteal (L) = −12 to −4 (**Fig. 2**). Average daily seizure frequency for each phase was calculated and compared among phases, separately for ovulatory and anovulatory cycles. The seizures recorded during ovulatory cycles occurred with significantly greater average daily frequency during the menstrual and ovulatory phases than during the follicular and luteal phases, in patterns labeled perimenstrual (C1) and periovulatory (C2). For the anovulatory cycles, seizures occurred with lower frequency during the follicular phase than during all other phases, in a pattern labeled C3 by the authors (see **Fig. 3**). The authors went on to plot the percentage of women with greater seizure frequency according the three patterns of catamenial epilepsy and evaluated points of inflection of the S-shaped distribution curves for optimal distinction between women with high and low susceptibility to hormonal influence. Based on these findings, these authors proposed a twofold increase in average daily seizure frequency during these phases in one of the three patterns for the designation of catamenial epilepsy. In their patient cohort, one-third of women showed at least one of the three patterns of catamenial epilepsy.

A follow-up study by Herzog and colleagues[70] in 87 women found that 39% of women enrolling in a PROG treatment trial demonstrated a catamenial pattern. This study assessed 87 women over a few menstrual cycles rather than just one cycle. Catamenial epilepsy designation was made if two of three cycles showed at least one of the three catamenial patterns. Another study by El-Khayat and colleagues[68] of 42 Egyptian women with epilepsy (and 21 controls) evaluated the pattern of seizure occurrence and hormone levels. Additionally, pelvic ultrasound was performed near the time of ovulation. A catamenial pattern of seizures occurred in 31% of patients (53.8% C1 pattern; 46.15% C3 pattern). Patients with the C3 pattern showed lower PROG levels in the midluteal phase compared with patients with the noncatamenial pattern, to those with the C1 pattern or to controls. Patients with the C1 pattern had lower progesterone levels than controls in the menstrual phase. The patients with a catamenial pattern also had higher estradiol/progesterone ratios.

Although approximately one-third of women with localization-related epilepsy have a catamenial pattern, this cyclic pattern is often underrecognized or underacknowledged by physicians treating women with epilepsy. Often the woman is the one to bring it up to her physician, but still too often her concerns are met with indifference or even doubt.[71] Perhaps one of the reasons is the perceived lack of treatment options. No similarly rigorous studies have been performed in women with idiopathic generalized epilepsy, but such studies would be more difficult given that seizures are often more readily controlled. Patients will often report, however, that their rare seizures only occur during the perimenstrual phase.

Epilepsy During Other Reproductive Life Stages

Alterations in seizure patterns can occur with other major hormonal shifts, such as during puberty, pregnancy, and perimenopause. Some epilepsy syndromes are first expressed or worsen during puberty.[72] Perimenopause is marked by erratic and frequently high estrogen levels, whereas postmenopause is characterized by stable, low estrogen levels. A retrospective questionnaire study suggested that seizure frequency can increase with perimenopause and can improve once the menopausal transition is complete.[73] This alteration in seizure pattern was more likely to occur in women who experienced a catamenial pattern during their reproductive years. In the postmenopausal group, HRT was significantly associated with an increase in seizures.

The latter finding led to design and implementation of a multicenter, double-blind, randomized, placebo-controlled trial of the effects of 2 doses of Prempro (CEE/MPA) (0.625 mg of conjugated equine estrogens, plus medroxyprogesterone acetate, 2.5 mg) on seizure control.[53] Subjects received placebo, single-dose CEE/MPA, or double-dose CEE/MPA. Twenty-one subjects were randomized after completing baseline. Five (71%) of seven subjects on double-dose CEE/MPA had a worsening seizure frequency of at least one seizure type, compared with four (50%) of eight on single-dose CEE/MPA and one (17%) of six on placebo ($P = .05$). Increasing CEE/MPA dose was also associated with an increase in the frequency of the subject's most severe seizure type ($P = .008$) and of complex partial seizures ($P = .05$). Despite the limited enrollment of this study, the conclusion could still be made that CEE/MPA was associated with a dose-related increase in seizure frequency in postmenopausal women with epilepsy.

This study in postmenopausal women with epilepsy was halted early because of findings from the Women's Health Initiative (WHI) study: overall health risks after 5 years of follow-up clearly exceeded benefits from use of single-dose CEE/MPA in healthy postmenopausal US women.[74] Although the released findings from the WHI study have resulted in decreased long-term HRT use for preventive health measures, HRT is still frequently used as treatment for perimenopausal symptom relief. The findings from the study by the Harden and colleagues[53] raise caution even for the short-term use of CEE/MPA in women with epilepsy. However, synthetic progestins such as medroxyprogesterone acetate are not metabolized to the active neurosteroid allopregnanolone. Future studies of whether an estrogen with natural PROG could circumvent the risk for increased seizures would be beneficial for women with epilepsy.

HORMONES AS THERAPIES IN PEOPLE WITH EPILEPSY

The benefit of hormonal therapy in the form of adrenocorticotropic hormone (ACTH) has long been recognized for infantile spasms, but it is only recently that investigation has extended to the use of sex steroid hormones or their analogs for the treatment of other epilepsies. An understanding of the effects of hormones on seizure susceptibility may provide an opportunity to use hormones as therapy in women with intractable epilepsy.

Cyclic Progesterone

Open-label studies of PROG supplementation have shown promising results (**Table 2**). Herzog[75] studied eight women with localization-related epilepsy and inadequate luteal phase cycles with catamenial exacerbation. Progesterone was administered as vaginal suppositories during the premenstrual phase or entire second half of the cycle in doses of 50 to 400 mg twice daily as adjunctive therapy to standard AEDs. The average monthly seizure frequency declined by 68% in the 3-month treatment period compared with the 3 months before therapy, with six of the eight women experiencing decreased seizure frequency. Adverse effects included mild sleepiness and symptoms of depression, but resolved with lowering of the dose.

A later open-label trial by Herzog[76] of 25 women with medically refractory temporal lobe epilepsy included women with either anovulatory or ovulatory cycles and with the associated catamenial patterns. PROG was administered as oral lozenges, 200 mg three times a day, in relation to the pattern of seizure exacerbation. For perimenstrual exacerbation (C1 pattern) they were given for days 23 to 25 of each menstrual cycle and then tapered to discontinuation by day 28. For luteal phase exacerbation (C3 pattern) progesterone lozenges were given for days 15 to 25 of each menstrual cycle followed by the same taper schedule. The dosage of progesterone dosage was adjusted if needed to produce physiologic luteal range progesterone serum levels between 5 and 25 ng/mL 4 hours after taking a lozenge. Over 3 months of treatment, overall average monthly decline was 54% for complex partial and 58% for secondarily generalized tonic clonic seizures. Overall, 72% of the patients experienced a reduction of seizures. The investigators noted that PROG was more efficacious when administered during the entire second half of the cycle for both groups with the different catamenial patterns, followed by gradual taper over 3 to 4 days. This observation formed the basis for future treatment trials.

Fifteen women from the treatment group in this open-label study were followed for more than 3 years and continued to show improved seizure control.[77] Three of the women maintained seizure freedom and four had seizure reduction of more than 75%, whereas another eight had 50% to 75% seizure reduction. It is encouraging that despite a likely primary action at the GABA$_A$-BDZ receptor complex (via

Table 2
Summary of open-label trials of progesterone in women with catamenial epilepsy

	Medroxy-progesterone[a]	Progesterone Suppositories[b]	Progesterone Lozenges[c]	Progesterone Lozenges[d]
Regimen	5 mg to 10 mg qd days 15 to 28 of cycle	100 mg to 200 mg tid days 15 to 28 of cycle	100 mg to 200 mg tid days 15 to 28 of cycle	100 mg to 200 mg tid days 15 to 28 of cycle
Assessment	At 3 months	At 3 months	At 3 months	At 3 years
Subjects	24	8	25	15 of original 25
Number improved	10 (42%)	6 (75%)	18 (72%)	15 (100%/60% overall)
Seizure frequency	10%	68%[e]	- 54%[f] CPS - 58%[e] SGMS	- 62%[f] CPS - 74%[f] SGMS

Abbreviations: CPS, complex partial seizure; qd, daily; SGMS, secondary generalized motor seizure; tid, 3 times a day.

[a] Results of 1983 study published in Herzog AG. Progesterone therapy in women with epilepsy: a 3-year follow-up. Neurology 1999;52(9);1917–8.

[b] Data from Herzog AG. Intermittent progesterone therapy and frequency of complex partial seizures in women with menstrual disorders. Neurology 1986;36(12);1607–10.

[c] Data from Herzog AG. Progesterone therapy in women with complex partial and secondary generalized seizures. Neurology 1995;45(9):1660–2.

[d] Data from Herzog AG. Progesterone therapy in women with epilepsy: a 3-year follow-up. Neurology 1999; 52(9):1917–8.

[e] $P < .05$.

[f] $P < .01$.

Data from Herzog AG. AAN CONTINUUM: lifelong learning in neurology. Neuroendocrinology 2009;15(2):37–66.

conversion to allopregnanolone), tolerance to adjunctive PROG does not appear to occur and the efficacy is maintained.

The findings from these open-label trials, including details about which regimen seems to most effective for all patterns of catamenial epilepsy, have led to a prospective, double-blind, randomized, placebo-controlled, multicenter trial of cyclic adjunctive progesterone lozenges. Enrollment recently ended and analysis of the data is pending. The population enrolled included women with medically refractory focal-onset seizures, and included a group with a noncatamenial pattern and another group with any of the three catamenial patterns.[70]

PROG lozenges can be obtained from almost all compounding pharmacies. It can be initiated, as was the case in the treatment trials, as 200 mg twice daily on days 15 to 25, with a taper to 100 mg twice daily for 2 days, then 50 mg three times a day for 1 day, then off. However, it is often helpful to later individualize the dose based on response and PROG levels with a target concentration of 20 to 40 ng/mL drawn 4 hours after dosing. Some women may require an even slower taper or addition of topical PROG cream during other phases of the menstrual cycle to prevent withdrawal effects. PROG is also available in a micronized form in an oral capsule preparation that may be effective, but it has not been studied formally. One concern by experts is the possible large first-pass effect of hepatic metabolism that occurs following swallowing of the capsule. In addition to possible sedation, and changes in mood, PROG can also be associated with breast tenderness, weight gain, irregular vaginal bleeding, and sometimes constipation. Higher PROG dosages may be required to achieve luteal-range levels in women who take EIAEDs.

If the currently ongoing multicenter, double-blind, randomized, placebo-controlled trial of cyclic progesterone lozenges in the treatment of women with localization-related epilepsy is positive, physicians will not only be able to acknowledge the effect of cycling hormones on seizures, but be able to use this relationship to the advantage of their patients in selecting treatment options.

Other Hormone Strategies for Catamenial Epilepsy

In addition to standard AED regimens, treatment strategies can include increasing the AED dose or adding another AED around the time of increased seizure susceptibility, or avoiding the cyclic variation in endogenous hormones by a continuous dosing of OCP or MPA acetate injections.

The use of adjusting conventional AED therapy during periods of seizure exacerbation has not been studied in a systematic manner or reported on, but is occasionally used by practitioners for women with catamenial seizure patterns. Intermittent benzodiazepines have been used for treatment of catamenial seizures, despite very few studies. One group reported on use of clobazam in a small group of patients a few decades ago, with moderately successful results.[78,79] Clobazam, 20 or 30 mg/day, was given for 10 days around menstruation in successive menstrual cycles to 13 women who had responded favorably to this drug in the earlier short-term placebo-controlled cross-over study. A little over one-third did very well with seizure freedom around menstruation with retained benefit for more than 3 years, another one-third had a moderate response, and another one-third had seizures or side effects leading to discontinuation of the clobazam. The most common adverse effects were sedation and depression.

Clobazam is not available in the United States but can be obtained from pharmacies outside the United States. Despite the lack of rigorous trials, it is a fairly popular treatment regimen for women with catamenial epilepsy in Europe, and is purported to be better tolerated than other benzodiazepines.

Another option is use of contraceptive hormones to eliminate the effect of cycling endogenous hormone concentrations. Again, although this may be used in clinical practice as a treatment strategy, clinical trials are lacking. There have been isolated case reports, but a paucity of systematic trials or even observational studies reported in the literature.[69] Taking this theoretical benefit one step further, there may be an additional advantage of continuous dosing of OCPs, with rare to no weeks of placebo administration.

MPA is a synthetic progestin and is available as an oral form and as an intramuscular injection every 3 months. This suppresses normal ovulatory hormone cycling, and thus could theoretically improve catamenial epilepsy. Mattson and colleagues[80] studied 14 women with medically refractory epilepsy for the effects of MPA. They were given the oral or depot-intramuscular form to achieve amenorrhea. Half the women were responders with seizure reduction and the group overall had a 39% reduction in seizure frequency. As is common for all women receiving depot-MPA, they had a 3- to 12-month delay in resumption of regular menses after treatment. In addition to this problem, in the general population, reported side effects are common with irregular menstrual bleeding, breast tenderness, weight gain, and depression. Another concern for women with epilepsy, especially if they are on an EIAED, is that depot-MPA is associated with increased risk for osteoporosis.

Other treatment strategies reported by experts include antiestrogens such as clomiphene citrate and gonadotropin-releasing hormone analogs, which suppress ovarian and testicular steroidogenesis.[69] Although there are small pilot studies demonstrating some benefit for seizure control, they have not been studied in any series of more than

15 patients and they carry significant gynecologic, metabolic, and bone health risks. When considered for seizure control, they should be administered in collaboration with a gynecologist or endocrinologist.

Other Neuroactive Steroids

Ganaxolone (GNX) is a neuroactive steroid analog, and is the synthetic 3β-methyl derivative of allopregnanolone.[59] It has a positive allosteroic modulatory effect at the neurosteroid binding site on the GABA$_A$ receptor complex, which is distinct from the benzodiazepine binding site (see **Fig. 3**). It has beneficial activity in a broad range of animal models of epilepsy. Ganaxolone also has the advantage that it lacks hormonal activity, and thus can more readily be applied as a therapeutic agent across both genders and all ages than PROG. Another advantage is that tolerance does not develop to GNX unlike the benzodiazepines, despite working at the same receptor complex.

The findings from a nonrandomized, open-label, pilot study in pediatric and adolescent subjects with refractory epilepsy have been reported.[81] Of the 15 subjects enrolled, 8 completed the trial and 3 continued in the compassionate-use extension period. The responder rate (> 50% reduction in seizure frequency) was 25%, and another 13% had a moderate response (25%–50% reduction in seizure frequency). Of the three who entered the extension phase, one remained seizure-free for more than 3.5 years of GNX administration. The medication was tolerated well, with somnolence being the most frequent side effect.

To date, 961 human subjects (135 children) have been exposed to GNX in safety and pharmacokinetic studies and in clinical trials (most of the latter in early Phase II studies).[59] GNX has been well tolerated in adults and children, and has appeared to have promising therapeutic benefits in adult patients with localization-related epilepsy and children with infantile spasms. Sedation and somnolence were the most commonly reported side effects, but are dose-related and reversible. Additionally, preliminary reports suggest that women with catamenial epilepsy are particularly responsive to GNX, perhaps because it provides neurosteroid replacement in these women.[59] It is currently undergoing further development in infants with newly diagnosed infantile spasms, in women with catamenial epilepsy, and in adults with refractory partial-onset seizures.[82]

SUMMARY

The relationships among hormones, epilepsy, and the medications used to treat epilepsy are complex, with tridirectional interactions that affect both men and women in various ways. Abnormalities of baseline endocrine status occur more commonly in people with epilepsy. Abnormalities are most often described for the sex steroid hormone axis, commonly presenting as sexual dysfunction in men and women with epilepsy and lower fertility. Other signs and symptoms in women with epilepsy include menstrual irregularities, premature menopause, and polycystic ovarian syndrome.

The evaluation and care of adult patients with epilepsy should include considerations of the common hormonal aberrations that occur in this patient population. Questions about reproductive health disorders, sexual function, symptoms of thyroid disorders, and bone health should be part of the evaluation of all adult patients with epilepsy. Further laboratory or radiologic testing and referral to other specialists to participate in collaborative care may be warranted if underlying disorders are suspected, especially given that many of these hormone abnormalities can result in long-term health risks as well as negatively affect quality of life.

AEDs and hormones have a bidirectional interaction that can impair the efficacy of contraceptive hormone treatments and of the AEDs. Endogenous hormones can influence seizure severity and frequency, resulting in catamenial patterns of epilepsy. However, this susceptibility to hormonal influences can be used to develop hormonal strategies to improve seizure control in women with epilepsy with use of cyclic PROG supplementation or alteration of the endogenous hormone release. Additionally, development of the neurosteroid analog ganaxolone provides a novel approach that can potentially be used across both genders and all age groups.

REFERENCES

1. Herzog AG. Neuroendocrinology: epilepsy. AAN Continuum 2009;15:37. Available at: http://www.aan.com/go/elibrary/continuum. Accessed September, 2009.
2. Herzog AG. Disorders of reproduction in patients with epilepsy: primary neurological mechanisms. Seizure 2008;17:101–10.
3. Herzog A, Seibel M, Schomer D, et al. Reproductive endocrine disorders in women with partial seizures of temporal lobe origin. Arch Neurol 1986;43: 341–6.
4. Herzog AG. A relationship between particular reproductive endocrine disorders and the laterality of epileptiform discharges in women with epilepsy. Neurology 1993;43:1907–10.
5. Kalinin VV, Zheleznova EV. Chronology and evolution of temporal lobe epilepsy and endocrine reproductive dysfunction in women: relationships to side of focus and catameniality. Epilepsy Behav 2007;11:185–91.
6. Bilo L, Meo R, Valentino R, et al. Abnormal pattern of luteinizing hormone pulsatility in women with epilepsy. Fertil Steril 1991;55:705–11.
7. Quigg M, Kiely JM, Johnson ML, et al. Interictal and postictal circadian and ultradian luteinizing hormone secretion in men with temporal lobe epilepsy. Epilepsia 2006;47:1452–9.
8. Lossius MI, Tauboll E, Mowinckel P, et al. Reversible effects of antiepileptic drugs on reproductive endocrine function in men and women with epilepsy—a prospective randomized double-blind withdrawal study. Epilepsia 2007;48:1875–82.
9. Herzog AG, Drislane FW, Schomer DL, et al. Differential effects of antiepileptic drugs on sexual function and hormones in men with epilepsy. Neurology 2005; 65:1016–20.
10. Kuba R, Pohanka M, Zakopcan J, et al. Sexual dysfunctions and blood hormonal profile in men with focal epilepsy. Epilepsia 2006;47:2135–40.
11. Morrell MJ, Flynn KL, Done S, et al. Sexual dysfunction, sex steroid hormone abnormalities, and depression in women with epilepsy treated with antiepileptic drugs. Epilepsy Behav 2005;6:360–5.
12. Molleken D, Richter-Appelt H, Stodieck S, et al. Sexual quality of life in epilepsy: correlations with sex hormone blood levels. Epilepsy Behav 2009;14:226–31.
13. Schupf N, Ottman R. Reproduction among individuals with idiopathic/cryptogenic epilepsy: risk factors for reduced fertility in marriage. Epilepsia 1996;37:833–40.
14. Dansky LV, Andermann E, Andermann F. Marriage and fertility in epileptic patients. Epilepsia 1980;21:261–71.
15. Artama M, Isojarvi JI, Raitanen J, et al. Birth rate among patients with epilepsy: a nationwide population-based cohort study in Finland. Am J Epidemiol 2004; 159:1057–63.
16. Olafsson E, Hallgrimsson JT, Hauser WA, et al. Pregnancies of women with epilepsy: a population-based study in Iceland. Epilepsia 1998;39:887–92.

17. Crawford P, Hudson S. Understanding the information needs of women with epilepsy at different lifestages: results of the 'Ideal World' survey. Seizure 2003; 12:502–7.
18. Klein P, Serje A, Pezzullo JC. Premature ovarian failure in women with epilepsy. Epilepsia 2001;42:1584–9.
19. Harden CL, Koppel BS, Herzog AG, et al. Seizure frequency is associated with age at menopause in women with epilepsy. Neurology 2003;61:451–5.
20. Gold EB, Bromberger J, Crawford S, et al. Factors associated with age at natural menopause in a multiethnic sample of midlife women. Am J Epidemiol 2001;153: 865–74.
21. Balen A. Pathogenesis of polycystic ovary syndrome—the enigma unravels? Lancet 1999;354:966–7.
22. Bauer J, Cooper-Mahkorn D. Reproductive dysfunction in women with epilepsy: menstrual cycle abnormalities, fertility, and polycystic ovary syndrome. Int Rev Neurobiol 2008;83:135–55.
23. Knochenhauer ES, Key TJ, Kahsar-Miller M, et al. Prevalence of the polycystic ovary syndrome in unselected black and white women of the southeastern United States: a prospective study. J Clin Endocrinol Metab 1998;83:3078–82.
24. Meo R, Bilo L. Polycystic ovary syndrome and epilepsy: a review of the evidence. Drugs 2003;63:1185–227.
25. Bilo L, Meo R, Nappi C, et al. Reproductive endocrine disorders in women with primary generalized epilepsy. Epilepsia 1988;29:612–9.
26. Isojarvi JI, Laatikainen TJ, Pakarinen AJ, et al. Polycystic ovaries and hyperandrogenism in women taking valproate for epilepsy. N Engl J Med 1993;329: 1383–8.
27. Isojarvi JI, Rattya J, Vv M, et al. Valproate, lamotrigine, and insulin-mediated risks in women with epilepsy. Ann Neurol 1998;43:446–51.
28. Lofgren E, Mikkonen K, Tolonen U, et al. Reproductive endocrine function in women with epilepsy: the role of epilepsy type and medication. Epilepsy Behav 2007;10:77–83.
29. Morrell MJ, Hayes FJ, Sluss PM, et al. Hyperandrogenism, ovulatory dysfunction, and polycystic ovary syndrome with valproate versus lamotrigine. Ann Neurol 2008;64:200–11.
30. Harden CL, Meador KJ, Pennell PB, et al. Practice parameter update: management issues for women with epilepsy—focus on pregnancy (an evidence-based review): teratogenesis and perinatal outcomes: report of the Quality Standards Subcommittee and Therapeutics and Technology Assessment Subcommittee of the American Academy of Neurology and American Epilepsy Society. Neurology 2009;73:133–41.
31. Isojarvi JI, Turkka J, Pakarinen AJ, et al. Thyroid function in men taking carbamazepine, oxcarbazepine, or valproate for epilepsy. Epilepsia 2001;42:930–4.
32. Verrotti A, Laus M, Scardapane A, et al. Thyroid hormones in children with epilepsy during long-term administration of carbamazepine and valproate. Eur J Endocrinol 2009;160:81–6.
33. Gomez JM, Cardesin R, Virgili N, et al. [Thyroid function parameters and TSH in patients treated with anticonvulsant drugs]. An Med Interna 1989;6:235–8 [in Spanish].
34. Isojarvi JI, Pakarinen AJ, Myllyla VV. Thyroid function in epileptic patients treated with carbamazepine. Arch Neurol 1989;46:1175–8.

35. Tiihonen M, Liewendahl K, Waltimo O, et al. Thyroid status of patients receiving long-term anticonvulsant therapy assessed by peripheral parameters: a placebo-controlled thyroxine therapy trial. Epilepsia 1995;36:1118–25.
36. Bauer J. Epilepsy and prolactin in adults: a clinical review. Epilepsy Res 1996;24: 1–7.
37. Collins WC, Lanigan O, Callaghan N. Plasma prolactin concentrations following epileptic and pseudoseizures. J Neurol Neurosurg Psychiatr 1983; 46:505–8.
38. Pritchard PB 3rd, Wannamaker BB, Sagel J, et al. Serum prolactin and cortisol levels in evaluation of pseudoepileptic seizures. Ann Neurol 1985;18:87–9.
39. Pack A. Bone health in people with epilepsy: is it impaired and what are the risk factors? Seizure 2008;17:181–6.
40. Pack AM, Morrell MJ, Marcus R, et al. Bone mass and turnover in women with epilepsy on antiepileptic drug monotherapy. Ann Neurol 2005;57:252–7.
41. Pack AM. Should patients with epilepsy be routinely screened for low bone mineral density? Nat Clin Pract Neurol 2008;4:354–5.
42. Guberman A. Hormonal contraception and epilepsy. Neurology 1999;53:S38–40.
43. Report of the Quality Standards Subcommittee of the American Academy of Neurology: practice parameter: management issues for women with epilepsy (summary statement). Neurology 1998;51:944–8.
44. Krauss GL, Brandt J, Campbell M, et al. Antiepileptic medication and oral contraceptive interactions: a national survey of neurologists and obstetricians. Neurology 1996;46:1534–9.
45. Davis AR, Pack AM, Kritzer J, et al. Reproductive history, sexual behavior and use of contraception in women with epilepsy. Contraception 2008;77:405–9.
46. Vessey M, Painter R, Yeates D. Oral contraception and epilepsy: findings in a large cohort study. Contraception 2002;66:77–9.
47. Pennell PB, Hovinga CA. Antiepileptic drug therapy in pregnancy I: gestation-induced effects on AED pharmacokinetics. Int Rev Neurobiol 2008;83:227–40.
48. Pennell PB. Antiepileptic drug pharmacokinetics during pregnancy and lactation. Neurology 2003;61:S35–42.
49. Pennell PB, Peng L, Newport DJ, et al. Lamotrigine in pregnancy: clearance, therapeutic drug monitoring, and seizure frequency. Neurology 2008;70: 2130–6.
50. Sabers A, Ohman I, Christensen J, et al. Oral contraceptives reduce lamotrigine plasma levels. Neurology 2003;61:570–1.
51. Reimers A, Helde G, Brodtkorb E. Ethinyl estradiol, not progestogens, reduces lamotrigine serum concentrations. Epilepsia 2005;46:1414–7.
52. Christensen J, Petrenaite V, Atterman J, et al. Oral contraceptives induce lamotrigine metabolism: evidence from a double-blind, placebo-controlled trial. Epilepsia 2007;48:484–9.
53. Harden CL, Herzog AG, Nikolov BG, et al. Hormone replacement therapy in women with epilepsy: a randomized, double-blind, placebo-controlled study. Epilepsia 2006;47:1447–51.
54. EURAP Study Group. Seizure control and treatment in pregnancy: observations from the EURAP epilepsy pregnancy registry. Neurology 2006;66:354–60.
55. Galimberti CA, Mazzucchelli I, Arbasino C, et al. Increased apparent oral clearance of valproic acid during intake of combined contraceptive steroids in women with epilepsy. Epilepsia 2006;47:1569–72.

56. Herzog AG, Blum AS, Farina EL, et al. Valproate and lamotrigine level variation with menstrual cycle phase and oral contraceptive use. Neurology 2009;72:911–4.

57. Frye CA. Hormonal influences on seizures: basic neurobiology. Int Rev Neurobiol 2008;83:27–77.

58. Reddy DS. Role of neurosteroids in catamenial epilepsy. Epilepsy Res 2004;62:99–118.

59. Reddy DS, Rogawski MA. Neurosteroid replacement therapy for catamenial epilepsy. Neurotherapeutics 2009;6:392–7.

60. Scharfman HE, MacLusky NJ. The influence of gonadal hormones on neuronal excitability, seizures, and epilepsy in the female. Epilepsia 2006;47:1423–30.

61. Herzog AG. Catamenial epilepsy: definition, prevalence, pathophysiology and treatment. Seizure 2008;17:151–9.

62. Reddy DS, Rogawski MA. Enhanced anticonvulsant activity of neuroactive steroids in a rat model of catamenial epilepsy. Epilepsia 2001;42:337–44.

63. Reddy DS, Kim HY, Rogawski MA. Neurosteroid withdrawal model of perimenstrual catamenial epilepsy. Epilepsia 2001;42:328–36.

64. Rhodes ME, Frye CA. Androgens in the hippocampus can alter, and be altered by, ictal activity. Pharmacol Biochem Behav 2004;78:483–93.

65. Backstrom T. Epileptic seizures in women related to plasma estrogen and progesterone during the menstrual cycle. Acta Neurol Scand 1976;54:321–47.

66. Herzog AG, Klein P, Ransil BJ. Three patterns of catamenial epilepsy. Epilepsia 1997;38:1082–8.

67. Duncan S, Read CL, Brodie MJ. How common is catamenial epilepsy? Epilepsia 1993;34:827–31.

68. El-Khayat HA, Soliman NA, Tomoum HY, et al. Reproductive hormonal changes and catamenial pattern in adolescent females with epilepsy. Epilepsia 2008;49:1619–26.

69. Foldvary-Schaefer N, Falcone T. Catamenial epilepsy: pathophysiology, diagnosis, and management. Neurology 2003;61:S2–15.

70. Herzog AG, Harden CL, Liporace J, et al. Frequency of catamenial seizure exacerbation in women with localization-related epilepsy. Ann Neurol 2004;56:431–4.

71. Morrell MJ, Sarto GE, Shafer PO, et al. Health issues for women with epilepsy: a descriptive survey to assess knowledge and awareness among healthcare providers. J Womens Health Gend Based Med 2000;9:959–65.

72. Cramer JA, Gordon J, Schachter S, et al. Women with epilepsy: hormonal issues from menarche through menopause. Epilepsy Behav 2007;11:160–78.

73. Harden CL, Pulver MC, Ravdin L, et al. The effect of menopause and perimenopause on the course of epilepsy. Epilepsia 1999;40:1402–7.

74. Rossouw JE, Anderson GL, Prentice RL, et al. Risks and benefits of estrogen plus progestin in healthy postmenopausal women: principal results from the Women's Health Initiative randomized controlled trial. JAMA 2002;288:321–33.

75. Herzog AG. Intermittent progesterone therapy and frequency of complex partial seizures in women with menstrual disorders. Neurology 1986;36:1607–10.

76. Herzog AG. Progesterone therapy in women with complex partial and secondary generalized seizures. Neurology 1995;45:1660–2.

77. Herzog AG. Progesterone therapy in women with epilepsy: a 3-year follow-up. Neurology 1999;52:1917–8.

78. Feely M, Calvert R, Gibson J. Clobazam in catamenial epilepsy. A model for evaluating anticonvulsants. Lancet 1982;2(8299):71–3.

79. Feely M, Gibson J. Intermittent clobazam for catamenial epilepsy: tolerance avoided. J Neurol Neurosurg Psychiatr 1984;47:1279–82.
80. Mattson RH, Cramer JA, Caldwell BV, et al. Treatment of seizures with medroxy-progesterone acetate: preliminary report. Neurology 1984;34:1255–8.
81. Pieribone VA, Tsai J, Soufflet C, et al. Clinical evaluation of ganaxolone in pediatric and adolescent patients with refractory epilepsy. Epilepsia 2007;48:1870–4.
82. Nohria V, Giller E. Ganaxolone. Neurotherapeutics 2007;4:102–5.

Selection of Antiepileptic Drugs in Adults

Linda J. Stephen, MBChB, MRCGP, Martin J. Brodie, MBChB, MD*

KEYWORDS

- Epilepsy • Antiepileptic drug selection • Seizures
- Treatment • Adults

Epilepsy affects approximately 50 million people worldwide, with an annual incidence of 50 to 70 cases per 100,000 population.[1] The condition can strike at any time of life, with an immediate impact on everyday activities and routine. Key to optimal management is swift referral to an epilepsy specialist, appropriate investigation, and timely institution of antiepileptic drug (AED) therapy. In the past 20 years, the explosion of 13 new agents into the marketplace has greatly increased the potential for therapeutic intervention. This article explores the rationale for treatment selection in adults with epilepsy.

STARTING ANTIEPILEPTIC DRUG TREATMENT

The decision to start AED treatment can be based on several criteria, including the likelihood of seizure recurrence, the consequences of continuing seizures for patients, and the beneficial and adverse effects of the pharmacologic agent chosen.

Relative risk of recurrence can vary depending on the seizure type or syndrome.[2] Patients with epileptiform discharges on an electroencephalogram or congenital neurologic defects are at high risk (up to 90%) of recurrence. Risk of seizure recurrence is also increased in people with previous symptomatic seizures, in those with cerebral lesions, and in patients with Todd's paralysis.[3]

Patients' views of the situation and those of their family should be taken into consideration when instituting AED treatment.[4] For people who are anxious not to have another seizure, early introduction of therapy may be the best option. Further seizure activity may be unacceptable for those who need to drive, continue in employment, or are responsible for vulnerable family members. Once two or more unprovoked seizures have occurred, the decision to start treatment is usually more clear-cut.

Division of Cardiovascular and Medical Sciences, Epilepsy Unit, Western Infirmary, Glasgow G11 6NT, Scotland, UK
* Corresponding author.
E-mail address: mjb2k@clinmed.gla.ac.uk (M. J. Brodie).

Neurol Clin 27 (2009) 967–992
doi:10.1016/j.ncl.2009.06.007
0733-8619/09/$ – see front matter © 2009 Elsevier Inc. All rights reserved.

neurologic.theclinics.com

Some patients, however, choose not to take AEDs, even after several seizures, because they dislike taking medication or view the diagnosis of epilepsy as a stigma. Treatment may be difficult in people who abuse drugs or alcohol or who have a problem complying with any therapeutic regimen. These individuals should be counseled appropriately and made aware of the implications of further seizure activity, including the risk of sudden unexpected death in epilepsy.[5]

EVIDENCE-BASED GUIDELINES

The number of available AEDs has increased rapidly in the past 20 years, giving more choice when initiating therapy. Major evidence-based guidelines have been developed during this time, assisting clinicians and patients in making appropriate treatment choices in newly diagnosed epilepsy. These include those issued by the National Institute for Clinical Excellence in the United Kingdom,[6] the Scottish Intercollegiate Guidelines Network,[2,7] the American Academy of Neurology/American Epilepsy Society,[8] and the International League Against Epilepsy.[9] These guidelines are based on the best available evidence but may not be a substitute for knowledge, skill, and experience in managing individual patients.

TREATMENT GOALS

The goals of treatment should be complete freedom from seizures with no (or acceptable) side effects and the maintenance of a normal lifestyle. When starting medication, AED monotherapy is preferred over combination regimens, as treatment with a single drug is usually associated with better compliance, fewer adverse effects, reduced likelihood of drug interactions, and lower teratogenic potential and is more cost effective.[10] The choice of drug should have efficacy for the given seizure type or syndrome, with other important properties comprising safety, tolerability, pharmacokinetic properties, and formulation.[11]

EFFICACY

The profile of activity against different seizure types and syndromes varies among the different AEDs (**Table 1**). Accurate classification, therefore, is of paramount importance. Certain epilepsy syndromes are found particularly responsive to specific agents. For example, juvenile myoclonic epilepsy responds well to sodium valproate,[12] and vigabatrin is regarded by many clinicians as the treatment of choice for infantile spasms secondary to tuberous sclerosis.[13] Conversely, narrow spectrum drugs, such as carbamazepine,[14] phenytoin,[15] gabapentin,[16] and oxcarbazepine,[17] can worsen myoclonic jerks and absence seizures.

With the emergence of many new AEDs in recent years, there is a growing evidence base of randomized trials (**Tables 2** and **3**) and systematic reviews (**Table 4**) comparing initial monotherapy treatments for different seizure types and syndromes. AEDs currently licensed for use as monotherapy in the United Kingdom include carbamazepine, phenytoin, phenobarbital, ethosuximide, sodium valproate, lamotrigine, topiramate, oxcarbazepine, and levetiracetam. There is, however, currently no overwhelming efficacy evidence supporting the use of a particular drug. This is due to differences in study design and the absence of comparative adverse effects data at equivalent dosage. There is a dearth of properly conducted randomized controlled trials, particularly in patients with generalized tonic-clonic seizures. Recent data from the levetiracetam versus controlled-release carbamazepine trial suggest that most adults with newly diagnosed epilepsy respond to a modest dose of any

Table 1
Efficacy of antiepileptic drugs against common seizure types and epilepsy syndromes

Antiepileptic Drug	Focal-Onset Seizures	Primary Generalized Seizures			Lennox-Gastaut Syndrome	Infantile Spasms
		Tonic Clonic	Absence	Myoclonic		
Carbamazepine	+	+	↓	↓	0	0
Phenytoin	+	+	↓	↓	0	0
Phenobarbital	+	+	+	0	?	?
Primidone	+	+	0	?	?	?
Ethosuximide	0	0	+	0	0	0
Sodium valproate	+	+	+	+	+	+
Clobazam	+	+	?	+	+	?+
Clonazepam	+	+	?	+	?+	?+
Vigabatrin	+	?+	↓	↓	?	+
Lamotrigine	+	+	+	+[a]	+	?+
Gabapentin	+	?+	↓	↓	?	?
Topiramate	+	+	?	+	+	?
Tiagabine	+	?	↓	?	?	?+
Oxcarbazepine	+	+	↓	↓	0	0
Levetiracetam	+	+	?+	+	?	?
Pregabalin	+	?	?	?	?	?
Stiripentol	+	+	?+	+	?+	?+
Zonisamide	+	?+	?+	?+	?+	?+
Rufinamide	+	+	?+	?+	+	?
Lacosamide	+	?	?	?	?	?

[a] Lamotrigine may worsen myoclonic seizures in some patients.

first-line AED.[36] The more pragmatic standard and new antiepileptic drugs (SANAD) trials assessing effectiveness favored lamotrigine over carbamazepine, gabapentin, topiramate, and oxcarbazepine for partial epilepsy[37] and sodium valproate over lamotrigine or topiramate for generalized and unclassifiable epilepsy.[38]

SAFETY

Establishing acceptable tolerability is a crucial function of regulatory studies performed by pharmaceutical companies for licensing purposes. On occasion, an important safety issue emerges once a drug becomes available for general clinical use. This was the case with felbamate, which was found to cause hepatic failure and aplastic anemia, severely limiting its use,[58] and with vigabatrin, where peripheral visual field defects were first documented 8 years after the drug was licensed.[59] Other AEDs, such as phenobarbital, carbamazepine, phenytoin, lamotrigine, oxcarbazepine, and zonisamide, are associated with a range of rashes and hypersensitivity reactions.[60] These can be minimized by a low starting dose and slow titration schedule. The presence of a previous allergic reaction might guide clinicians away from prescribing one of the AEDs described previously.[61] Recent data support a particular association

Table 2
Randomized controlled trials comparing antiepileptic drug monotherapies in patients with newly diagnosed partial-onset seizures

Reference	AEDs Compared	Study Population	Conclusions	Comments
Mikkelsen et al, 1981[18]	Carbamazepine Clonazepam	36 adults with complex partial seizures	No significant difference was found between the 2 drugs during 6 months' treatment.	Small cohorts
Ramsay et al, 1983[19]	Carbamazepine Phenytoin	87 adults with newly diagnosed partial-onset and primary GTCS	Efficacy and tolerability were the same for both drugs.	Double-blind study; small patient numbers
Mattson et al, 1985[20]	Carbamazepine Phenobarbital Phenytoin Primidone	622 adults with partial and secondary generalized seizures	Control of tonic-clonic seizures did not differ between the drugs. Carbamazepine more often controlled partial seizures compared with phenobarbitone or primidone. Primidone had efficacy similar to phenobarbital, but was tolerated less well.	Multicenter study
Dam et al, 1989[21]	Carbamazepine Oxcarbazepine	235 adults with newly diagnosed partial-onset and primary GTCS	No significant differences in efficacy were found between the two drugs. There was a trend toward better tolerability with oxcarbazepine.	Double-blind multicenter study
Mattson et al, 1992[22]	Carbamazepine Sodium valproate	480 adults with complex partial or secondary GTCS	Carbamazepine was superior to valproate in controlling complex partial seizures. Carbamazepine is as effective as sodium valproate in controlling secondary GTCS.	Double-blind multicenter study

Study	Drugs	Patients	Results	Study type
Richens et al, 1994[23]	Carbamazepine, Sodium valproate	300 adults with newly diagnosed partial-onset or primary GTCS	The drugs controlled seizures equally effectively. Significantly more patients continued on valproate than carbamazepine for at least 6 months.	Open-label study
Brodie et al, 1995[11]	Carbamazepine, Lamotrigine	260 patients aged >13 years with untreated partial-onset or primary GTCS	Similar efficacy results were obtained for both drugs. Lamotrigine was significantly better tolerated.	Double-blind multicenter study
Christie et al, 1997[25]	Oxcarbazepine, Sodium valproate	249 adults with partial or GTCS	No significant differences in efficacy or tolerability found between the two drugs.	Double-blind multicenter study
Bill et al, 1997[26]	Phenytoin, Oxcarbazepine	287 adults with untreated partial-onset and primary GTCS	No significant differences in efficacy found between the two drugs. Oxcarbazepine was significantly better tolerated than phenytoin.	Double-blind multicenter study
Guerreiro et al, 1997[27]	Phenytoin, Oxcarbazepine	193 children and adolescents with epilepsy	No significant differences in efficacy found between the two drugs. Oxcarbazepine was tolerated and retained significantly better.	Double-blind multicenter study
Chadwick et al, 1998[28]	Gabapentin 300 mg, 900 mg, and 1800 mg, Carbamazepine	292 patients aged 12–86 years with newly diagnosed partial-onset seizures	Gabapentin at 900 mg or 1800 mg/d is as effective and as safe as carbamazepine.	Open-label study
Steiner et al, 1999[29]	Phenytoin, Lamotrigine	181 newly diagnosed adults with partial-onset or primary GTCS	Efficacy results were similar for the two drugs. There was a trend toward better tolerability with lamotrigine.	Double-blind study; the high rash rate with lamotrigine probably was due to high starting doses

(continued on next page)

Table 2
(continued)

Reference	AEDs Compared	Study Population	Conclusions	Comments
Brodie et al, 1999[30]	Carbamazepine Lamotrigine	150 patients aged ≥65 years with newly diagnosed epilepsy	No difference was found between the 2 drugs in time to first seizure. More patients continued with lamotrigine than with carbamazepine.	Lamotrigine: carbamazepine treatment ratio was 2:1
Chadwick, 1999[31]	Carbamazepine Vigabatrin	459 patients aged 12–65 years with partial-onset seizures	All efficacy outcomes favored carbamazepine and failed to show equivalence between the two drugs. Time to first seizure was significantly greater with carbamazepine. Vigabatrin was associated with more psychiatric symptoms.	Double-blind multicenter study
Brodie et al, 2002[11]	Lamotrigine Gabapentin	309 adults with partial-onset seizures or primary GTCS	The drugs were similar in efficacy and tolerability.	Double-blind multicenter study
Privitera et al, 2003[32]	Carbamazepine Sodium valproate Topiramate	621 children and adults with newly diagnosed partial-onset seizures or primary GTCS	No significant differences in efficacy were found between the three drugs.	Double-blind multicenter study
Gilliam et al, 2003[33]	Topiramate 50 mg/d, 200 mg/d, or 500 mg/d	Patients aged ≥3 years with partial-onset seizures	Seizure-free rates were significantly higher and time to first seizure was significantly longer with 200 mg/d and 500 mg/d.	Double-blind multicenter study
Arroyo et al, 2005[34]	Topiramate 50 mg/d or 400 mg/d	Patients ≥6 years old with untreated partial-onset or GTCS	The higher dose was significantly more likely to produce seizure freedom than the lower dose. More patients on the higher dose discontinued treatment.	Multicenter study

Study	Patients	Drugs	Findings	Study type
Rowan et al, 2005[35]	593 patients aged ≥65 years with newly diagnosed epilepsy	Carbamazepine Lamotrigine Gabapentin	Seizure control outcomes were similar for the three drugs. Significantly more patients came off carbamazepine due to adverse events compared with gabapentin and lamotrigine.	Double-blind multicenter study
Brodie et al, 2007[36]	579 patients ≥16 years with ≥2 partial-onset or GTCS in the past year	Controlled release carbamazepine Levetiracetam	Seizure free rates were equivalent for both drugs.	Double-blind multicenter study
Marson et al, 2007[37]	1721 adults with partial-onset seizures	Carbamazepine Gabapentin Lamotrigine Oxcarbazepine Topiramate	For time to treatment failure, lamotrigine was significantly better tolerated than carbamazepine, gabapentin or topiramate. For time to 12-month remission, carbamazepine was significantly better tolerated than gabapentin.	Multicenter study
Marson et al, 2007[38]	716 adults with newly diagnosed epilepsy	Sodium valproate Lamotrigine Topiramate	Valproate was significantly better than topiramate in time to treatment failure. For patients with idiopathic generalized epilepsies, valproate had significantly better efficacy than topiramate or lamotrigine. Valproate was significantly better tolerated than topiramate.	Multicenter study
Saetre et al, 2007[39]	186 patients aged ≥65 years with newly diagnosed epilepsy	Controlled release carbamazepine Lamotrigine	Effectiveness was comparable for both drugs. There was a trend toward higher seizure free rates with carbamazepine and for better tolerability with lamotrigine.	Double-blind multicenter study

Abbreviation: GTCS, generalized tonic-clonic seizures.

Table 3
Randomized controlled trials comparing antiepileptic drug monotherapies in patients with generalized tonic-clonic seizures

Reference	AEDs Compared	Study Population	Conclusions	Comments
Shakir et al, 1981[40]	Sodium valproate Phenytoin	33 adults with epilepsy	Sodium valproate was as effective as phenytoin.	Small cohort
Turnbull et al, 1982[41]	Phenytoin Sodium valproate	88 adults with untreated partial-onset or primary GTCS	No significant differences in efficacy between the drugs. Both were more effective for GTCS than partial seizures.	
Ramsay et al, 1983[19]	Carbamazepine Phenytoin	87 adults with newly diagnosed partial-onset and primary GTCS	Efficacy and tolerability were the same for both drugs.	Small patient numbers
Turnbull et al, 1985[42]	Phenytoin Sodium valproate	140 patients aged >16 years with partial or tonic-clonic seizures	No significant differences in efficacy between the two drugs.	Single-center study
Callaghan et al, 1985[43]	Carbamazepine Phenytoin Sodium valproate	181 adults with untreated epilepsy	All the drugs were highly effective in controlling generalized seizures but less effective in controlling partial seizures.	Single-center study
Dam et al, 1989[21]	Carbamazepine Oxcarbazepine	235 adults with newly diagnosed partial-onset and primary GTCS	No significant differences in efficacy were found between the two drugs. There was a trend toward better tolerability with oxcarbazepine.	Double-blind multicenter study
Aikia et al, 1992[44]	Phenytoin Oxcarbazepine	37 adult patients with newly diagnosed epilepsy	No significant differences in efficacy between the drugs.	Single-center double-blind study; small cohort

Placencia et al, 1993[45]	Carbamazepine Phenobarbital	192 patients aged aged between 2 and 60 years with 2 or more untreated seizures	Both drugs had equal efficacy.	Community-based study
Richens et al, 1994[23]	Carbamazepine Sodium valproate	300 adults with newly diagnosed partial-onset or primary GTCS	The drugs controlled seizures equally effectively. Significantly more patients continued on valproate than carbamazepine for at least 6 months.	Multicenter open-label study
Pulliainen et al, 1995[46]	Carbamazepine Phenytoin	43 adults with newly diagnosed partial-onset or primary GTCS	No significant differences in efficacy between the drugs.	Single-center open-label study
Heller et al, 1995[47]	Phenobarbital Phenytoin Carbamazepine Sodium valproate	243 patients aged >16 years with untreated epilepsy	No significant differences in efficacy between the drugs. More patients stopped phenobarbital due to side effects.	Two-center randomized study
Kalviainen et al, 1995[48]	Carbamazepine Vigabatrin	100 patients aged 15 to 64 years with untreated epilepsy	Significantly more patients remained seizure-free with carbamazepine than with vigabatrin. The former was withdrawn more often due to adverse effects. The latter was statistically more often stopped due to lack of efficacy.	Single-center open-label study
Brodie et al, 1995[24]	Carbamazepine Lamotrigine	260 patients aged >13 years with untreated partial-onset or primary GTCS	Similar efficacy results were obtained for both drugs. Lamotrigine was significantly better tolerated.	Double-blind multicenter study

(continued on next page)

Table 3
(continued)

Reference	AEDs Compared	Study Population	Conclusions	Comments
Reunanen et al, 1996[49]	Carbamazepine Lamotrigine	343 patients aged >12 years with untreated partial or GTCS	Carbamazepine and lamotrigine were equally efficacious, with a trend to better tolerability with lamotrigine.	Multicenter randomized study
Bill et al, 1997[26]	Phenytoin Oxcarbazepine	287 adults with untreated partial-onset and primary GTCS	No significant differences in efficacy between the drugs. Oxcarbazepine was significantly better tolerated than phenytoin.	Double-blind multicenter study
Christie et al, 1997[25]	Oxcarbazepine Sodium valproate	249 adults with partial or generalized seizures	No significant differences in efficacy or tolerability found between the two drugs.	Double-blind multicenter study
Steiner et al, 1999[29]	Phenytoin Lamotrigine	181 untreated adults with partial-onset or primary GTCS	Efficacy results were similar for the two drugs. There was a trend toward better tolerability with lamotrigine.	The high rash rate with lamotrigine probably was due to high starting doses.
Brodie and Kwan, 2002[50]	Lamotrigine Gabapentin	309 adults with partial-onset seizures or primary GTCS	The drugs were similar in efficacy and tolerability.	Double-blind multicenter study

Privitera et al, 2003[32]	Carbamazepine Sodium valproate Topiramate	621 children and adults with newly diagnosed partial-onset seizures or primary GTCS	No significant differences in efficacy were found between the three drugs.	Double-blind multicenter study
Arroyo et al, 2005[34]	Topiramate 50 mg/d, or 400 mg/d	487 patients aged ≥ 6 years with untreated partial-onset or GTCS	The higher dose was significantly more likely to produce seizure freedom than the lower dose. More patients on the higher dose discontinued treatment.	
Marson et al, 2007[37]	Sodium valproate Lamotrigine Topiramate	716 adults with newly diagnosed epilepsy	Valproate was significantly better than topiramate in time to treatment failure. For patients with IGEs, valproate had significantly better efficacy than topiramate or lamotrigine. Valproate was significantly better tolerated than topiramate.	Multicenter, randomized study

Abbreviations: GTCS, generalized tonic-clonic seizures; IGEs, idiopathic generalized epilepsies.

Table 4
Systematic reviews of antiepileptic drug monotherapy comparison studies

Reference	Antiepileptic Drugs Compared	Study Population	Conclusions	Comments
Marson et al, 2000[51]	Carbamazepine Sodium valproate	Children and adults with partial-onset seizures or generalized-onset tonic-clonic seizures	Some evidence supported use of carbamazepine for partial-onset seizures. No evidence to support use of valproate in generalized-onset seizures.	Misclassification of epilepsy may have confounded results.
Tudur Smith et al, 2001[52]	Phenytoin Sodium valproate	Children and adults with partial-onset or primary generalized tonic-clonic seizures	No significant differences in efficacy outcomes between the two drugs.	
Tudur Smith et al, 2003[53]	Carbamazepine Phenobarbital	Adults and children with partial-onset or primary generalized tonic-clonic seizures	Drugs were equally effective at controlling focal-onset and primary generalized tonic-clonic seizures.	
Taylor et al, 2003[54]	Phenobarbital Phenytoin	Adults and children with partial-onset or primary generalized tonic-clonic seizures	Phenobarbital was significantly more likely to be discontinued than phenytoin. No difference in time to 12-month remission or first seizure.	Differences in study design made comparisons difficult.
Posner et al, 2005[55]	Ethosuximide Sodium valproate Lamotrigine	Children and adolescents with absence seizures	Evidence was insufficient to make conclusions regarding efficacy.	Trials included were of poor methodologic quality with small patient numbers.
Muller et al, 2006[56]	Phenytoin Oxcarbazepine	Children and adults with epilepsy	For patients with partial-onset seizures, oxcarbazepine is significantly less likely to be withdrawn. Data did not allow efficacy comparisons.	Misclassification of epilepsy types may have confounded results.
Gamble et al, 2006[57]	Carbamazepine Lamotrigine	Children and adults with partial-onset seizures or generalized seizures with or without other seizure types	Carbamazepine may be superior to lamotrigine in terms of seizure control for time to first seizure.	Studies of a longer duration are required to assess long-term outcomes.

between the HLA-B* 1502 allele and AED-induced cutaneous reactions in Han Chinese.[62]

TERATOGENICITY

The incidence of minor and major fetal malformations is higher in women with epilepsy than in the general population, even if they are untreated.[63] Commonly cited percentages are 3% to 6% for women with epilepsy compared with 2% to 3% in the general population.[64] The risk increases disproportionately with the number of AEDs taken, approximately 3% for one drug (similar to background risk), 5% for two, 10% for three, and greater than 20% in women taking more than three AEDs. A syndrome initially ascribed to hydantoins, including phenytoin (fetal hydantoin syndrome), but now known to occur with other AEDs, including carbamazepine and valproate, consists of facial dimorphism, cleft lip and palate, cardiac defects, digital hypoplasia, and nail dysplasia.[64]

Current evidence suggests that the risk of major congenital malformations is 2 to 4 times higher with the use of valproic acid compared with other AEDs, such as carbamazepine and lamotrigine, although this may be minimized by keeping the daily dose at or below 1000 mg.[65] Absolute rates have ranged from 6% to 11%. Exposure to high-dose valproic acid in utero may impair later cognitive function.[66] The risk of major malformations with high-dosage lamotrigine remains to be resolved.[67]

TOLERABILITY

For an AED to be effective, it must be well tolerated and have efficacy. AEDs are commonly associated with unwanted dose-related central nervous system effects, such as dizziness, drowsiness, and ataxia. As with idiosyncratic reactions, these can be minimized by a low starting dose and slow titration schedule. Several of the newer agents show superior tolerability over established AEDs,[21,24,26,48,49] although seizure freedom may still be unattainable due to the development of dose-related adverse effects in some patients.

Cognitive impairment is common in patients with epilepsy, particularly in those with focal epilepsies.[68] Of the established AEDs, phenobarbital perhaps has the greatest potential for cognitive and behavioral toxicity. Dose-related impairment occurs in attention and vigilance, reaction time, short-term memory, and performance IQ.[69,70] Phenobarbital also may produce hyperactivity and aggravation of behavioral disorders.[71] Phenytoin can cause a decline in concentration, memory, mental speed, visuomotor functions, and intelligence.[72] The adverse cognitive and psychomotor effects found with carbamazepine likely are caused partly by the active metabolite carbamazepine-epoxide.[72] When studied in older patients, valproic acid generally had minimal cognitive impact,[73-75] although the drug occasionally can impair attention, visuomotor function, complex decision making, and psychomotor speed. Comparing the cognitive effects of carbamazepine, phenobarbital, phenytoin, and primidone, a Department of Veterans Affairs cooperative study found few pre- to post-AED treatment neuropsychologic changes in patients with new-onset epilepsy.[20] A second Veterans Administration study found mild cognitive changes using carbamazepine and valproic acid as monotherapy for the initial treatment of partial-onset seizures, although there were no significant differences between the two drugs.[74]

Some of the newer AEDs with multiple mechanisms of action have a poorer neuropsychiatric profile than drugs that block voltage-dependent sodium channels, such as phenytoin, carbamazepine, oxcarbazepine, and lamotrigine. Vigabatrin is associated with agitation, ill temper, disturbed behavior, and depression.[76] Levetiracetam can increase irritability in some patients,[77] although others may experience positive behavioral effects.[78] Depression also may be more common with this AED.[36] Topiramate produces somnolence, slowing, memory problems, and language difficulties.[79] When the cognitive effects of levetiracetam and topiramate were compared in patients with refractory epilepsy, no significant differences were found between the two drugs.[80] Lamotrigine has mood-stabilizing properties as adjunctive and monotherapy in patients with bipolar depressive disorder.[81–83] Adjunctive lamotrigine significantly improved anger-hostility subscale scores compared with adjunctive levetiracetam in patients with partial seizures.[84] Zonisamide may impair learning[85] and is associated with aggression, depression, or mood swings in some patients.[86] Animal studies suggest the drug may have antiparkinsonian properties, linked to its facilitation of dopamine transmission.[87] A few patients taking each of these drugs have developed paranoid and psychiatric symptoms, although this seems most likely to occur in patients treated with topiramate.[88]

Awareness of a patient's medical history may bring to light endocrine signs and symptoms that can influence choice of AED monotherapy. Epilepsy itself may be responsible for reproductive endocrine abnormalities.[89] The situation surrounding metabolic influences of AEDs is complex and not yet fully understood. Because many of the data are derived from research conducted in small cohorts, with designs that may bias outcomes, results need to be interpreted with caution. Weight gain is associated with sodium valproate,[90] vigabatrin,[31] gabapentin,[91] and pregabalin.[92] Conversely, treatment with topiramate[79] and zonisamide[93] may result in weight loss in some patients.

There is particular interest in the relationship between polycystic ovary syndrome (PCOS) and epilepsy. Changes associated with PCOS occurred in up to 64% of Finnish women taking valproic acid.[94,95] Indian researchers reported weight gain (40%), hirsutism (20%), and PCOS (20%) in 25 women taking valproic acid for 1 year.[96] Similar results were reported in a Korean study, affecting 42% of women.[97] In other studies, PCOS has been found in 7.7%,[98] 9.1%,[99] 11.1%,[100] 28%,[101] and 48.6%[102] of women with epilepsy. Some researchers report PCOS changes in 5.7% to 16.7% of patients with carbamazepine monotherapy.[99–102] A recent Finnish analysis found sodium valproate a predictor for development of PCOS, polycystic ovaries, and hyperandrogenism.[103]

A history of sexual dysfunction may also affect choice of AED. Hepatic enzyme-inducing AEDs, such as carbamazepine, phenytoin, and phenobarbital, can stimulate production of sex hormone–binding globulin, a binding site for testosterone, where the latter, testosterone, is physiologically inactive.[104] These drugs also may induce the metabolism of testosterone. Daily doses of oxcarbazepine greater than 900 mg exert a similar effect on sex hormone–binding globulin as carbamazepine.[105] Erectile dysfunction also is reported with pregabalin.[106]

Osteomalacia and osteoporosis are linked with chronic AED treatment.[107–109] Phenobarbital, primidone, phenytoin, and carbamazepine increase the breakdown of vitamin D, leading to secondary hyperparathyroidism, osteomalacia, and increased bone turnover, although not all studies back such a hypothesis.[107] Other mechanisms include a direct effect of AEDs on osteoblasts, osteocytes, and osteoclasts; resistance to parathyroid hormone; inhibition of calcitonin secretion; and impaired calcium absorption.[110] Research has shown an association between elevated homocysteine, reduction in bone mineral density, and increased fracture incidence.[111] In all, six AEDs (phenytoin, carbamazepine, phenobarbital, primidone, oxcarbazepine, and lamotrigine) have known antifolate properties, thus, the potential to increase homocysteine concentrations.

Chronic dosing with phenytoin can produce gum hypertrophy,[112] which is mini-mized with continuing attention to dental hygiene. Long-term treatment with pheno-barbital may be associated with a range of fibrosing disorders, such as reflex sympathetic dystrophy, shoulder-hand syndrome, frozen shoulder, and Dupuytren's contracture.[113]

PHARMACOKINETIC PROPERTIES

Ideally, an AED should be absorbed fully, have low protein binding, and undergo linear pharamacokinetics, with clearance unaffected by renal impairment.[114] It should neither induce nor inhibit hepatic monooxygenase or conjugating enzymes, interact with concomitant medication, or produce neurotoxic or other adverse effects. A long elimination half-life is advantageous, allowing once or twice daily dosing. A well-established target dose should be achievable without or with limited titration. Many older AEDs undergo hepatic metabolism with renal elimination of inactive metabolites (**Table 5**). Phenytoin pharmacokinetics are complex. With increasing doses, the eliminating enzyme system becomes progressively saturated. Thus, a small increase in dose can result in a large rise in plasma concentration and neurotoxicity.[115]

Phenobarbital, primidone, phenytoin, and carbamazepine induce the metabolism of lipid-soluble drugs, such as the combined oral contraceptive pill,[116] cytotoxic agents, antiretrovirals, statins, warfarin, and cardiac antiarrhythmics.[114] Newer AEDs are less

Table 5
Pharmacokinetic interactions between antiepileptic drugs

AED	Undergoes Hepatic Metabolism	Affects Hepatic Cytochrome P450 Enzymes	Affects Metabolism of Other AEDs	Metabolism Affected by Other AEDs
Established AEDs				
Carbamazepine	Yes	Yes	Yes	Yes
Clobazam	Yes	No	No	Yes
Clonazepam	Yes	No	No	Yes
Ethosuximide	Yes	No	No	Yes
Phenobarbital	Yes	Yes	Yes	Yes
Phenytoin	Yes	Yes	Yes	Yes
Primidone	Yes	Yes	Yes	Yes
Valproate	Yes	Yes	Yes	Yes
Modern AEDs				
Felbamate	Yes	Yes	Yes	Yes
Gabapentin	No	No	No	No
Lacosamide	Yes	No	No	No
Lamotrigine	Yes	No	No	Yes
Levetiracetam	No	No	No	Yes[a]
Oxcarbazepine	Yes	Yes	Yes[a]	Yes
Pregabalin	No	No	No	No
Tiagabine	Yes	No	No	Yes
Topiramate	Yes	Yes	Yes[a]	Yes
Vigabatrin	No	No	Yes[a]	No
Zonisamide	Yes	No	No	Yes

[a] Effect modest; see text.

likely to interfere with hepatic metabolism, although oxcarbazepine,[117,118] felbamate,[119] and higher doses of topiramate[120] can induce the oestrogenic component of the combined oral contraceptive pill.[121,122] Lamotrigine reduces levonorgestrel concentrations by an, as yet, unknown mechanism.[123]

Where there is a linear relationship between dose and plasma concentration, concentration monitoring can be helpful in assessing side effects and compliance and in establishing the most effective concentration in seizure-free patients.[124] Routine measurement of plasma levels of newer AEDs is not recommended, as they do not correlate well on a population basis with efficacy or side effects.[121] Therapeutic drug monitoring can play a useful role in individualizing clinical management, provided that drug concentrations are measured at an appropriate time in appropriate patients with a clear indication and are interpreted correctly. The availability of concentration monitoring may be the reason that one AED is chosen over another for a particular patient.

FORMULATION

Readily identifiable and palatable formulations can help to improve adherence, thus seizure control. Several AEDs are available in alternative formulations to tablets, such as syrup and sprinkles, which can be useful in patients with swallowing difficulties and for those with percutaneous endoscopic gastrostomy tubes. Parenteral formulations are invaluable in the rapid treatment of status epilepticus and in other circumstances where oral access is not available. The use of rectal diazepam to abolish prolonged seizure activity is now superceded by the administration of buccal or nasal midazolam.[125,126] Intravenous formulations are available for sodium valproate, levetiracetam, and lacosamide in addition to phenytoin, fosphenytoin, phenobarbital, and the benzodiazepines, clonazepam, diazepam, lorazepam, and midazolam.

COST

Despite the introduction of several novel agents, price remains a factor in determining the global use of antiepileptic medication. With few differences in efficacy amongst AEDs, the low costs of older drugs, such as phenobarbital and phenytoin, make these agents an attractive option for developing nations. One thousand generic 100-mg phenobarbital tablets currently cost $6.16.[127] This is considerably less than treatment with any of the new AEDs.

COMBINING ANTIEPILEPTIC DRUGS

Approximately 59% of people with newly diagnosed epilepsy become seizure-free on a single AED.[128] Another 5% require combination therapy to gain complete control of their seizures. Patients with symptomatic or cryptogenic epilepsy more likely are medication resistant than those with idiopathic epilepsy.[129–131] The British National General Practice Study of Epilepsy reported 69% of people with idiopathic generalized epilepsies as having 5 years' seizure freedom at 9-year follow-up compared with 61% for those with remote symptomatic epilepsy.[132]

There may be several different rationales for choosing drug combinations for patients not responding to AED monotherapy. Along with considering seizure type and syndrome classification, factors such as age, gender, comedication, and comorbidity should be taken into account.[133] It also seems sensible to combine drugs with different mechanisms of action, although it is becoming increasingly apparent that several AEDs act in multiple ways that are not yet understood fully.[134] There is, however, clinical and laboratory evidence to suggest that additive or synergistic effects are seen with regimens, such as sodium valproate with ethosuximide for absence seizures,[135] sodium valproate with lamotrigine for focal-onset and generalized seizures,[136,137] and lamotrigine with topiramate[138] for a range of seizure types. In patients with localization-related epilepsy, higher seizure freedom rates were reported in adults taking combination therapy.[139] Of 135 patients taking duotherapy, 37 (27%) were controlled, whereas 5 (10%) of 50 patients taking three AEDs were seizure-free.

With more information becoming available on seizure pathophysiology, three broad mechanisms of AED action are recognized: (1) modulation of voltage-dependent ion channels, (2) enhancement of inhibitory neurotransmission, and (3) attenuation of excitatory neurotransmission (**Table 6**). It is becoming increasingly apparent, however, that many AEDs have multiple cellular effects.[140] Exploration of these mechanisms will allow better understanding of the pathophysiology of seizure propagation and spread and should lead ultimately to improved management of people with refractory epilepsy.[140]

Table 6
Perceived mechanisms of action of antiepileptic drugs

Antiepileptic Drug	↓Na$^+$ Channels	↓Ca^{2+} Channels^c	↑GABA Transmission	↓Glutamate Transmission
Established				
Benzodiazepines			++	
Carbamazepine	++			
Ethosuximide		++ (T-type)		
Phenobarbital		?	++	?
Phenytoin	++			
Valproate	?	? (T-type)	+	?
Modern				
Felbamate	+	?	+	+
Gabapentin	?	++ (α2δ)	+	
Lacosamide	+^{a}			
Lamotrigine	++	?		
Levetiracetam^b		?	?	?
Oxcarbazepine	++			
Pregabalin		++ (α2δ)		
Rufinamide	++			
Stiripentol			?+	
Tiagabine			++	
Topiramate	+	+	+	+
Vigabatrin			++	
Zonisamide	+	+ (T-type)		

Abbreviations: GABA, gamma-aminobutyric acid; ++, primary action; + probable action; ?, possible action.
^{a} Lacosamide also binds to collapsin-response mediator protein 2.
^{b} Levetiracetam acts by binding to synaptic vesicle protein 2A.
^{c} Unless otherwise stated, action on high-voltage–activated calcium channels.

PRACTICAL CONSIDERATIONS

The first consideration when choosing a monotherapy in newly diagnosed epilepsy is that the drug of choice has efficacy for a patient's seizure type or syndrome (**Table 1**). If the classification is unclear, an AED with a broad spectrum of action, such as sodium valproate or levetiracetam, may be selected. For patients taking other drugs, the possibility of pharmacokinetic interactions may come into play. Enzyme inducers are probably best avoided in patients taking other lipid-soluble agents, as discussed previously. For the majority of patients, AEDs are started in a low dose and slowly titrated according to efficacy and tolerability. In those who develop adverse effects, or with compliance issues, plasma concentration monitoring can aid decision making.[121] For untreated patients with a high seizure density, a drug that can be rapidly titrated to therapeutic dosing, such as levetiracetam, should be preferred. For patients with swallowing difficulties, AEDs marketed in formulations, such as syrups, liquids, crushable tablets, and sprinkles, can make adherence easier.

Sodium valproate is associated with fetal malformations,[141] cognitive problems in offspring,[66] weight gain,[95] and PCOS.[94] This drug, therefore, generally is not recommended in girls and women of childbearing age. There are, however, some young women with difficult-to-control idiopathic epilepsy syndromes, whose seizures seem responsive to sodium valproate only.

Older people generally respond well to AED therapy, with seizure freedom rates of up to 80% in individuals who develop seizures later in life.[142] When starting an older person on treatment, a slow titration schedule should be used with a low target dose, given that there are age-related changes in pharmacokinetics and pharmacodynamics, together with the likelihood of complications from comorbidities and interactions with comedications.[143] Well-tolerated AEDs with a low potential for drug interactions, such as lamotrigine, levetiracetam, and gabapentin, are generally selected for these individuals.[144]

In some patients, an AED can be used with the aim of ameliorating more than one problem. For example, in patients with partial-onset seizures and generalized anxiety disorder, adjunctive pregabalin may have efficacy for both conditions.[145,146] Clobazam also can be a useful adjunctive therapy in this setting.[147] Pregabalin and gabapentin can be prescribed in patients with partial-onset seizures and neuropathic pain.[148,149] For individuals with seizures and migraine, treatment with topiramate is an option.[79,150,151]

Using these strategies, a seizure-freedom rate of 60% to 70% can be attained in patients with newly diagnosed epilepsy.[128] With accurate classification of seizure type or syndrome, timely investigation, and appropriate pharmacologic management, the outlook for individuals with newly diagnosed epilepsy has never been more positive. In coming years, genomic research may shed further light on seizure pathophysiology and the reasons underlying refractoriness and adverse drug reactions. As such, it is hoped this may allow a more precise selection of AED treatment, and greater potential for seizure freedom.

REFERENCES

1. Hauser WA, Annegers JF, Rocca WA. Descriptive epidemiology of epilepsy: contributions of population-based studies from Rochester, Minnesota. Mayo Clin Proc 1996;71:576–86.
2. SIGN Guideline 70. Diagnosis and management of epilepsy in adults. Scottish Intercollegiate Guidelines Network. Edinburgh. 2003. Available at: www.sign.ac.uk. Accessed April 2009.

3. Dulac O, Leppik IE, Chadwick DW, et al. Starting and stopping treatment. In: Engel J Jr, Pedley TA, editors. Epilepsy: a comprehensive textbook. 2nd edition. Philadelphia: Wolter Kluwer/Lippincott Williams and Wilkins; 2008. p. 1301–9.

4. Stephen LJ, Brodie MJ. The management of a first seizure. Still a major debate. Special problems: adults and elderly. Epilepsia 2008;49(Suppl 1):45–9.

5. Mohanraj R, Norrie J, Stephen LJ, et al. Mortality in adults with newly diagnosed and chronic epilepsy: a retrospective comparative study. Lancet Neurol 2006;5: 481–7.

6. National Institute for Clinical Excellence. Clinical guideline 20. The epilepsies. The diagnosis and management of the epilepsies in adults and children in primary and secondary care. Available at: http://www.nice.org.uk/nicemedia/pdf/CG020NICEguideline.pdf. 2004. Accessed April 2009.

7. SIGN Guideline 81. Diagnosis and management of epilepsies in children and young people. Scottish Intercollegiate Guidelines Network. Edinburgh.www.sign.ac.uk. 2005.

8. American Academy of Neurology. Efficacy and tolerability of the new antiepileptic drugs. I. Treatment of new-onset epilepsy: report of the TTA and QSS subcommittees of the American Academy of Neurology and of the American Epilepsy Society. 2004. Available at: http://www.aesnet.org/go/practice/guidelines. Accessed April 2009.

9. Glauser T, Ben-Menachem E, Bourgeois B, et al. ILAE Treatment Guidelines: evidence-based analysis of antiepileptic drug efficacy and effectiveness as initial monotherapy for epileptic seizures and syndromes. Epilepsia 2006;47: 1094–120.

10. Leppik IE. Rational monotherapy for epilepsy. In: Brodie MJ, Treiman DM, editors. Modern management of epilepsy, Balliere's clinical neurology, vol. 5. London: Balliere-Tindall; 1996. p. 749–55 England.

11. Brodie MJ, Chadwick DW, Anhut H, et al. Gabapentin versus lamotrigine monotherapy: a double-blind comparison in newly diagnosed epilepsy. Epilepsia 2002;43:993–1000.

12. Sundqvist A, Tomson T, Lundkvist B. Valproate as monotherapy for juvenile myoclonic epilepsy: dose-effect study. Ther Drug Monit 1998;21:91–6.

13. Elterman RD, Shields WD, Mansfield KA, et al. Randomized trial of vigabatrin in patients with infantile spasms. Neurology 2001;57:1416–21.

14. Liporace JD, Sperling MR, Dichter MA. Absence seizures and carbamazepine in adults. Epilepsia 1994;35:1026–8.

15. Duarte J, Sempere AP, Cabezas MC, et al. Postural myoclonus induced by phenytoin. Clin Neuropharmacol 1996;19:536–8.

16. Ascapone J, Diedrich A, DellaBadia J. Myoclonus associated with the use of gabapentin. Epilepsia 2000;41:479–81.

17. Gelisse P, Genton P, Kuate C, et al. Worsening of seizures by oxcarbazepine in juvenile idiopathic generalized epilepsies. Epilepsia 2004;45:1282–6.

18. Mikkelsen B, Berggreen P, Joensen P, et al. Clonazepam (Rivotril) and carbamazepine (Tegretol) in psychomotor epilepsy: a randomized multicenter trial. Epilepsia 1981;22:415–20.

19. Ramsay RE, Wilder BJ, Berger JR, et al. A double-blind study comparing carbamazepine with phenytoin as initial seizure therapy in adults. Neurology 1983;33: 904–10.

20. Mattson RH, Cramer JA, Collins JF, et al. Comparison of carbamazepine, phenobarbital, phenytoin and primidone in partial and secondarily generalized tonic-clonic seizures. N Engl J Med 1985;313:145–51.

21. Dam M, Ekberg R, Løying Y, et al. A double-blind study comparing oxcarbazepine and carbamazepine in patients with newly diagnosed, previously untreated epilepsy. Epilepsy Res 1989;3:70–6.

22. Mattson RH, Cramer JA, Collins JF. A comparison of valproate with carbamazepine for the treatment of complex partial seizures and secondarily generalized tonic-clonic seizures in adults. N Engl J Med 1992;327:765–71.

23. Richens A, Davidson DL, Cartlidge NE, et al. A multicentre comparative trial of sodium valproate and carbamazepine in adult onset epilepsy. J Neurol Neurosurg Psychiatry 1994;57:682–7.

24. Brodie MJ, Richens A, Yuen AW. Double-blind comparison of lamotrigine and carbamazepine in newly diagnosed epilepsy. The UK Lamotrigine/Carbamazepine Monotherapy Trial Group. Lancet 1995;345:476–9.

25. Christie W, Kramer G, Vigonius U, et al. A double-blind controlled clinical trial: oxcarbazepine versus sodium valproate in adults with newly diagnosed epilepsy. Epilepsy Res 1997;26:451–60.

26. Bill PA, Vigonius U, Pohlmann H, et al. A double-blind controlled clinical trial of oxcarbazepine versus phenytoin in adults with previously untreated epilepsy. Epilepsy Res 1997;27:195–204.

27. Guerreiro MM, Vigonius U, Pohlmann H, et al. A double-blind, controlled clinical trial of oxcarbazepine versus phenytoin in children and adolescents with epilepsy. Epilepsy Res 1997;27:205–13.

28. Chadwick DW, Anhut H, Greiner MJ, et al. A double-blind trial of gabapentin monotherapy for newly diagnosed partial seizures: International Gabapentin Monotherapy Study Group 945–77. Neurology 1998;51:1282–8.

29. Steiner TJ, Dellaportas CI, Findley LJ, et al. Lamotrigine monotherapy in newly diagnosed untreated epilepsy: a double-blind comparison with phenytoin. Epilepsia 1999;40:601–7.

30. Brodie MJ, Overstall PW, Giorgi L. Multicentre, double-blind, randomised comparison between lamotrigine and carbamazepine in elderly patients with newly diagnosed epilepsy. The UK Lamotrigine Elderly Study Group. Epilepsy Res 1999;37:81–7.

31. Chadwick DW. Safety and efficacy of vigabatrin and carbamazepine in newly diagnosed epilepsy: a multicentre randomised DB study: Vigabatrin European Monotherapy Study Group. Lancet 1999;354:13–9.

32. Privitera MD, Brodie MJ, Mattson RH, et al. Topiramate, carbamazepine and valproate monotherapy: double-blind comparison in newly diagnosed epilepsy. Acta Neurol Scand 2003;107:165–75.

33. Gilliam FG, Veloso F, Bomhof MA, et al. A dose-comparison trial of topiramate as monotherapy in recently diagnosed partial epilepsy. Neurology 2003;60:196–202.

34. Arroyo S, Dodson WE, Privitera MD, et al. A randomized dose-controlled study of topiramate as first-line therapy in epilepsy. Acta Neurol Scand 2005;112:214–22.

35. Rowan AJ, Ramsay RE, Collins JF, et al. New onset geriatric epilepsy: a randomized study of gabapentin, lamotrigine and carbamazepine. Neurology 2005;64:1868–73.

36. Brodie MJ, Perucca E, Ryvlin P, et al. Comparison of levetiracetam and controlled-release carbamazepine in newly diagnosed epilepsy. Neurology 2007;68:402–8.

37. Marson A, Al-Kharusi A, Alwaidh M, et al. The SANAD study of effectiveness of carbamazepine, gabapentin, lamotrigine, oxcarbazepine, or topiramate for treatment of partial epilepsy: an unblinded randomised controlled trial. Lancet 2007;369:1000–15.

38. Marson A, Al-Kharusi A, Alwaidh M, et al. The SANAD study of effectiveness of valproate, lamotrigine, or topiramate for generalised and unclassifiable epilepsy: an unblinded randomised controlled trial. Lancet 2007;369:1016–26.

39. Saetre E, Perucca E, Isojärvi J, et al. An international multicentre randomized double-blind controlled trial of lamotrigine and sustained-release carbamazepine in the treatment of newly diagnosed epilepsy in the elderly. Epilepsia 2007;48:1292–302.

40. Shakir RA, Johnson RH, Lambie DG, et al. Comparison of sodium valproate and phenytoin as single drug treatment in epilepsy. Epilepsia 1981;22:27–33.

41. Turnbull DM, Rawlins MD, Weightman D, et al. A comparison of phenytoin and valproate in previously untreated adult epileptic patients. J Neurol Neurosurg Psychiatry 1982;45:55–9.

42. Turnbull DM, Howel D, Rawlins MD, et al. Which drug for the adult epileptic patient: phenytoin or valproate? Br Med J 1985;313:145–51.

43. Callaghan N, Kenny RA, O'Neill B, et al. A prospective study between carbamazepine, phenytoin, and sodium valproate as monotherapy in previously untreated and recently diagnosed patients with epilepsy. J Neurol Neurosurg Psychiatry 1985;48:639–44.

44. Aikia M, Kalviainen R, Sivenius J, et al. Cognitive effects of oxcarbazepine and phenytoin monotherapy in newly diagnosed epilepsy: one year follow-up. Epilepsy Res 1992;11:199–203.

45. Placencia M, Sander JW, Shorvon SD, et al. Antiepileptic drug treatment in a community health care setting in northern Ecuador: a prospective 12-month assessment. Epilepsy Res 1993;14:237–44.

46. Pulliainen V, Jokelainen M. Comparing the cognitive effects of phenytoin and carbamazepine in long-term monotherapy: a two-year follow-up. Epilepsia 1995;36:1195–202.

47. Heller AJ, Chesterman P, Elwes RD, et al. Phenobarbitone, phenytoin, carbamazepine, or sodium valproate for newly diagnosed adult epilepsy: a randomised comparative monotherapy trial. J Neurol Neurosurg Psychiatry 1995;57:682–7.

48. Kalviainen R, Aikia M, Saukkonen AM, et al. Vigabatrin vs carbamazepine monotherapy in patients with newly diagnosed epilepsy: a randomized, controlled study. Arch Neurol 1995;52:989–96.

49. Reunanen M, Dam M, Yuen AWC. A randomised open multicentre comparative trial of lamotrigine and carbamazepine as monotherapy in patients with newly diagnosed or recurrent epilepsy. Epilepsy Res 1996;345:149–55.

50. Brodie MJ, Kwan P. Staged approach to epilepsy management. Neurology 2002;58(Suppl 5):S2–8.

51. Marson AG, Williamson PR, Hutton JL, et al. Carbamazepine versus valproate monotherapy for epilepsy (Cochrane Review). Cochrane Database Syst Rev 2000;(3):CD001030. doi:10.1002/14651858.

52. Tudur Smith C, Marson AG, Williamson PR. Phenytoin versus valproate monotherapy for partial onset seizures and generalized onset tonic-clonic seizures. Cochrane Database Syst Rev 2001;(4):CD001769. doi:10.1002/14651858.

53. Tudur Smith C, Marson AG, Williamson PR. Carbamazepine versus phenobarbitone monotherapy for epilepsy. The Cochrane Database Syst Rev 2003;(1):CD001904. doi:10.1002/14651858.

54. Taylor S, Tudur Smith C, Williamson PR, et al. Phenobarbitone versus phenytoin monotherapy for partial onset seizures and generalized onset tonic-clonic seizures. Cochrane Database Syst Rev 2003;(2):CD002217. doi:10.1002/14651858.

55. Posner EB, Mohamed K, Marson AG. Ethosuximide, sodium valproate or lamotrigine for absence seizures in children and adolescents. Cochrane Database Syst Rev 2005;(4):CD003032. doi:10.1002/14651858.

56. Muller M, Marson AG, Williamson PR. Oxcarbazepine versus phenytoin monotherapy. CD003615. The Cochrane Database Syst Rev 2006;(2)10.1002/14651858.

57. Gamble CL, Williamson PR, Marson AG. Lamotrigine versus carbamazepine monotherapy for epilepsy. Cochrane Database Syst Rev 2006;(1):CD001031. doi:10.1002/14651858.

58. Pellock JM, Brodie MJ. Felbamate: an update. Epilepsia 1997;38:1261–4.

59. Willmore LJ, Abelson MB, Ben-Menachem E, et al. Vigabatrin: 2008 update. Epilepsia 2009;50:163–73.

60. Arif H, Buchbaum R, Weintraub D, et al. Comparison and predictors of rash associated with 15 antiepileptic drugs. Neurology 2007;68:1701–9.

61. Hirsch LJ, Arif H, Nahm EA, et al. Cross-sensitivity of skin rashes with antiepileptic drug use. Neurology 2008;71:1527–34.

62. Man CLB, Kwan P, Baum L, et al. Association between HLA-B*1502 allele and antiepileptic drugs-induced cutaneous reactions in Han Chinese. Epilepsia 2007;48:1015–8.

63. Holmes LB, Harvey EA, Coull BA, et al. The teratogenicity of antiepileptic drugs. N Engl J Med 2001;344:1132–8.

64. Tomson T, Perucca E, Battino D. Navigating toward fetal and maternal health: the challenge of treating epilepsy in pregnancy. Epilepsia 2004;45:1171–5.

65. Harden C, Meador KJ, Pennell PB, et al. Management issues for women with epilepsy—focus on pregnancy (an evidence-based review): II. Teratogenesis and perinatal outcomes. Epilepsia 2009;50:1237–46.

66. Meador K, Baker G, Browning N, et al. Cognitive function at 3 years of age after fetal exposure to antiepileptic drugs. N Engl J Med 2009;360:1597–605.

67. Morrow J, Russell A, Guthrie E, et al. Malformation risks of antiepileptic drugs in pregnancy: a prospective study from the UK Epilepsy and Pregnancy Register. J Neurol Neurosurg Psychiatry 2006;77:193–8.

68. Dodrill CB. Neuropsychological aspects of epilepsy. Psychiatr Clin North Am 1992;15:383–94.

69. Camfield CS, Chaplin S, Doyle AB, et al. Side effects of phenobarbital in toddlers. J Pediatr 1979;95:361–5.

70. Sulzbacher S, Farwell JR, Temkin N, et al. Late cognitive effects of early treatment with phenobarbital. Clin Pediatr 1999;38:387–94.

71. Kwan P, Brodie MJ. Phenobarbital for the treatment of epilepsy in the 21st century: a critical review. Epilepsia 2004;45:1141–9.

72. Gillham RA, Williams N, Wiedmann KD, et al. Concentration-effect relationships with carbamazepine and its epoxide on psychomotor and cognitive function in epileptic patients. J Neurol Neurosurg Psychiatry 1988;51:655–60.

73. Craig I, Tallis R. Impact of valproate and phenytoin on cognitive function in elderly people: results of a single-blind, randomized, comparative study. Epilepsia 1994;35:381–90.

74. Prevey ML, Delaney RD, Cramer JA, et al. Effect of valproate on cognitive functioning: comparison with carbamazepine. Arch Neurol 1996;53:1008–16.

75. Read CL, Stephen LJ, Stolarek IH, et al. Cognitive effects of anticonvulsant monotherapy in elderly patients: a placebo-controlled study. Seizure 1998;7:159–62.

76. Kwan P, Brodie MJ. Neuropsychological effects of epilepsy and antiepileptic drugs. Lancet 2001;357:216–22.

77. Mula M, Trimble MR, Yuen A, et al. Psychiatric adverse events during levetiracetam therapy. Neurology 2003;61:704–8.
78. Bootsma HPR, Ricker L, Diepman L, et al. Long-term effects of levetiracetam and topiramate in clinical practice: a head-to-head comparison. Seizure 2008; 17:19–26.
79. Ben-Menachem E, Henriksen O, Dam M, et al. Double-blind, placebo-controlled trial of topiramate as add-on therapy in patients with refractory partial seizures. Epilepsia 1996;37:539–43.
80. Huang C-W, Pai M-C, Tsai J-J. Comparative cognitive effects of levetiracetam and topiramate in intractable epilepsy. Psychiatry Clin Neurosci 2008;62: 548–53.
81. Geddes JR, Calabrese JR, Goodwin GM. Lamotrigine for treatment of bipolar depression: independent meta-analysis and meta-regression of individual patient data from five randomised trials. Br J Psychiatry 2009;194:4–9.
82. Van der Loos ML, Mulder P, Hartong GH, et al. Efficacy and safety of lamotrigine as add-on treatment to lithium in bipolar depression: a multicenter, double-blind, placebo-controlled trial. J Clin Psychopharmacol 2009;70:223–31.
83. Vernillo AT, Rifkin BR, Hauschka PV. Phenytoin affects osteocalcin secretion from osteoblastic rat osteosarcoma 17/2.8 cells in culture. Bone 1990;11:309–12.
84. Labiner DM, Ettinger AB, Fakhoury TA, et al. Effects of lamotrigine compared with levetiracetam on anger, hostility, and total mood in patients with partial epilepsy. Epilepsia 2009;50:434–42.
85. Berent S, Sackellares JC, Giordani B, et al. Zonisamide (CI-912) and cognition: results from preliminary study. Epilepsia 1987;28:61–7.
86. Miyamoto T, Kohsaka M, Tsukasa K. Psychotic episodes during zonisamide treatment. Seizure 2000;9:65–70.
87. Asanuma M, Miyazaki I, Diaz-Corrales FJ, et al. Preventing effects of a novel anti-parkinsonian agent zonisamide on dopamine quinine formation. Neurosci Res 2008;60:106–13.
88. Loring DW, Marino S, Meador KJ. Neuropsychological and behavioural effects of antiepileptic drugs. Neuropsychol Rev 2007;17:413–25.
89. Herzog AG, Seibel MM, Schomer DL, et al. Reproductive endocrine disorders in women with partial seizures of temporal lobe origin. Arch Neurol 1986;43:341–6.
90. Dinesen H, Gram L, Anderson T, et al. Weight gain during treatment with valproate. Acta Neurol Scan 1984;70:65–9.
91. DeToledo JC, Toledo C, DeCerce J, et al. Changes in body weight with chronic, high-dose gabapentin therapy. Ther Drug Monit 1997;19:394–6.
92. Brodie MJ, Wilson EA, Wesche DL, et al. Pregabalin drug interaction studies: lack of effect on the pharmacokinetics of carbamazepine, phenytoin, lamotrigine and valproate in patients with partial epilepsy. Epilepsia 2005;46: 1407–13.
93. Schmidt D, Jacob R, Loiseau P, et al. Zonisamide for add-on treatment of refractory partial epilepsy: a European double-blind trial. Epilepsy Res 1993;15:67–73.
94. Isojärvi JI, Laatikainen TJ, Pakarinen AJ, et al. Polycystic ovaries and hyperandrogenism in women taking valproate for epilepsy. N Engl J Med 1993;329: 1383–8.
95. Isojärvi JI, Laatikainen TJ, Knip M, et al. Obesity and endocrine disorders in women taking valproate for epilepsy. Ann Neurol 1996;39:579–84.
96. Prabhakar S, Sahota P, Kharbanda PS, et al. Sodium valproate, hyperandrogenism and altered ovarian function in Indian women with epilepsy: a prospective study. Epilepsia 2007;48:1371–7.

97. Kim JY, Lee HW. Metabolic and hormonal disturbances in women with epilepsy on antiepileptic drug monotherapy. Epilepsia 2007;48:1366–70.
98. Luef G, Abraham I, Trinka E, et al. Hyperandrogenism, post-prandial hyperinsulinaemia and the risk of PCOS in a cross sectional study of women with epilepsy treated with valproate. Epilepsy Res 2002;48:91–102.
99. Luef G, Abraham I, Haslinger M, et al. Polycystic ovaries, obesity and insulin resistance in women with epilepsy: a comparative study of carbamazepine and valproic acid in 105 women. J Neurol 2002;249:835–41.
100. Bauer J, Jarre A, Klingmuller D, et al. Polycystic ovary syndrome in patients with focal epilepsy: a study in 93 women. Epilepsy Res 2000;41:163–7.
101. Betts T, Dutton N, Yarrow H. Epilepsy and the ovary (cutting out the hysteria). Seizure 2001;10:220–8.
102. Isojärvi JI, Tauboll E, Pakarinen AJ, et al. Altered ovarian function and cardiovascular risk factors in valproate-treated women. Am J Med 2001;111:290–6.
103. Löfgren E, Mikkonen K, Tolonen U, et al. Reproductive endocrine function in women with epilepsy: The role of epilepsy type and medication. Epilepsy Behav 2007;10:77–83.
104. Isojärvi JI, Tauboll E, Herzog AG. Effect of antiepileptic drugs on reproductive endocrine function in individuals with epilepsy. CNS Drugs 2005;19:207–23.
105. Patsalos PN, Zakrewska JM, Elyas AA. Dose dependent enzyme induction by oxcarbazepine. Eur J Clin Pharmacol 1990;39:187–8.
106. Hitiris N, Barrett JA, Brodie MJ. Five case reports: erectile dysfunction association with pregabalin add-on treatment in patients with partial seizures. Epilepsy Behav 2006;8:418–21.
107. Farhat G, Yamout B, Mikati MA, et al. Effect of antiepileptic drugs on bone density in ambulatory patients. Neurology 2002;58:1348–53.
108. Souverein PC, Webb DJ, Weil JG, et al. Use of antiepileptic drugs and risk of fractures. Case-control study among patients with epilepsy. Neurology 2006;66:1318–24.
109. Stephen LJ, McLellan AR, Harrison JH, et al. Bone density and antiepileptic drugs: a case-controlled study. Seizure 1999;8:339–42.
110. Fitzpatrick LA. Pathophysiology of bone loss in patients receiving anticonvulsant therapy. Epilepsy Behav 2004;5(Suppl 2):3–15.
111. Elliot J, Jacobson M, Haneef Z. Homocysteine and bone loss in epilepsy. Seizure 2007;16:22–34.
112. Angelopolous AP, Goaz PW. Incidence of diphenylhydantoin gingival hyperplasia. Oral Surg Oral Med Oral Oncol 1972;34:898–906.
113. Falasca GF, Toly TM, Reginato AJ, et al. Reflex sympathetic dystrophy associated with antiepileptic drugs. Epilepsia 1994;35:394–9.
114. Perucca E. Clinically relevant drug interactions with antiepileptic drugs. Br J Clin Pharmacol 2005;61:246–55.
115. Valodia PN, Seymour SA, McFadyen ML, et al. Validation of population pharmacokinetic parameters of phenytoin using a parallel Michaelis-Menten and first-order elimination model. Ther Drug Monit 2000;22:313–9.
116. Back D, Bates M, Bowden A, et al. The interaction of phenobarbital and other anticonvulsants with oral contraceptive steroid therapy. Contraception 1980;22:495–503.
117. Fattore C, Cipolla G, Gatti G, et al. Induction of ethinyloestradiol and levonorgestrel metabolism by oxcarbazepine in healthy women. Epilepsia 1999;40:783–7.
118. Klosterskov Jensen P, Saano V, Haring P, et al. Possible interaction between oxcarbazepine and an oral contraceptive. Epilepsia 1992;33:1149–52.

119. Saano V, Glue P, Banfield CR, et al. Effects of felbamate on the pharmacokinetics of a low-dose combination oral contraceptive. Clin Pharmacol Ther 1995;58:523–31.
120. Rosenfeld WE, Doose DR, Walker SA, et al. Effect of topiramate on the pharmacokinetics of an oral contraceptive containing norethindrone and ethinyl estradiol in patients with epilepsy. Epilepsia 1997;38:317–23.
121. Patsalos PN, Berry DJ, Bourgeois BFD, et al. Antiepileptic drugs—best practice guideline for therapeutic drug monitoring. Epilepsia 2008;49:1239–76.
122. Pellock JM. Carbamazepine side effects in children and adults. Epilepsia 1987; 28(Suppl 3):S64–70.
123. O'Brien MD, Guillebaud J. Contraception for women with epilepsy. Epilepsia 2006;47:1419–22.
124. Johannessen SI, Tomson T. General principles. Laboratory monitoring of antiepileptic drugs. In: Levy RH, Mattson RH, Meldrum BS, et al, editors. Antiepileptic drugs. 5th edition. Philadelphia: Lippincott, Williams and Wilkins; 2002. p. 103–11.
125. Scott RC, Besag FM, Neville BG. Buccal midazolam and rectal diazepam for treatment of prolonged seizures in childhood and adolescence: a randomised trial. Lancet 1999;353:623–6.
126. Wilson MT, Macleod S, O'Regan ME. Nasal/buccal midazolam use in the community. Arch Dis Child 2004;89:50–1.
127. International drug price indicator guide. Management sciences for health. 2009. Available at: http://erc.msh.org/mainpage.cfm?file=1.0.htm&module=DMP& language=English. Accessed April 2009.
128. Mohanraj R, Brodie MJ. Diagnosing refractory epilepsy: response to sequential treatment schedules. Eur J Neurol 2006;8:434–7.
129. Annegers JF, Hauser WA, Elveback LR. Remission of seizures and relapse in patients with epilepsy. Epilepsia 1979;20:729–37.
130. Devinsky O. Patients with refractory seizures. N Engl J Med 1999;340:1565–70.
131. Kwan P, Brodie MJ. Early identification of refractory epilepsy. N Engl J Med 2000;342:314–9.
132. Cockerell OC, Johnson AL, Sander JW, et al. Prognosis of epilepsy: a review and further analysis of the first nine years of the British National General Practice Study of Epilepsy, a prospective population-based study. Epilepsia 1997;38:31–46.
133. Stefan H, Loes da Silva FH, Löscher W, et al. Epileptogenesis and rational therapeutic strategies. Acta Neurol Scand 2006;113:139–55.
134. Kwan P, Brodie MJ. Combination therapy in epilepsy. When and what to use. Drugs 2006;66:1817–29.
135. Rowan AJ, Meijer JWA, de Beer-Pawlikowski N, et al. Valproate ethosuximide combination therapy for refractory absence seizures. Arch Neurol 1983;40: 797–802.
136. Brodie MJ, Yuen AW. Lamotrigine substitution study: evidence for synergism with sodium valproate? The 105 Study Group. Epilepsy Res 1997;26:423–32.
137. Pisani F, Oteri G, Russo MF, et al. The efficacy of valproate-lamotrigine comedication in refractory complex partial seizures: evidence for a pharmacodynamic interaction. Epilepsia 1999;40:1141–6.
138. Stephen LJ, Sills GJ, Brodie MJ. Lamotrigine and topiramate may be a useful combination. Lancet 1998;351:958–9.
139. Peltola J, Peltola M, Raitanen J, et al. Seizure-freedom with combination therapy in localization-related epilepsy. Seizure 2008;17:276–80.
140. Kwan P, Brodie MJ. Emerging drugs for epilepsy. Exp Opinion Emerg Drugs 2007;12:407–22.

141. Meador K, Reynolds MW, Crean S, et al. Pregnancy outcomes in women with epilepsy: a systematic review and meta-analysis of published pregnancy registries and cohorts. Epilepsy Res 2008;81:1–13.

142. Stephen LJ, Kelly K, Mohanraj R, et al. Pharmacological outcomes in older people with newly diagnosed epilepsy. Epilepsy Behav 2006;13:277–82.

143. Stephen LJ, Brodie MJ. Epilepsy in elderly people. Lancet 2000;355:1441–6.

144. Brodie MJ, Kwan P. Epilepsy in the elderly. Br Med J 2005;331:1317–22.

145. Beydoun A, Uthman BM, Kugler AR, et al. Safety and efficacy of two pregabalin regimens for add-on treatment of partial epilepsy. Neurology 2005;64:475–80.

146. Pande AC, Crockatt JG, Feltner DE, et al. Pregabalin in generalized anxiety disorder: a placebo-controlled trial. Am J Psychiatry 2003;160:533–40.

147. Michael B, Marson AG. Clobazam as an add-on in the management of refractory epilepsy. Cochrane Database Syst Rev 2008;(2):CD004154. doi:10.1002/14651858.

148. Freynhagen R, Strojek K, Griesing T, et al. Efficacy of pregabalin in neuropathic pain evaluated in a 12-week, randomised, double-blind, multicentre, placebo-controlled trial of flexible- and fixed-dose regimens. Pain 2005;115:254–63.

149. Serpell MG. Neuropathic pain study group. Gabapentin in neuropathic pain syndromes: a randomised, double-blind, placebo-controlled trial. Pain 2002;99:557–66.

150. Ashtari F, Shaygannejad V, Akbari M. A double-blind, randomized trial of low-dose topiramate vs propranolol in migraine prophylaxis. Acta Neurol Scand 2008;113:301–5.

151. Privitera M, Fincham R, Penry J, et al. Topiramate placebo-controlled dose-ranging trial in refractory partial epilepsy using 600-, 800- and 1000-mg daily dosages. Neurology 1996;46:1678–82.

Teratogenic Effects of Antiepileptic Medications

Torbjörn Tomson, MD, PhD[a,b],*, Dina Battino, MD[c]

KEYWORDS

- Epilepsy • Pregnancy • Antiepileptic drugs
- Teratogenicity • Birth defects

It has been estimated that 0.3% to 0.5% of all children are born to mothers with epilepsy,[1,2] corresponding to approximately 25 000 children each year in the United States alone.[3] With increasing use of antiepileptic drugs (AEDs) for other indications, such as psychiatric conditions, migraines, and pain disorders, the number of women using AEDs during pregnancy is likely to be considerably higher. Although the focus of this article is on the potential teratogenic effects of AEDs, it is important to underline that the potential adverse outcomes in the offspring because of maternal use of AEDs need to be weighed and balanced against the risks associated with the underlying disease itself. In epilepsy, the maternal and fetal risks with uncontrolled major convulsive seizures generally necessitate continued drug treatment during pregnancy.[4] The challenge to physicians is to prescribe a treatment that effectively controls generalized tonic-clonic seizures in particular while minimizing the risk of adverse AED effects on the fetus. This is a realistic goal because most women with epilepsy have uneventful pregnancies and give birth to perfectly normal children.

The first report suggesting an association between use of AEDs and major congenital malformations was published more than 40 years ago.[5] This short report described oral clefts and some other abnormalities in 6 children who were exposed to phenytoin, phenobarbital, and primidone in different combinations.[5] Subsequent studies during the following decade, mainly retrospective case series, confirmed that use of all the major older generation AEDs, such as phenobarbital, phenytoin, valproate, and carbamazepine, was associated with an increased risk of birth defects.[6] Later, prospective cohort studies tried to distinguish between the contributions of AEDs versus the underlying epilepsy to the adverse fetal outcome, and case-control studies analyzed specific birth defects in relation to individual AEDs. The last decade has seen the

---

[a] Department of Clinical Neuroscience Karolinska Institutet, Stockholm Sweden
[b] Department of Neurology, Karolinska Hospital, SE-171 76 Stockholm, Sweden
[c] Department of Neurophysiopatology, Fondazione I.R.C.C.S. Istituto Neurologico "Carlo Besta", 20133 Milan, Italy
* Corresponding author. Department of Neurology, Karolinska Hospital, SE-171 76 Stockholm, Sweden.
E-mail address: torbjorn.tomson@karolinska.se (T. Tomson).

establishment of epilepsy and pregnancy registries. These prospective observational studies aim at enrollment of large numbers of pregnant women with the ultimate goal of comparing the teratogenic potential of different AEDs.[7] These data are reviewed in this article with emphasis on findings that have emerged during the last 5 to 10 years.

SOME METHODOLOGIC ASPECTS

The methodologies that have been applied vary with the specific objectives of the studies. Case-control designs are useful for uncommon outcomes and have been used to analyze the association between specific types of malformations and exposure to AEDs. The risk of recall bias is a problem shared by case-control and other types of retrospective studies. A woman with unfavorable outcome of her pregnancy is more likely to remember various exposures during pregnancy than a woman with a normal pregnancy outcome. A prospective design with enrollment in the study and recording of exposure before pregnancy outcome is known is important to avoid recall and selection bias. With the more widespread use of early prenatal diagnostic tests, it is becoming increasingly difficult to enroll purely prospective pregnancies.

It must be kept in mind that even properly conducted prospective clinical studies of teratogenic outcomes are observational. For ethical and practical reasons, no randomized controlled trials compare the teratogenicity of different AEDs. Women have not been allocated to their AED, dosage, and dosage schedule by chance but rather based on various individual characteristics, including seizure type and epilepsy classification, educational level, other socioeconomic circumstances, comorbidities, and family history of birth defects. Some of these factors that contribute to the AED selection also might affect pregnancy outcome. An association between a particular drug and high malformation prevalence does not necessarily mean a causal relationship. Observational studies need to consider these potential confounding factors, obtain such information, and try to control for those in the analyses.

An additional concern relates to the generalizability of the observations. There is a spectrum of different methods used to enroll pregnant women. Each method affects differently the representativeness of the cohort. This must be kept in mind when study results are interpreted and translated into general treatment recommendations. Until recently, most cohort studies recruited patients from single or a few collaborating epilepsy centers, thus generally selecting more severe cases. For obvious reasons, the cohorts were small, each rarely exceeding 500 pregnancies.[6,8] They were not powered to analyze specific types of malformations, compare different AEDs, or to include important confounding factors in their analyses. Because of these shortcomings, pregnancy registries have been designed to prospectively enroll larger cohorts of pregnant women and enable more refined analyses of teratogenic effects. Some registries are not specifically established for assessment of AEDs but have been used for that purpose. Examples are national drug prescription databases that are cross-linked with registries of birth defects.[9,10] Such registries may have the advantage of being population-based and sometimes nationwide and representative. They generally lack information on other factors that could contribute to the outcome, however, including the indication for treatment drug dosage.

Specific AED and pregnancy registries have been operational for approximately 10 years. Some are organized by pharmaceutical companies and only collect data on the manufacturers' own product, which makes the results difficult to interpret in the absence of a comparator.[11] Others are organized by independent research groups and include information on all AED exposures.[7] They may be regional (eg, Australia, United Kingdom, North America) or international (European and International Registry of Antiepileptic Drugs in Pregnancy, EURAP). Using slightly different methodologies, each of these groups has been successful in enrolling thousands of pregnancies with AED exposure. Each group records the type of drug exposure in an unbiased way without prior knowledge of teratogenic outcome, and detailed data on other relevant patient characteristics are obtained. The internal validity of the risk assessments is likely to be high, whereas the possibility to generalize from the results depends on how pregnancies were enrolled. Many of these registries have released results that are discussed later.

The pregnancy registries focus on major congenital malformations—or birth defects—as teratogenic outcome. Other types of cohort studies have assessed possible adverse effects of AED exposure in utero on postnatal cognitive development. Sample sizes are considerably smaller, but because they also are observational, controlling for confounding factors remains an important issue.

MAJOR CONGENITAL MALFORMATIONS
Epilepsy or Antiepileptic Drugs

The prevalence of major congenital malformations in offspring of women with epilepsy has ranged from 4% to 10%, corresponding to a 2- to 4-fold increase from the expected prevalence in the general population.[4,7,12] Available data strongly suggest that this risk increase is caused mainly by AED exposure rather than epilepsy or seizures. Pooled data from 26 studies, including outcomes in treated and untreated women with epilepsy and healthy women, revealed a malformation rate of 6.1% in offspring of women with epilepsy who were treated with AEDs, 2.8% among children of women with untreated epilepsy, and 2.2% in the healthy control group.[12] These observations are in line with a meta-analysis based on 10 studies reporting rates of congenital malformations in offspring of untreated women with epilepsy.[13] The malformation rate in this group was not higher than among offspring of healthy controls without epilepsy (odds ratio [OR] 1.92; 95% CI 0.92–4.00). Although untreated women with epilepsy are different in many respects from women who are under treatment during pregnancy, these data convincingly demonstrate that treatment is the major cause of increased risks of birth defects, although epilepsy-related factors should not be totally disregarded.

Polytherapy with AEDs is associated with a higher malformation rate (6.8%) than monotherapy (4%) in a pooled analysis.[12] This has been a consistent finding throughout most studies. Although alternative interpretations are possible because of confounding factors, this observation provides supportive evidence for the contribution of drug treatment to the increased risk of birth defects in children of women with epilepsy. It should be acknowledged that these conclusions are based mainly on studies reflecting the use of AEDs 10 to 25 years ago, when drug selection, dosing, treatment strategies, and monitoring were different compared with today.

Patterns of Malformations

The pattern of malformations in children born to women with epilepsy is mostly the same as seen in the general population, with cardiac defects being the most common followed by facial clefts and hypospadia.[8] The pattern may vary with the type of AED, however. Neural tube defects and hypospadias are more common among offspring of mothers who used valproate during pregnancy; the risk of neural tube defects in association with use of valproate has been estimated at 1% to 2%.[14] An increased risk of neural tube defects of 0.5% to 1% has been reported after carbamazepine exposure.[15,16] Recent data from the North American AED Pregnancy Registry suggested a 10-fold increase in risk of oral clefts among lamotrigine-exposed infants,[17] but this specific association has not been confirmed in other registries.[17,18]

Comparative Teratogenic Potential

For the woman with epilepsy who needs treatment and for her physician, the important question is whether AEDs differ in their teratogenic potential. Malformation rates reported from pregnancy registries for the 5 most frequently used AEDs (valproate, carbamazepine, lamotrigine, phenobarbital, and phenytoin) are summarized in **Table 1**.

GlaxoSmithKline's International Lamotrigine Pregnancy Registry[11] reported a malformation rate of 2.9% based on 802 monotherapy exposures, which is difficult to interpret in the absence of a comparator. The Finnish drug prescription database is a population-based nationwide registry. It has been cross-linked with the National Medical Birth Registry to identify 1411 pregnancies with AED exposure.[9] The risk of malformations was higher in children exposed to valproate monotherapy than in untreated patients (malformation rate 10.6%; OR = 4.18; 2.31–7.57). In contrast, the risk of malformations was not elevated in association with exposure to carbamazepine, oxcarbazepine, or phenytoin monotherapy. Another population-based nationwide registry, the Swedish Medical Birth Registry, reported 1398 pregnancies with exposure to AEDs.[10] The risk for severe malformations in offspring was greater after exposure to valproate compared with carbamazepine monotherapy (OR = 2.59; 95% CI: 1.43–4.68).[9] Updated malformation rates for the 4 most frequently used AEDs in this registry are provided in **Table 1**.[19]

The largest AED and pregnancy registries are The North American Antiepileptic Drugs and Pregnancy Registry (NAAPR), the United Kingdom Epilepsy and Pregnancy Register, and EURAP, an international registry enrolling pregnancies from more than 40 countries, in Europe, Australia, Asia, Oceania, and South America.[7] These registries have enrolled 6000 to 13 000 pregnancies; 2 of them—NAAPR and the UK register—have published results on teratogenic outcome. NAAPR initially disclosed malformation rates associated with specific treatments when found to differ significantly from the background rate. Increased malformation rates in comparison with the general population have so far been identified with phenobarbital (relative risk [RR] 4.2; 95% CI 1.5–9.4)[20] with a malformation rate of 6.5% based on 77 monotherapy exposures and valproate (RR 7.3; 95% CI 4.4–12.2),[21] malformation rate 10.7% (149 exposed). Subsequently, and based on new criteria, NAAPR reported malformation rates of

Table 1
Malformation rates and percentage (number of exposures) with different antiepileptic drugs in monotherapy in different registries

Registry	Valproate	Carbamazepine	Lamotrigine	Phenobarbital	Phenytoin
GlaxoSmithKline[11]	—	—	2.9% (802)	—	—
Finnish Drug prescription[9]	10.6% (263)	2.7% (805)	—	—	—
Swedish Medical Birth Registry[19]	7.7% (507)	5.4% (1199)	4.9% (400)	—	7.6% (145)
UK Register[24]	6.2% (715)	2.2% (900)	3.2% (647)	—	3.7% (82)
North American Registry[17,20–23]	10.7% (149)	2.5% (873)	2.8% (684)	6.5% (77)	2.6% (390)
Australian Register[25]	13.3% (166)	3.0% (234)	1.4% (146)	—	3.2% (31)

2.8% (n = 684) with lamotrigine monotherapy,[17] 2.5% (n = 873) with carbamazepine,[22] and 2.6% (n = 390) with phenytoin monotherapy.[23]

The UK register published their first report based on 3607 cases.[24] The rate of major congenital malformations for pregnancies exposed to valproate monotherapy was 6.2% (4.6%–8.2%) compared with 2.2% (1.4%–3.4%) for carbamazepine. The malformation rate with lamotrigine monotherapy was 3.2% (2.1%–4.9%) based on 647 pregnancies. Interestingly, the malformation rate in offspring of 227 untreated women with epilepsy was 3.5% (1.8%–6.8%), which was similar to the 3.7% rate (3.0%–4.5%) among the pregnancies with monotherapy exposure in general (n = 2468). **Table 1** indicates that malformation rates across studies vary considerably for the same AED in monotherapy. Carbamazepine exposure was associated with rates ranging from 2.2% to 5.4%, lamotrigine had rates from 1.4% to 4.9%, phenytoin from 2.6% to 7.6 %, and valproate had rates ranging from 6.2% to 13.3% (**Table 1**). The wide ranges in malformation rates reflect differences in study populations, criteria, and methodology. Prevalences of malformations with different AEDs should not be compared across studies. There seems to be a consistent pattern within studies with higher rates with valproate and lower rates with carbamazepine and lamotrigine, however (**Table 1**). Even within-study comparisons should be made with caution considering the possible effects of confounding factors.

Data on pregnancy outcomes with other new generation AEDs than lamotrigine are still scarce. Reports on malformation rates in prospective pregnancies with monotherapy exposure to gabapentin, topiramate, levetiracetam, oxcarbazepine, and zonisamide are summarized in **Table 2**. The table is based on data from peer-reviewed publications with an exception made for the latest release from NAAPR, so far available only as abstract.[9,19,23–37] Even when pregnancies from several different studies are added up, the total number of monotherapy exposures for each of gabapentin, topiramate, levetiracetam, and oxcarbazepine ranges are approximately 240 up to

Table 2
Monotherapy exposures and number with major malformations with some newer generation antiepileptic drugs

Reference	Gabapentin	Topiramate	Levetiracetam	Oxcarbazepine	Zonisamide
Kondo et al.[26]	—	—	—	—	4 (0)
Samrén et al.[27]	—	—	—	2 (0)	—
Fonager et al.[28]	1 (0)	—	—	14 (0)	—
Hvas et al.[29]	—	—	—	7 (0)	—
Long[30]	—	—	3 (0)	—	—
Montouris[31]	16 (1)	—	—	—	—
Kaaja et al.[32]	—	—	—	9 (1)	—
Meischenguiser et al.[33]	—	—	—	35 (0)	—
Källen[19]	68 (5)	—	—	4 (0)	—
Artama et al.[9]	—	—	—	99 (1)	—
UK registry[24,36,37]	31 (1)	42 (1)	39 (0)	—	—
Ornoy et al.[34]	—	29 (1)	—	—	—
ten Berg et al.[35]	—	—	11 (0)	—	—
Holmes et al.[23]	127 (1)	197 (8)	197 (4)	121 (2)	—
TOTAL	**243 (8)**	**268 (10)**	**250 (4)**	**291 (4)**	**4 (0)**

290. For zonisamide exposure, only four pregnancies were reported. Clearly these numbers are too small for a reliable assessment of the risks.

EFFECTS ON POSTNATAL COGNITIVE DEVELOPMENT

In 2004, a Cochrane Review concluded that most studies on developmental effects of AEDs are of limited quality and that there was little evidence about which drugs carry more risks than others to the development of children exposed.[38] More recently, some studies suggested that exposure to valproate might be associated with a risk of adverse cognitive development.[39–43] A retrospective survey from the United Kingdom indicated that additional educational needs were more common among children who were exposed to valproate or carbamazepine than controls.[39] A follow-up investigation of partly the same cohort revealed significantly lower verbal IQ in children exposed to valproate monotherapy (mean 83.6; 95% CI 78.2–89.0; n = 41) than in unexposed children (90.9; 95% CI 87.2–94.6; n = 80) and children exposed to carbamazepine (94.1; 95% CI 89.6–98.5; n = 52) or phenytoin (98.5; 95% CI 90.6–106.4; n = 21).[40] Multiple regression analysis found exposure to valproate, 5 or more tonic-clonic seizures in pregnancy, and low maternal IQ to be associated with lower verbal IQ. Doses of more than 800 mg/d were associated with lower verbal IQ than lower doses, for which no differences were seen compared with other monotherapies. These results should be interpreted with caution given the small numbers, the retrospective nature of the study, and the fact that only 40% of eligible mothers agreed to participate.

Two small population-based prospective studies from Finland, each including only 13 children who were exposed to valproate in utero, reported similar trends with worse cognitive outcome compared with other exposures.[41,42] Findings were not statistically significant, however, which may be explained by the small sample size and existence of confounding factors.[42] The first reasonably powered prospective comparative study of cognitive effects of children exposed to AEDs recently published interim results of the children 3 years of age.[43] Women taking valproate, carbamazepine, lamotrigine, or phenytoin were enrolled in early pregnancy, and the cognitive development of their children was assessed at 3 years. Children exposed to valproate (n = 53) had significantly lower IQs (92; 95% CI 88%–97%) than children exposed to the other AEDs (carbamazepine 98 [n = 73]; lamotrigine 101[n = 84]; phenytoin 99 [n = 48]), whereas IQ scores did not differ significantly among children exposed to the other 3 AEDs. There was a significant correlation between the valproate dose in pregnancy and a child's IQ. In fact, children exposed to valproate doses of less than 1000 mg/d did not differ in IQ from children exposed to other AEDs.

These observations are intriguing, and the results are in line with those of previous retrospective and smaller studies. It should be noted, however, that IQs in children exposed to valproate were in the normal range. Because of the observational design, one cannot completely exclude some influence of confounding factors, such as possible differences in seizure control during and after pregnancy and breast-feeding. This is an interim analysis of a study for which the primary outcome is at 6 years.

DOSE DEPENDENCY

A dose-effect relationship has so far been shown most consistently for teratogenicity in association with valproate. Dosages of more than 800 to 1000 mg/d have been associated with significantly greater risks than lower dosages, as summarized in **Table 3**.[9,24,25,27,44,45] Data on cognitive outcome reveal a similar pattern. The retrospective study from Liverpool found that verbal IQ was no different from unexposed controls among children exposed to valproate doses of less than 800 mg/d.[40]

Table 3
Studies reporting a dose–effect relationship with malformations and valproate exposure

Reference	High Risk (mg/d)	Low Risk (mg/d)	Malformation Rate Low VPA Dose	Malformation Rate Other Monotherapy
Samrén et al[44]	>1000	<600	Not available	Not available
Samrén et al[27]	>1000	<600	Not available	Not available
Kaneko et al[45]	>1000	<1000	1.9%	7.2%
Artama et al[9]	>1500	<1500	9.5%	2.5%
Vajda et al[25]	>1100	<1100	5.4%	3.0%
Morrow et al[24]	>1000	<600	4.1%	2.7%

Likewise, the prospective NEAD study found the IQ of children whose mothers took valproate in doses less than 1000 mg/d to be similar to IQs in children exposed to other AEDs.[43] The UK Epilepsy and Pregnancy Register also reported a positive dose response for major congenital malformations for lamotrigine. Doses more than 200 mg/d were associated with higher risks.[24] This pattern was not found in the International Lamotrigine Registry of GlaxoSmithKline, however, and the North American pregnancy registry did not find lamotrigine doses to be significantly higher in mothers of children with malformations compared with mothers of healthy children.[11]

SUMMARY

Data on clinical teratogenicity are at best derived from carefully conducted observational studies, whereas randomized, controlled trials have no place in this research area. We can only expect level B recommendations and lower. New relevant information has become available during the last 5 years on pregnancy outcomes with 3 of the most frequently used AEDs: carbamazepine, valproate, and lamotrigine. It seems that birth defect rates with carbamazepine monotherapy are lower than previously thought. In some large studies rates are only marginally increased compared with different control populations. More recent data do not suggest adverse effects of carbamazepine on cognitive development.

The overall prevalence of malformations in association with lamotrigine exposure seems to be similar to that of carbamazepine. The only available prospective study on cognition does not indicate any adverse effects of lamotrigine.[43] Malformation rates with valproate have consistently been found to be 2 to 3 times higher compared with carbamazepine or lamotrigine. More limited data also suggest adverse effects of high doses of valproate on cognitive development of the exposed child. For newer generation AEDs other than lamotrigine, data are still too limited to determine the risks for birth defects and are nonexisting with respect to possible adverse effects on cognitive development. Doses are important, and evidence is lacking for higher risks with valproate compared with other AEDs if doses are less than 800 to 1000 mg/d. Confounding factors contribute to some of the apparent differences between AEDs in pregnancy outcomes, and more data are needed, particularly concerning cognitive outcomes and specific birth defects.

Based on these observations, valproate should not be a first-line AED for women who are considering pregnancy. In this situation this drug is best avoided if other effective but safer AEDs can be found for each individual woman's seizure disorder. Based on pregnancy outcome data, carbamazepine seems comparatively safe and a reasonable first-line choice in localization-related epilepsy. Alternatives are less clear in idiopathic generalized epilepsies. Lamotrigine seems comparatively safe, but its use in pregnancy is complicated by pharmacokinetic changes and risks of breakthrough seizures.[46] The experience with use of levetiracetam and topiramate during pregnancy is still insufficient.

Any attempt to change drugs should be completed and evaluated before conception; withdrawals or other major changes should be avoided during pregnancy. These conclusions are largely in line with the recently published report of the Quality Standards Subcommittee and Therapeutics and Technology Subcommittee of the American Academy of Neurology and the American Epilepsy Society.[47]

REFERENCES

1. Gaily E. Development and growth in children of epileptic mothers: a prospective controlled study. Acta Obstet Gynecol Scand 1991;70(7–8):631–2.
2. Holmes LB, Harvey EA, Coull BA, et al. The teratogenicity of anticonvulsant drugs. N Engl J Med 2001;344(15):1132–8.
3. Meador KJ, Pennell PB, Harden CL, et al. Pregnancy registries in epilepsy: a consensus statement on health outcomes. Neurology 2008;71(14):1109–17.
4. Tomson T, Hiilesmaa V. Epilepsy in pregnancy. BMJ 2007;335:769–73.
5. Meadow SR. Anticonvulsant drugs and congenital abnormalities. Lancet 1968; 2(7581):1296.
6. Tomson T, Battino D. Teratogenicity of antiepileptic drugs: state of the art. Curr Opin Neurol 2005;18:135–40.
7. Tomson T, Battino D, French J, et al. Antiepileptic drug exposure and major congenital malformations: the role of pregnancy registries. Epilepsy Behav 2007;11(3):277–82.
8. Battino D, Tomson T. Management of epilepsy during pregnancy. Drugs 2007; 67(18):2727–46.
9. Artama M, Auvinen A, Raudaskoski T, et al. Antiepileptic drug use of women with epilepsy and congenital malformations in offspring. Neurology 2005;64(11): 1874–8.
10. Wide K, Winbladh B, Kallen B. Major malformations in infants exposed to antiepileptic drugs in utero, with emphasis on carbamazepine and valproic acid: a nation-wide, population-based register study. Acta Paediatr 2004;93(2):174–6.
11. Cunnington M, Ferber S, Quarteny G. Effect of dose on frequency of major birth defects following fetal exposure to lamotrigine monotherapy in an international observational study. Epilepsia 2007;48(6):1207–10.
12. Tomson T, Battino D. The management of epilepsy in pregnancy. In: Shorvon S, Pedley TA, editors. The blue books of neurology: the epilepsies 3. Philadelphia: Saunders Elsevier; 2009. p. 241–64.
13. Fried S, Kozer E, Nulman I, et al. Malformation rates in children of women with untreated epilepsy: a meta-analysis. Drug Saf 2004;27(3):197–202.
14. Lindhout D, Schmidt D. In-utero exposure to valproate and neural tube defects. Lancet 1986;1(8494):1392–3.
15. Rosa FW. Spina bifida in infants of women treated with carbamazepine during pregnancy. N Engl J Med 1991;324(10):674–7.
16. Kallen AJ. Maternal carbamazepine and infant spina bifida. Reprod Toxicol 1994; 8(3):203–5.
17. Holmes LB, Baldwin EJ, Smith CR, et al. Increased frequency of isolated cleft palate in infants exposed to lamotrigine during pregnancy. Neurology 2008;70: 2152–218.

18. Dolk H, Jentink J, Loane M, et al. Does lamotrigine use in pregnancy increase or-ofacial cleft risk relative to other malformations? Neurology 2008;71:714–22.
19. Available at: www.janusinfo.org. Accessed February 10, 2009.
20. Holmes LB, Wyszynski DF, Lieberman E, The AED (antiepileptic drug) pregnancy registry: a 6-year experience. Arch Neurol 2004;61(5):673–8.
21. Wyszynski DF, Nambisan M, Surve T, et al. Antiepileptic drug pregnancy registry: increased rate of major malformations in offspring exposed to valproate during pregnancy. Neurology 2005;64(6):961–5.
22. Hernandez-Diaz S, Smith CR, Wyszynski DF, et al. Risk of major malformations among infants exposed to carbamazepine during pregnancy. Birth Def Res (Part A): Clin Mol Teratol 2007;79:357.
23. Holmes LB, Smith CR, Hernandez-Diaz S. Pregnancy registries: larger sample sizes essential. Birth Defects Res 2008;82:307.
24. Morrow J, Russell A, Guthrie E, et al. Malformation risks of antiepileptic drugs in pregnancy: a prospective study from the UK epilepsy and pregnancy register. J Neurol Neurosurg Psychiatr 2006;77(2):193–8.
25. Vajda FJ, Hitchcock A, Graham J, et al. The Australian register of antiepileptic drugs in pregnancy: the first 1002 pregnancies. Aus NZ J Obstet Gynecol 2007;47:468–74.
26. Kondo T, Kaneko S, Amano Y, et al. Preliminary report on teratogenic effects of zonisamide in the offspring of treated women with epilepsy. Epilepsia 1996;37:1242–4.
27. Samren EB, van Duijn CM, Christiaens GC, et al. Antiepileptic drug regimens and major congenital abnormalities in the offspring. Ann Neurol 1999;46(5):739–46.
28. Fonager K, Larsen H, Pedersen L, et al. Birth outcomes in women exposed to anticonvulsant drugs. Acta Neurol Scand 2000;101(5):289–94.
29. Hvas CL, Henriksen TB, Ostergaard JR, et al. Epilepsy and pregnancy: effect of antiepileptic drugs and lifestyle on birthweight. BJOG 2000;107(7):896–902.
30. Long L. Levetiracetam monotherapy during pregnancy: a case series. Epilepsy Behav 2003;4:447–8.
31. Montouris G. Gabapentin exposure in human pregnancy: results from the Gabapentin Pregnancy Registry. Epilepsy Behav 2003;4(3):310–7.
32. Kaaja E, Kaaja R, Hiilesmaa V. Major malformations in offspring of women with epilepsy. Neurology 2003;60(4):575–9.
33. Meischenguiser R, D'Giano CH, Ferraro SM. Oxcarbazepine in pregnancy: clinical experience in Argentina. Epilepsy Behav 2004;5(2):163–7.
34. Ornoy A, Cohen E. Outcome of children born to epileptic mothers treated with carbamazepine during pregnancy. Arch Dis Child 1996;75(6):517–20.
35. ten Berg K, Samrén EB, van Oppen AC, et al. Levetiracetam use and pregnancy outcome. Reprod Toxicol 2005;20:175–8.
36. Hunt S, Craig J, Russell A, et al. Levetiracetam in pregnancy: preliminary experience from the UK epilepsy and pregnancy register. Neurology 2006;67(10):1876–9.
37. Hunt S, Russell A, Smithson WH, et al. Topiramate in pregnancy: preliminary experience from the UK epilepsy and pregnancy register. Neurology 2008;71(4):272–6.
38. Adab N, Tudur SC, Vinten J, et al. Common antiepileptic drugs in pregnancy in women with epilepsy. Cochrane Database Syst Rev 2004;(3):CD004848.
39. Adab N, Jacoby A, Smith D, et al. Additional educational needs in children born to mothers with epilepsy. J Neurol Neurosurg Psychiatr 2001;70(1):15–21.

40. Vinten J, Adab N, Kini U, et al. Neuropsychological effects of exposure to anticonvulsant medication in utero. Neurology 2005;64(6):949–54.
41. Gaily E, Kantola-Sorsa E, Hiilesmaa V, et al. Normal intelligence in children with prenatal exposure to carbamazepine. Neurology 2004;62(1):28–32.
42. Eriksson K, Viinikainen K, Monkkonen A, et al. Children exposed to valproate in utero: population based evaluation of risks and confounding factors for long-term neurocognitive development. Epilepsy Res 2005;65(3):189–200.
43. Meador KJ, Baker GA, Browning N, et al. NEAD Study Group. Cognitive function at 3 years of age after fetal exposure to antiepileptic drugs. N Engl J Med 2009; 360(16):1597–605.
44. Samren EB, van Duijn CM, Koch S, et al. Maternal use of antiepileptic drugs and the risk of major congenital malformations: a joint European prospective study of human teratogenesis associated with maternal epilepsy. Epilepsia 1997;38(9): 981–90.
45. Kaneko S, Battino D, Andermann E, et al. Congenital malformations due to antiepileptic drugs. Epilepsy Res 1999;33(2–3):145–58.
46. Pennell PB, Peng L, Newport DJ, et al. Lamotrigine in pregnancy: clearance, therapeutic drug monitoring and seizure frequency. Neurology 2008;70:2130–216.
47. Harden CL, Meador KJ, Pennell PB, et al. Practice parameter update: management issues for women with epilepsy. Focus on pregnancy (an evidence-based review): teratogenesis and perinatal outcomes. Report of the Quality Standards Subcommittee and Therapeutics and Technology Subcommittee of the American Academy of Neurology and American Epilepsy Society. Neurology 2009;73(2): 126–32.

Identification of Pharmacoresistant Epilepsy

Anne T. Berg, PhD

KEYWORDS

- Antiepileptic drugs • Surgery • Methodology • Natural history
- Epileptic encephalopathy • Definitions

Until recently, the epilepsy literature regarding seizure prognosis has been divided between epidemiologic studies of remission and studies focused on experimental pharmacologic therapies and surgical treatment of refractory epilepsy. In the first case, the epidemiologic studies were not specifically interested in pharmacoresistance. At best, there was a tacit assumption that not being in remission was the complement of pharmacoresistance. Hence, by studying remission, one was, for all intents and purposes, studying pharmacoresistance. In the second case, experimental and surgical therapies were targeted at patients whose seizures were clearly refractory to standard pharmacologic treatments. Pharmacoresistance was established well before patients entered such treatment studies. The pertinent questions considered whether a new approach could offer any hope where the standard ones had already failed.

These studies offer no clear definition of pharmacoresistance. In the case of epidemiologic studies, defining pharmacoresistance is irrelevant to the outcome. Remission is defined as the absence of seizures,[1–5] and the reason for not being in remission is immaterial. For studies of surgical therapy and randomized trials of new drugs, the definition is also not especially relevant, as patients treated in these settings are selected to be some of the most extreme cases in whom no doubt remains regarding their seizures' resistance to therapy. For example, in one surgical study, the median number of different antiepileptic drugs (AEDs) tried before referral to surgery was 5.[6]

In broad and general terms, pharmacoresistance is the failure of seizures to come under complete control or acceptable control in response to AED therapy. Different specific conceptual definitions have been summarized previously.[7] In theory, one could use all possible drugs in all possible combinations to determine pharmacoresistance.[8] Practically, this is an impossible standard to meet and likely also dangerous for

This work was supported by Grant R37-31146 from the NIH-NINDS.
Department of Biology, Northern Illinois University, DeKalb, IL 60115, USA
E-mail address: atberg@niu.edu

Neurol Clin 27 (2009) 1003–1013
doi:10.1016/j.ncl.2009.06.001
neurologic.theclinics.com

patients. This leaves important questions regarding how best to define pharmacoresistance in a way that it can be meaningfully studied.

To date, only a few studies have defined pharmacoresistance separately from lack of remission.[1,9–15] In these definitions, common elements are (1) the number of drugs that need to be failed, (2) the seizure frequency, and (3) factors related to time (**Table 1**). The consensus regarding number of drug failures seems to be 2 or 3. For other aspects, there is somewhat greater variability. Some require a specified period during which a minimum seizure frequency is observed. Others require that a seizure has occurred within a specified period of time (eg, the last 6 months). The absolute agreement among these various definitions tended to be high (83%–96%), although agreement corrected for chance (κ) ranged from a low of 0.35 (poor) to a high of 0.79 (excellent).[16]

Many of the definitions are designed for identifying the prevalence of pharmacoresistance at a given point in time (eg, 2 years after diagnosis,[13] 5 years after diagnosis,[1] or as of last contact).[11] Prevalence is a useful concept in epidemiology and public health. It provides an estimate of the number of individuals who have a specific condition at a specified point in time . The prevalence of intractable epilepsy in a geographically defined population in France was estimated using 2 slightly different definitions to determine the number of people in the population who met each definition and the proportion of people with epilepsy who were pharmacoresistant.[17] Both definitions required the failure of 2 AEDs. Defining intractability as any seizure in the past year yielded a population prevalence of 1.4 per 1000 and accounted for 26% of people with epilepsy. The second definition required an average of 1 seizure per month during the past year and yielded a population prevalence of 0.9 per 1000, accounting for 17% of people with epilepsy. This information is valuable in understanding the types of medical and other services that might be required to care for patients with epilepsy in the population. This was the first, and quite a successful, effort to quantify the population burden of refractory epilepsy with a definition that included drug failure.

RECOGNIZING PHARMACORESISTANCE AS IT OCCURS

Although the prevalence of pharmacoresistance at a given point in time is important for public health and needs assessments, it is not necessarily the subject of greatest clinical relevance when considering treatment and management of individual patients. Identifying which patients are at high risk of pharmacoresistance and prospectively identifying drug resistance as soon as it becomes evident are arguably more important. This corresponds to the clinical situation in which a case is followed from day to day, the patient reports his seizures to his physician, the physician adjusts the doses upwards and monitors for side effects, both decide to try a new AED, and so forth. On which day and based on which criteria can a patient's seizures be deemed pharmacoresistant? Implicit in this question is that once someone has met criteria for pharmacoresistance, it is time to consider a new approach or pursue other options.

The substitution of prevalent pharmacoresistance for incident pharmacoresistance in many of the cohort studies that have examined this issue is, in part, based on 2 common assumptions. Firstly, there seems to be an implicit assumption that pharmacoresistance, when it occurs, will be evident from the onset of epilepsy. Secondly, there is another implicit assumption that the course of epilepsy is a static or stable phenomenon: patients whose seizures are controlled remain so; patients whose seizures are pharmacoresistant have seizures at a fairly constant rate. Neither of these assumptions turns out to be the case, at least not for all patients, and this has important implications for how we define pharmacoresistance and study it. In addition, prevalence measures ignore the role of increased mortality among patients with

Table 1
Components of selected definitions of pharmacoresistant or intractable epilepsy

Author	Study Methods	Drug Failures	Seizure Frequency	Other Criteria
Huttenlocher and Hapke[14]	Retrospective cohort, chart review	2	1 seizure per month	For ≥ 2 years
Berg et al[9]	Retrospective case-control, chart review	3	1 seizure per month	For ≥ 2 years
Casetta et al[12]	Nested case-control study in prospective cohort	3	1 seizure per month	For ≥ 2 years
Arts et al[1]	Prospective, chart review	2	Any	<3 months seizure-free during fifth year of follow-up
Dlugos et al[13]	Retrospective, chart review	2	Any	<6 months seizure-free 19–24 months after initial diagnosis and treatment
Camfield and Camfield[11]	Prospective, chart review	3	1 seizure every 2 months	During most recent year
Berg[10] (2 definitions)	Prospective, direct patient contact & chart review	2	Average ≥ 1 seizure per month	For 18 months, no more than 3 months seizure-free
		2	No minimal frequency requirement	Explicitly excluded uninformative trials as "failures"
Spooner et al[15]	Prospective, chart review	2	No minimal frequency requirement	—

uncontrolled seizures.[18–21] People with pharmacoresistant epilepsy who die tend to be undercounted in prevalence estimates.

To date, only 2 studies have examined the development of pharmacoresistance prospectively from the time of initial diagnosis of epilepsy. Information about drug use and failure as well as seizure occurrence was evaluated on an ongoing basis (every 3–4 months) in 1 study from the United States[10] and at 7 and 14 years after initial diagnosis in another study from Australia.[15] Study subjects were considered pharmacoresistant once they met the criteria of the definitions used in the study. In both instances, the investigators observed that pharmacoresistance did not necessarily occur immediately and could first be preceded by a period of seizure remission. The Australian study enrolled children with only temporal lobe epilepsy (TLE). In the American study, children with all forms of epilepsy were enrolled. The finding of delayed expression of pharmacoresistance was largely a phenomenon observed in the focal epilepsies. Retrospective accounts from surgical series have also documented that a proportion of patients undergoing evaluations for resective surgery have histories of significant remission periods before referral to surgery (either before or after the initial appearance of pharmacoresistance).[6,22]

Children with epileptic encephalopathies and other secondary generalized epilepsies tended to express their pharmacoresistance very early in the course of their epilepsy. These disorders tend to start explosively with multiple daily seizures that are quickly demonstrated to be refractory to standard treatments. In focal epilepsies, high initial seizure frequency is also associated with an increased risk of early expression of pharmacoresistance.[23] This tendency may reinforce the perception that intractability is necessarily apparent from the outset.

SEIZURE FREQUENCY AND DURATION OF TREATMENT

Patient characteristics, in particular seizure frequency, may play a role in how quickly drug efficacy or inefficacy can be determined. In patients who typically have multiple daily seizures, determination of a drug's efficacy or lack thereof may be made in a matter of a week in many cases, although for complete control of seizures (success) there is no specific criterion. In one study, a year of seizure freedom was required before considering a drug trial successful.[10] Trials of drugs that stopped after less than a year, even if the patient was seizure-free, were considered uninformative. For patients with seizures occurring on a weekly or monthly basis, more time will be required to determine failure. For those with truly infrequent seizures, for example a few per year, there is no clear way to determine efficacy versus failure, at least not quickly.

Several studies, including the Australian[15] and American[10] studies discussed earlier, have documented the occurrence of brief remissions after having met various criteria for pharmacoresistance.[1,14,24] For the most part, the remissions were not long lasting, and patients frequently relapsed. For most patients with otherwise poorly differentiated focal epilepsy, it seems that pharmacoresistance may not always be evident from the outset. Furthermore, once criteria for pharmacoresistance are met, the course of seizures may not necessarily be inexorably refractory but may be punctuated by periods of relative seizure quiescence. In an extension of the US study,[25] 57% of patients whose seizures had failed trials of 2 different AEDs subsequently had at least a 1-year period of remission. Repeated remissions and relapses were common. After a median period of 10 years of follow-up from the second AED failure, 37% were seizure-free for at least a year and 23% were seizure-free for at least 3 years.

A disproportionate number of patients who were seizure-free at last contact were those with traditional idiopathic syndromes. Overall, 50% of the idiopathic group, compared with only 20% of the focal and 18% of the epileptic encephalopathy group, were in remission at last contact.

PREDICTORS OF PHARMACORESISTANCE

Prognostic information about who will develop pharmacoresistance is limited. In adult-onset epilepsy, there are no adequate studies based on well-defined and characterized cohorts and using a meaningful definition of pharmacoresistance. In childhood-onset epilepsy, three large prospective and representative cohort studies provide a mixed message on this matter. All three studies found that the epileptic encephalopathy or secondary generalized syndromes had higher risks than other forms of epilepsy; however, the levels of risks varied considerably. Two studies found that about half the children in this group developed pharmacoresistance.[10,11] The third study reported that only about 10% were pharmacoresistant.[1] In the US study, traditional idiopathic syndromes had the lowest risk of pharmacoresistance, and other focal epilepsies had an intermediate risk. This was not the case in the other two studies.

The Australian study, limited to TLE, found that the strongest discriminator between pharmacoresistant and controlled patients was an abnormal MRI finding.[15] An earlier study based on a 2-year follow-up period, also focused on pediatric TLE, reported highly comparable results.[13] These observations highlight an important concern with epidemiologic studies and with trying to study pharmacoresistance in a population-based setting. Although the population-based model provides good representation, it rarely has adequate clinical detail to provide information useful to studies regarding tertiary epilepsy care. The absence of neuroimaging, particularly MRI, in most epidemiologic studies is a limitation of this type of model for studying epilepsy. Studies of pharmacoresistance in the future should incorporate routine MRI examinations to the greatest extent practical and ethically possible.

CURRENT REFERRAL RECOMMENDATIONS

The pediatric epilepsy surgery subcommission of the International League against Epilepsy recommends that children whose seizures have failed fully to respond to trials of 2 or 3 AEDs be evaluated at a comprehensive epilepsy center.[26] The National Association of Epilepsy Centers recommends that patients whose seizures are not fully controlled after 1 year be evaluated at a specialized center.[27] This issue was also highlighted in a practice parameter that recognized that failure of 2 drugs was becoming a common criterion for pharmacoresistance, and it was recommended that adults whose seizures had failed significantly to improve with trials of appropriate AEDs be referred for evaluation to an epilepsy surgery center.[8] Part of the reason to recommend a comprehensive center is so that patients who might benefit from surgical procedures can be identified and properly evaluated. Other considerations are accuracy in diagnosis, starting with whether the patient has epilepsy or some other disorder whose symptoms are mistaken for seizures.[28–31] In addition, especially in the case of childhood epilepsy, accurate diagnosis of the specific type of epilepsy is key, to the extent that it may influence treatment and management decisions and provide information about likely prognosis.

In children, there is a large array of highly distinctive forms of epilepsy "syndromes" that tend to have specific implications for treatment and prognosis. Recognition of these particular forms of epilepsy, including specific causes, has been helpful in improving their pharmacologic management. This is seen in expert opinion of preferred first and second choices of therapy in various clinical scenarios[32,33] and addressed in newer practice guidelines.[34] There have also been a few examples of moderate success in the treatment of highly refractory forms and causes of epilepsy, in particular, vigabatrin for infantile spasms secondary to tuberous sclerosis,[35] stiripentol for Dravet syndrome,[36,37] and the ketogenic diet for epilepsy associated with glucose transporter 1 deficiency.[38]

Approximately 50% of childhood-onset epilepsy and closer to 90% of adult-onset epilepsy are of a focal nature and do not conform to any of the well-described genetic and developmental epilepsy syndromes (including the epileptic encephalopathies and the more typically tractable "idiopathic" syndromes).[39–41] These have been dubbed the "garden variety focal epilepsy."[42] It is to this group of focal epilepsies that most resective surgical patients belong.

These focal epilepsies are poorly characterized, and they are generally described solely with respect to the presence or absence of a demonstrable lesion or other condition (symptomatic vs cryptogenic) and the region of the brain from which the seizures appear to arise (eg, frontal or occipital lobe), based on varying degrees of clinical investigations. As previously proposed,[43] concerted efforts might profitably be applied to better "phenotyping" these garden variety focal epilepsies in an effort to identify specific forms. Factors such as specific electroencephalographic patterns and findings, age at onset, patterns of seizure occurrence, seizure duration (eg, status epilepticus), diurnal patterns, provoking or triggering factors, and other features might, if rigorously examined, provide some insights into subtypes of focal epilepsy that are currently not recognized. To the extent that this phenotyping may be relevant to choice of AED, it may serve to improve treatment and potentially decrease the number viewed as pharmacoresistant. One study examined the response to successive treatments with AEDs in patients whose seizures had failed to improve with previous AEDs. Although the chance of success of the next AED decreased with increasing numbers of previous failures, a proportion of patients did achieve seizure freedom. Whether this reflects true response to the drugs or some aspect of the natural history cannot be addressed by this study. To the extent that it reflects true drug response, it seems as if there is a certain random element in whose seizures responds to which drug. Ideally, one should be able to identify who will be most likely to respond to which drug, so that agents do not have to be tried at random.

WHY IS IT NECESSARY TO IDENTIFY PHARMACORESISTANCE AS SOON AS POSSIBLE?

Uncontrolled seizures can have a devastating effect on the individual and family. School, employment, driving, and all aspects of social functioning and activities can be adversely affected. Psychiatric complications, particularly depression and anxiety, may, in part, be consequences of uncontrolled seizures,[44] although there is clearly a complex and bidirectional association between epilepsy and depression.[45] Mortality is considerably increased in people with epilepsy.[46] This is of particular concern for mortality secondary to seizure-related accidents[47,48] and for sudden unexpected death associated with epilepsy.[49,50]

There is also a growing recognition of the toll that uncontrolled seizures take on cognition and developmental function. This is a concern for the intractable focal epilepsies in adults.[8] Hermann and colleagues[51] demonstrated declines in confrontational naming, memory function, and fine motor control over time in adults with refractory TLE compared with healthy controls without epilepsy. The phenomenon is perhaps most dramatic in a group of disorders with onset primarily during infancy and early childhood, the epileptic encephalopathies. The concept of epileptic encephalopathy is still in development.[52-54] The observation of developmental plateauing or even losses in children who, before the onset of seizures, appeared relatively if not entirely normal, has led to the hypothesis that it is the epileptic activity in the developing brain that may interfere with and possibly permanently derail the acquisition of normal brain function. The concern is greatest for those syndromes traditionally labeled as epileptic encephalopathies; however, some evidence raises the possibility that there may be a spectrum of dysfunction and that adverse effects may occur in association with other forms of epilepsy that are not necessarily counted among the epileptic encephalopathies. For example, Hermann and colleagues[55] found that earlier versus later (< 14 years vs >14 years) age at onset of TLE was associated with reduction in white matter volume and significantly decreased performance on an array of neurocognitive measures. Cormack and colleagues[56] studied a group of children undergoing resection for intractable TLE. They found that the earlier the age at onset, the greater the risk of intellectual disability. In fact, of those with onset when younger than 1 year, 82% were considered intellectually disabled (IQ< 70) compared to 12% of those with onset at 5 years or older. Even taking into account underlying lesions, seizure control, and treatment, one study reported evidence that earlier age at onset (< 5 years) was associated with evidence of lower level of intellectual ability compared to later age at onset (>5 years).[57] This was found even within groups of patients who had "cryptogenic" focal and "idiopathic" generalized epilepsy.

COGNITION AS A FACET OF INTRACTABLE EPILEPSY

The concerns with the adverse effect on cognition, especially in the developing brain, raise another issue: is control of seizures the full measure of whether a patient's epilepsy is drug-responsive or pharmacoresistant? On the one hand, there is reason to suspect that mechanisms underlying the developmental syndromes known as the epileptic encephalopathies may differ from those of garden variety focal epilepsy. It would be reasonable to investigate the mechanisms of pharmacoresistance and treatment separately within each of these broad groups and, more realistically, within specific subtypes and syndromes. On the other hand, there is the possibility that the effect of epileptic activity, especially in the developing brain, may occur along a continuum of severity that spans all forms of epilepsy, from the most intractable to the seemingly "benign." There may well be effects at all ages, including in adulthood; however, the effects may be more severe and less reversible when the epileptic activity disrupts neurodevelopmental processes during critical times in development. These complexities represent another facet in considering how best to define and understand pharmacoresistance and how to treat epilepsy most effectively in the short term and long term.

Limited but compelling data from surgical studies support the notion that early intervention, when feasible, may ultimately spare developmental function and improve long-term behavioral and cognitive outcomes.[58-61] Preliminary data on the treatment of cryptogenic infantile spasms also suggest that there may be some hope for rescued development.[62] Thus, accurate recognition of pharmacoresistance as soon as possible is not simply a methodological nicety but a clinical necessity.

Early intervention, however, requires early recognition. This in turn requires clear guidelines for drug use and definitions of treatment failure. It also requires that these guidelines and recommendations to be effectively disseminated to care providers of people who have epilepsy.

FUTURE CHALLENGES

There remains much to do at this point. First and foremost, the field needs a valid and robust operational definition of pharmacoresistance, one that can be meaningfully used in most, if not all, clinical research settings and that is relevant to clinical patient care. This definition must include explicit guidelines for what constitutes a drug's failure, and how many different drugs should be failed for a patient's epilepsy to be deemed pharmacoresistant. At this point, consensus seems to be converging on 2 AEDs. Systematic, prospective application of the definition in appropriately designed clinical investigations should replace retrospective chart review studies and secondary analyses of data sets that are not suited to address key questions surrounding pharmacoresistance. Although population-based studies are often touted as the gold standard approach to studying prognosis, such studies are often deficient in the areas most required for the study of pharmacoresistance and other clinically relevant issues. A hybrid design, in which some compromise is allowed in the recruitment and representativeness of patients in exchange for high-quality clinical information, is necessary. Some of the studies already follow this design but are criticized for not being population-based.[1,10] The emphasis must shift to how best to identify pharmacoresistance at its earliest possible presentation, who is at greatest risk, and how best to treat and manage those who appear pharmacoresistant. This is a serious problem that deserves concerted, methodologically sound, and clinically sophisticated efforts to resolve.

An important component of clinical management and research endeavors is teaching non–epilepsy-specialist clinicians who manage care for patients with epilepsy the importance of assessing treatment failure in a timely systematic manner. Emphasizing the risks and consequences of uncontrolled seizures from relatively minor cognitive effects to mental retardation, autism, and sudden death should be an important part of education for care providers, patients, and their families. Although not all patients who meet criteria for pharmacoresistance are surgical candidates, such a determination can often be made only after comprehensive evaluation by epilepsy specialists. Because the diagnosis of epilepsy is not always simple, a comprehensive assessment should also address the accuracy of the diagnosis of epilepsy and of the specific form of epilepsy when it can be identified.

REFERENCES

1. Arts WFM, Brouwer OF, Peters ACB, et al. Course and prognosis of childhood epilepsy: 5-year follow-up of the Dutch study of epilepsy in childhood. Brain 2004;127:1774–84.
2. Cockerell OC, Johnson AL, Sander JW, et al. Remission of epilepsy: results from the national general practice study of epilepsy. Lancet 1995;346:140–4.
3. Collaborative Group for the Study of Epilepsy. Prognosis of epilepsy in newly referred patients: a multicenter prospective study of the effects of monotherapy on the long-term course of epilepsy. Epilepsia 1992;33:45–51.
4. Hauser E, Freilinger M, Seidl R, et al. Prognosis of childhood epilepsy in newly referred patients. J Child Neurol 1996;11:201–4.
5. Lindsten H, Stenlund H, Forsgren L. Remission of seizures in a population-based adult cohort with a newly diagnosed unprovoked epileptic seizure. Epilepsia 2001;42:1025–30.
6. Berg AT, Langfitt J, Shinnar S, et al. How long does it take for partial epilepsy to become intractable? Neurology 2003;60:186–90.

7. Arzimanoglou A, Ryvlin P. Toward a clinically meaningful definition of drug resistance. In: Kahane P, Berg A, Loscher W, et al, editors. Drug resistant epilepsy. Montrouge: John Libbey Eurotext; 2008. p. 1–6.

8. Engel J, Wiebe S, French J, et al. Practice parameter: temporal lobe and localized neocortical resections for epilepsy. Neurology 2003;60:538–47.

9. Berg AT, Levy SR, Novotny EJ, et al. Predictors of intractable epilepsy in childhood: a case-control study. Epilepsia 1996;37:24–30.

10. Berg AT, Vickrey BG, Testa FM, et al. How long does it take epilepsy to become intractable? A prospective investigation. Ann Neurol 2006;60:73–9.

11. Camfield P, Camfield C. Nova Scotia pediatric epilepsy study. In: Jallon P, Berg A, Dulac O, editors. Prognosis of epilepsies. Montrouge, France: John Libbey, Eurotext; 2003. p. 113–26.

12. Casetta I, Granieri E, Monetti VC, et al. Early predictors of intractability in childhood epilepsy: a community-based case-control study in Copparo, Italy. Acta Neurol Scand 1999;99:329–33.

13. Dlugos D, Sammel M, Strom B, et al. Response to first drug trial predicts outcome in childhood temporal lobe epilepsy. Neurology 2001;57:2259–64.

14. Huttenlocher PR, Hapke RJ. A follow-up study of intractable seizures in childhood. Ann Neurol 1990;28:699–705.

15. Spooner CG, Berkovic SF, Mitchell LA, et al. New onset temporal lobe epilepsy in children: lesion on MRI predicts poor seizure outcome. Neurology 2006;67:2147–53.

16. Berg AT, Kelly MM. Defining intractability: comparisons among published definitions. Epilepsia 2006;47:431–6.

17. Picot MC, Baldy-Moulinier M, Daurest J-P, et al. The prevalence of epilepsy and pharmacoresistant epilepsy in adults: a population-based study in a Western European country. Epilepsia 2008;49:1230–8.

18. Berg AT, Shinnar S, Testa FM, et al. Mortality in childhood-onset epilepsy. Arch Pediatr Adolesc Med 2004;158:1147–52.

19. Callenbach PMC, Westendorb RGJ, Geerts AT, et al. Mortality risk in children with epilepsy: the Dutch study of epilepsy in childhood. Pediatrics 2001;107: 1259–63.

20. Lhatoo SD, Johnsons AL, Goodridge DM, et al. Mortality in epilepsy in the first 11 to 14 years after diagnosis: multivariate analysis of a long-term prospective, population-based cohort. Ann Neurol 2001;49:336–44.

21. Shackleton DP, Westendorp RGJ, Kasteleijn-Nolst Trenite DGA, et al. Mortality in patients with epilepsy: 40 years of follow up in a Dutch cohort study. J Neurol Neurosurg Psychiatr 1999;66:636–40.

22. French JA, Williamson PD, Thadani VM, et al. Characteristics of medial temporal lobe epilepsy: I. results of history and physical examination. Ann Neurol 1993;34:774–80.

23. Berg AT, Shinnar S, Levy SR, et al. Early development of intractable epilepsy in children: a prospective study. Neurology 2001;56:1445–52.

24. Takenaka J, Aso K, Watanabe K, et al. Transient remission in intractable localization-related epilepsy. Pediatr Neurol 2000;23:328–31.

25. Berg AT, Levy SR, Testa FM, et al. Remission of epilepsy after 2 drug failures in children: a prospective study. Ann Neurol 2009;65:510–9.

26. Cross JH, Jaykar P, Nordli D, et al. Proposed criteria for referral and evaluation of children for epilepsy surgery: recommendations of the subcomission for pediatric epilepsy surgery. Epilepsia 2006;47:953–9.

27. National Association of Epilepsy Centers. Guidelines for essential services, personnel, and facilities in specialized epilepsy centers in the United States. Epilepsia 2001;42:804–14.

28. Ghougassian DF, d'Souza W, Cook MJ, et al. Evaluating the utility of inpatient video-EEG monitoring. Epilepsia 2004;45:928–32.

29. Kanner AM, LaFrance WC, Betts T. Psychogenic non-epileptic seizures. In: Engel J, Pedley TA, editors. Epilepsy: a comprehensive textbook. Philadelphia: Lippincott Williams & Wilkins; 2008. p. 2795–810.

30. Pellock JM. Other nonepileptic paroxysmal disorders. In: Wyllie E, Gupta A, Lachhwani DK, editors. The treatment of epilepsy: principles and practice. Philadelphia: Lipincott Williams & Wilkins; 2006. p. 631–42.

31. Smolowitz JL, Hopkins SC, Perrine T, et al. Diagnostic utility of an epilepsy monitoring unit. Am J Med Qual 2007;22:117–22.

32. Wheless JW, Clarke DF, Arzimanoglou A, et al. Treatment of pediatric epilepsy: European expert opinion, 2007. Epileptic Disord 2007;9:353–412.

33. Wheless JW, Clarke DF, Carpenter D. Treatment of pediatric epilepsy: expert opinion, 2005. J Child Neurol 2005;20:S1–56.

34. Glauser T, Ben-Menachem E, Bourgeois B, et al. ILAE treatment guidelines: evidence-based analysis of antiepileptic drug efficacy and effectiveness as initial monotherapy for epileptic seizures and syndromes. Epilepsia 2006;47: 1094–120.

35. McKay MT, Weiss SK, Adams-Webber T, et al. Practice parameter: medical treatment of infantile spasms. Neurology 2004;62:1668–81.

36. Chiron C. Stiripentol. Neurotherapeutics 2007;4:123–5.

37. Chiron C, Marchand MC, Tran A, et al. Stiripentol in severe myoclonic epilepsy in infancy: a randomised placebo-controlled syndrome-dedicated trial. STICLO study group. Lancet 2000;356:1638–42.

38. Klepper J. GLUT1 deficiency syndrome - 2007 update. Dev Med Child Neurol 2007;49:707–16.

39. Berg AT, Shinnar S, Levy SR, et al. Newly diagnosed epilepsy in children: presentation at diagnosis. Epilepsia 1999;40:445–52.

40. Callenbach PM, Geerts AT, Arts WF, et al. Familial occurrence of epilepsy in children with newly diagnosed multiple seizures: Dutch study of epilepsy in childhood. Epilepsia 1998;39:331–6.

41. Jallon P, Loiseau P, Loiseau J. Newly diagnosed unprovoked epileptic seizures: presentation at diagnosis in CAROLE study. Epilepsia 2001;42:464–75.

42. Cross JH, Eltze C. Epileptic encephalopathies versus "garden variety focal epilepsies": can they be considered together? In: Kahane P, Berg A, Loscher W, et al, editors. Drug resistant epilepsies. Montrouge, France: John Libbey Eurotext; 2008. p. 199–211.

43. Berg AT. The risks, correlates, and temporal patterns of intractable epilepsy. In: Kahane P, Berg A, Loscher W, et al, editors. Drug resistant epilepsies. Montrouge, France: John Libbey Eurotext; 2008. p. 7–16.

44. Kanner AM. Depression in epilepsy: prevalence, clinical semiology, pathogenic mechanisms, and treatment. Biol Psychiatry 2003;54:388–98.

45. Kanner AM. Depression in epilepsy: a complex relation with unexpected consequences. Curr Opin Neurol 2008;21:190–4.

46. Lhatoo S, Sander J. The epidemiology of epilepsy and learning disablility. Epilepsia 2001;42:6–9.

47. Bell GS, Gaitatzis A, Bell CL, et al. Drowning in people with epilepsy: how great is the risk? Neurology 2008;71:578–82.

48. Sheth GS, Krauss G, Krumholz A, et al. Mortality in epilepsy: driving fatalities vs other causes of death in patients with epilepsy. Neurology 2004;63:1002–7.

49. Langan Y, Nashef L, Sander JW. Case-control study of SUDEP. Neurology 2005; 64:1131–3.
50. Walczak TS, Leppik IE, D'Amelio M, et al. Incidence and risk factors in sudden unexpected death in epilepsy: a prospective cohort study. Neurology 2001;56: 519–25.
51. Hermann BP, Seidenberg M, Dow C, et al. Cognitive prognosis in chronic temporal lobe epilepsy. Ann Neurol 2006;60:80–7.
52. Berg AT. Introduction to the epilepsies. In: Engel J, Pedley TA, editors. Epilepsy: a comprehensive text. 2nd edition. Philadelphia: Lippincott-Raven Press; 2008. p. 761–6.
53. Dulac O. Epileptic encephalopathy. Epilepsia 2001;42(Suppl 3):23–6.
54. Panayiotopoulos CP. The epilepsies: seizures, syndromes and management. Chipping Norton: Bladon Medical Publishing; 2005.
55. Hermann B, Seidenberg M, Bell B, et al. The neurodevelopmental impact of childhood-onset temporal lobe epilepsy on brain structure and function. Epilepsia 2002;43:1062–71.
56. Cormack F, Cross JH, Isaacs E, et al. The development of intellectual abilities in pediatric temporal lobe epilepsy. Epilepsia 2007;48:201–4.
57. Berg AT, Langfitt JT, Testa FM, et al. Global cognitive function in children with epilepsy: a community-based study. Epilepsia 2008;49:608–14.
58. Freitag H, Tuxhorn I. Cognitive function in preschool children after epilepsy surgery: rationale for early intervention. Epilepsia 2005;46:561–7.
59. Jonas R, Asarnow RF, LoPresti C, et al. Surgery for symptomatic infant-onset epileptic encephalopathy with and without infantile spasms. Neurology 2005; 64:746–50.
60. Thompson PJ, Duncan JS. Cognitive decline in severe intractable epilepsy. Epilepsia 2005;46:1780–7.
61. Weiner HL, Carlson C, Ridgway EB, et al. Epilepsy surgery in young children with tuberous sclerosis: results of a novel approach. Pediatrics 2006;117:1494–502.
62. Lux AL, Edwards SW, Hancock E, et al. The United Kingdom Infantile Spasms Study (UKISS) comparing hormone treatment with vigabatrin on developmental and epilepsy outcomes to age 14 months: a multicentre randomised trial. Lancet Neurol 2005;4:712–7.

Localization in Epilepsy

Dimitris G. Placantonakis, MD, PhD, Theodore H. Schwartz, MD*

KEYWORDS

- Epilepsy • Electroencephalography • MEG • FMR1
- PET • SPECT

Pharmacologic therapy represents the first line of treatment of epilepsy and is effective in most patients. However, about 20% to 30% of cases develop intractable seizures that cannot be controlled by medication alone. In such cases, surgical intervention, including resection of epileptogenic brain tissue, is considered for therapeutic, often curative, purposes. The concept of surgical management of epilepsy relies on the premise of precise localization of the epileptogenic focus, which gives rise to the seizures, and multiple techniques exist to identify epileptogenic tissue. However, to appreciate the value of each of these techniques, one must first gain an understanding of the organization of the epileptic focus, and a few terms must be defined.

ICTAL VERSUS INTERICTAL EVENTS

Seizures, or ictal events, consist of the paroxysmal, synchronous, rhythmic firing of a population of pathologically interconnected neurons capable of demonstrating high-frequency oscillatory activity called "fast ripples" (250–500 Hz).[1–3] These events are caused by an imbalance in excitatory and inhibitory mechanisms leading to hypersynchrony and hyperexcitability.[4] When seizures are not occurring, electroencephalographic (EEG) recordings from patients with chronic epilepsy show abnormal paroxysmal events in a large population of neurons called interictal spikes. These spikes generally consist of a high amplitude surface negativity (1–5 mV) lasting 50 to 200 ms followed by a slow wave, with no behavioral correlate.[5]

Ictal events can be understood in terms of 3 separate mechanisms: initiation, propagation, and termination.[6] A typical seizure event often develops from a "tonic" stage, characterized by recruitment of adjacent neurons in the face of disinhibition, to a "clonic" stage again characterized by periodic spike-and-wave events that may represent, in one theory, a return of inhibitory function that eventually terminates the ictal discharge.[7,8] Interictal and ictal events are not static phenomena, and their dynamic spatiotemporal evolution can make localization challenging.

Department of Neurological Surgery, Weill Medical College of Cornell University, New York-Presbyterian Hospital, New York, NY 10065, USA
* Corresponding author.
E-mail address: schwarh@med.cornell.edu (T.H. Schwartz).

Neurol Clin 27 (2009) 1015–1030
doi:10.1016/j.ncl.2009.08.004
0733-8619/09/$ – see front matter © 2009 Elsevier Inc. All rights reserved.

THE EPILEPTIC FOCUS

Engel[7,8] organized focal epilepsy into 3 distinct anatomico-functional regions: the epileptic focus, the epileptogenic lesion, and the epileptogenic region. The epileptic focus is the area of maximal electrophysiological interictal activity. This region is a dynamic spatiotemporal zone because interictal activity often shifts from one location to another. The epileptogenic lesion is the anatomic pathology thought to be responsible for the epileptic state. This structural lesion is generally adjacent to the epileptic focus but can also be distant.[9] The epileptogenic region is a theoretical concept defined as the area of brain that is necessary and sufficient for producing recurrent ictal events, or seizures. This concept is important for epilepsy surgeons because removal of this region should lead to cessation of seizures. In addition, several other important terms are discussed. The ictal onset zone (IOZ), defined electrographically as the area of brain from which a particular seizure arises, may also shift from seizure to seizure, and is usually smaller than the epileptic focus and contained within the epileptogenic region.[10] The IOZ is important in defining the epileptogenic region because it is usually the most critical target in successful surgical resections. However, removal of only the IOZ is often insufficient to completely eliminate seizures, and some percentage of surrounding epileptic focus must also be removed.[11,12]

IMPLICATIONS OF SPATIOTEMPORAL DYNAMICS AND VARIABILITY

Single-unit recordings from animals with experimental epilepsy indicate that the population of neurons participating in each epileptiform event fluctuates over time[13,14] and, in humans, the location of interictal spikes often has no relationship to the IOZ.[15] Hence, the size and boundaries between the IOZ and the epileptogenic focus, and their relationship with the epileptogenic lesion, are in a dynamic state of flux reflecting an underlying modulation of neuronal excitability, synchronization, and inhibition that is poorly understood.[15] Among clinicians there is intense disagreement as to what amount of electrographically abnormal tissue is critical for epileptogenesis and, subsequently, which areas need to be removed to obtain a surgical cure.[12,16–20] Although some investigators contend that removal of the anatomic lesion is sufficient,[19,21–25] others emphasize the importance of the IOZ[26] or the area with frequent interictal spikes.[11,12,27–29] This controversy highlights a lack of clear understanding of the location of the epileptogenic region as it relates to the causative structural abnormality and the electrographic markers of epileptogenicity. For this reason, there are multiple methods for localizing the epileptic focus, the epileptogenic lesion, and the epileptogenic region. To help facilitate the presentation of these modalities, the authors divide the diagnostic modalities into 2 categories: anatomic (structural and chemical) and functional.

ANATOMIC LOCALIZATION
Magnetic Resonance Imaging

Magnetic resonance imaging (MRI) remains the imaging modality of choice when structural or anatomic abnormalities are suspected (**Fig. 1**A, B).[30,31] Sequences of particular importance included T2-weighted and fluid attenuated inversion recovery (FLAIR) images, and gadolinium-enhanced T1-weighted images in lesional cases, such as tumors, vascular abnormalities, infectious or inflammatory nidi, and cortical dysplasia.[30–33] Although 1.5 T MRI is widely available, higher-field magnets, such as 3.0 T, are becoming increasingly used in the context of epilepsy. The use of 3.0 T MRI produces images with improved signal-to-noise ratios,[34] which can help localize

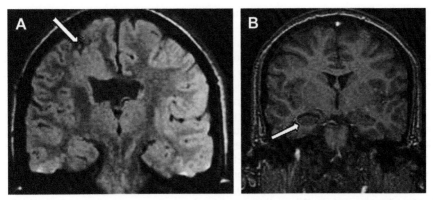

Fig. 1. Examples of epileptogenic anatomic abnormalities identified with MRI. (*A*) Coronal FLAIR sequences indicate focal cortical dysplasia (*arrow*). (*B*) Coronal T1 images demonstrate right hippocampal atrophy (*arrow*), consistent with MTS. (*Courtesy of* L. Heier, MD, Ithaca, NY.)

structural abnormalities that may underlie epileptogenesis. High-field MRI may be of particular importance in cases of cryptogenic epilepsy, in which subtle structural changes may be missed by conventional 1.5 T imaging. Although 3 T MRI may only identify brain abnormalities in 25% of previously normal 1.5 T scans,[35] the addition of surface coils can increase this rate to 65%, particularly in cases of cortical dysplasia.[36] Even with more modest numbers, the improved detection rate is critical, because detection of an imaging abnormality dramatically increases postsurgical freedom from seizures.[37,38]

MRI has been shown to be particularly sensitive in identifying the structural abnormalities related to mesial temporal sclerosis (MTS).[39,40] In 80% to 90% of MTS cases, MRI allows the detection of T2 and FLAIR hyperintensity in the mesial temporal structures, whereas coronal images can allow direct qualitative or volumetric comparison of the 2 hippocampi and the demonstration of unilateral hippocampal atrophy.

MR Spectroscopy

MR spectroscopy (MRS) has recently been used to help localize epileptogenic foci, particularly in the context of temporal lobe epilepsy.[30] Abnormalities revealed by MRS include reductions in *N*-acetyl aspartate (NAA) levels or the NAA to choline and creatine ratios.[41] Other findings may include an elevation in the Glx peak (Glx denotes a complex peak consisting of glutamate, glutamine and γ-aminobutyric acid [GABA]), or the Myo peak, attributed to a sugar representing an astroglial marker.[42] MRS remains a secondary diagnostic modality in the context of epilepsy, and any findings should be corroborated by other diagnostic modalities.

FUNCTIONAL LOCALIZATION

Although anatomic diagnostic modalities remain important in the workup of seizure disorders, and MRI is now almost always included in the diagnostic algorithm, the identification of epileptogenic foci relies heavily on functional studies in most cases.

Clinical Semiology

Seizure semiology can frequently provide important clues in the localization of seizure onset. Scalp electroencephalography (sEEG) is routinely combined with video recordings of patients during ictal events to help correlate electrographic seizures with clinical manifestations.

Overall, semiologic signs can be classified into positive or negative motor signs, automatisms, autonomic manifestations, and speech signs.[43] Although several semiologic manifestations of seizures can predict the hemispheric lateralization of seizures, they are generally not considered reliable predictors of lobar localization of foci within a hemisphere. Moreover, rapid secondary generalization of partial seizures can produce complex semiology. Finally, the interpretation of seizure semiology becomes less important in cases of multifocal seizures. Therefore, clinical semiology alone is not used for the localization of epileptogenic foci. It is most commonly coupled with sEEG in the form of video-EEG (vEEG) in an attempt to correlate the semiology to electrical discharges. As additional, more sophisticated, functional localization studies are introduced into clinical practice, the "art" of seizure semiology interpretation may become less important. Alternatively, patients' reports of aura symptoms and initial behavioral phenomena at seizure onset may provide clues to the localization of the onset zone that may be beyond the spatiotemporal resolution and spatial sampling abilities of many of the other modalities described in this article.

sEEG

sEEG remains the most commonly used, and the easiest to perform, functional study in epileptic patients (**Fig. 2**).[32] sEEG can identify ictal and interictal events, and, combined with vEEG, the electrographic events can be correlated with the clinical semiology. Although sEEG remains a powerful diagnostic tool, it has several limitations. First, muscle and eye movement artifacts may mask the neurophysiologic recordings and thus prevent the identification of epileptogenic foci. Second, electrical signals become attenuated due to limited conductivity through the cerebrospinal fluid (CSF), skull, and skin, thus affecting the quality of the recordings. Third, sEEG relies on a finite number of surface electrodes, which may limit the spatial resolution of the recordings. Fourth, volume conduction may impair spatial specificity. The use of current source density and dipole modeling are only 2 examples of techniques used to overcome these limitations.[44,45]

As mentioned earlier, continuous sEEG or vEEG can identify interictal epileptiform discharges, which are generally not seen in patients without seizures. Interictal spikes include periodic lateralized epileptiform discharges (PLEDs), which are strongly associated with clinical seizures.[46] Other interictal events that represent slow neuronal population oscillations rather than paroxysmal spikes include temporal intermittent rhythmic δ activity, which represents a reliable predictor of epileptic seizures, and focal polymorphic δ activity, which, on the contrary, is not generally linked to epilepsy.[46] Interictal discharges, although sometimes concordant with the localization of ictal events, may also be grossly discordant, as described in the earlier section.

The most important data obtained with sEEG pertains to the localization of ictal foci. Ictal events can begin in several ways, of which the most common are periodic spiking, low voltage fast activity, or an electrodecremental response. However, rapid seizure generalization or ictal origin in brain areas not adequately covered by scalp electrodes, such as the inferior aspect of the frontal lobes, may preclude localization. High-density arrays and complex methods for signal analysis, such as independent component analysis and phase congruency, may increase the sensitivity of sEEG.[47,48] Nevertheless, the spatial resolution of sEEG at determining the IOZ is limited to an area of several centimeters, which is hardly adequate for surgical planning.

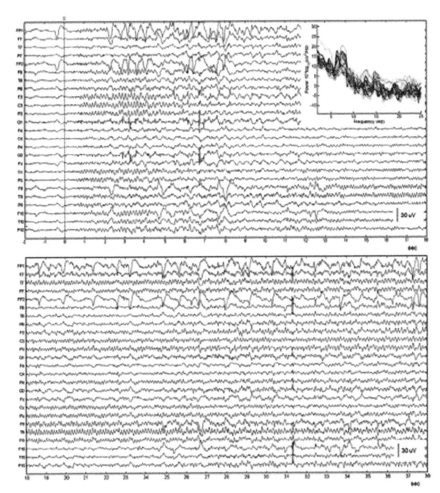

Fig. 2. Scalp EEG represents the most widely used functional diagnostic modality in epilepsy patients. In this example, the traces show the initiation (*red line*) and evolution of a clinical seizure. The inset in the upper panel shows the power spectrum of the Fourier transforms of the traces. (*Adapted from* Jung KY, Kang JK, Kim JH, et al. Spatiotemporospectral characteristics of scalp ictal EEG in mesial temporal lobe epilepsy with hippocampal sclerosis. Brain Res 2009;1287:206–19; with permission.)

Magnetoencephalography

Magnetoencephalography (MEG) is a novel technique used for localization of ictal foci. Its premise lies in the detection of magnetic fields generated by current flow occurring during synchronized neuronal discharges. Such current flow must be parallel to the surface of the brain and skull to produce magnetic fields in a perpendicular orientation that can then be detected extracranially. The technique is applicable not only to the identification and localization of epileptogenic foci (**Fig. 3**A, B) but also to the functional mapping of adjacent brain, which is essential for planning safe surgical resections of seizure foci.[49,50]

Compared with conventional sEEG, MEG has distinct advantages and issues associated with its use.[50] Advantages of MEG include a theoretically higher spatial

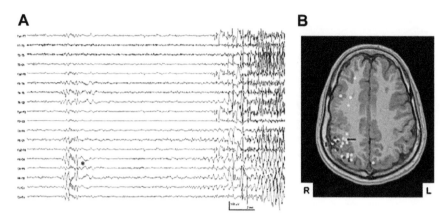

Fig. 3. MEG helps identify epileptogenic foci in conjunction with EEG. (*A*) The scalp EEG demonstrated a seizure that appeared to originate from the right centroparietal area. (*B*) Identification of spike sources with MEG and superimposition on MRI confirmed that the spikes originated predominantly from abnormal cortex surrounding the right central sulcus. Note the right hemispheric polymicrogyria evident in the MRI image. (*Adapted from* Galicia E, Imai K, Mohamed IS, et al. Changing ictal-onset EEG patterns in children with cortical dysplasia. Brain Dev 2009;31:569–76, with permission.)

discrimination related to lower detection thresholds; superior conductivity of magnetic fields through the CSF, skull, and skin; potentially improved signal-to-noise ratios; and the existence of algorithms for three-dimensional source modeling, which can allow for stereologic localization of ictal foci. Disadvantages associated with MEG include a much higher cost and limited availability; the need for extensive magnetic insulation to ensure an interpretable signal-to-noise ratio, limited to recording interictal rather than ictal events; and limited interpretation of data if head movement is involved during ictal events, because the MEG sensors are not fixed to the head.

Although several centers have recently implemented MEG technology in the context of localizing ictal foci, mapping eloquent brain, and planning epilepsy surgery,[51,52] the high cost of acquiring and maintaining the technology is prohibitive to most institutions. Moreover, a recent systematic review of the literature failed to demonstrate a benefit of MEG in seizure-free outcomes after epilepsy surgery.[53,54]

Positron Emission Tomography

Positron emission tomography (PET) is a neuroimaging modality that involves the metabolic use of a radioactive substrate as an index of brain metabolic changes that may be coupled to seizures.[30,55,56] The most commonly used tracer is [^{18}F]fluorodeoxyglucose (FDG). FDG is a glucose analog that is taken up by metabolically active cells. However, because it cannot be metabolized by glycolytic enzymes, it accumulates in the cytoplasm. FDG-PET has been particularly useful in cases of temporal lobe epilepsy, in which it has a sensitivity of approximately 90%.[30,31,57] Typically, interictal PET identifies focal areas of hypometabolism (**Fig. 4**A, B); however, such hypometabolic areas are generally considered to be larger than the actual epileptogenic foci. A possible explanation for the spatial discrepancy between the interictal FDG-PET and the ictal focus may be the phenomenon of surround inhibition following seizures. FDG-PET is currently being used for surgical planning in the resection of pediatric cortical dysplasia.[58]

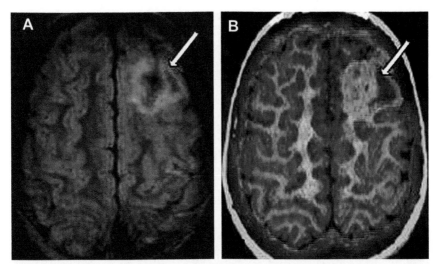

Fig. 4. Interictal PET helps identify hypometabolic areas that may contain epileptogenic foci. (*A*) FLAIR MRI images identify a left frontal area consistent with focal cortical dysplasia (*arrow*). (*B*) PET signal superimposed on the MRI indicates interictal hypometabolism of the dysplasia. (*Adapted from* Lee KK, Salamon N. [18F]Fluorodeoxyglucose-positron-emission tomography and MR imaging coregistration for presurgical evaluation of medically refractory epilepsy. AJNR Am J Neuroradiol 2009 [Epub ahead of print]; with permission. Copyright © 2009, American Society of Neuroradiology.)

Other substrates are now being developed for PET applications.[30] Notably, [11C]- or [18F]flumazenil, an antagonist at the benzodiazepine binding site of the ionotropic γ-aminobutyric acid A (GABA$_A$) receptor, has recently been used to image the relative distribution of GABA$_A$ receptors in the brains of patients with epilepsy.[59,60] Moreover, PET imaging with [11C]carfentanil, which selectively binds the μ-opioid receptor, has shown increased binding near temporal lobe epileptogenic foci.[61] Imaging with substrates that selectively bind the 5-HT$_{1A}$ serotonin receptor, nicotinic acetylcholine receptor (nAChR) and type 1 cannabinoid receptor (CB1R) is also being pursued.[55] PET imaging with [11C]methyl-L-tryptophan, a serotonin precursor, has been used to identify epileptogenic tissue in certain types of epilepsy.[62–64] These novel PET imaging applications can help identify foci with aberrant inhibition and neuromodulation, which may be somewhat colocalized with epileptogenesis.

Single Photon Emission Computed Tomography

Single photon emission computed tomography (SPECT) represents a functional imaging modality believed to represent cerebral perfusion.[30,55,56,65] The substrates that are imaged are usually 99mTc-labeled molecules, such as [99mTc]HMPAO or [99mTc]ECD. They are rapidly taken up by brain tissue within less than 1 minute after intravenous injection, and remain trapped within brain tissue for up to 4 additional hours. Because of such kinetics, SPECT can be used to acquire an ictal profile[66] if the substrate is injected at the time of the seizure (**Fig. 5**), even though the actual imaging may be obtained after the ictal event has subsided. Ictal SPECT can be compared with interictal SPECT to help identify the perfusion alterations during the ictal event. Subtraction ictal SPECT coregistered to MRI (SISCOM) refers to a combined imaging modality in which the interictal SPECT is subtracted from the ictal SPECT and the subtraction image is merged with an MRI to anatomically define the area with the

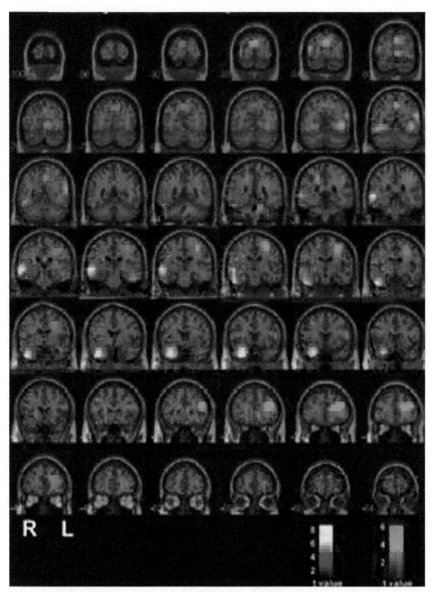

Fig. 5. Ictal SPECT superimposed on coronal T1-weighted MRI demonstrates hyperperfusion of the right temporal lobe, consistent with epileptogenic activity. (*Adapted from* McNally KA, Paige AL, Varghese G, et al. Localizing value of ictal-interictal SPECT analyzed by SPM (ISAS). Epilepsia 2005;46:1450–64; with permission.)

perfusion abnormality.[65,67–69] SISCOM was shown to be superior to ictal and interictal SPECT in localizing epileptogenic foci and predicting the outcome of epilepsy surgery.[70] In the case of temporal lobe epilepsy, SISCOM was shown to have a localization sensitivity of 97%.[71] The subtraction of ictal and interictal profiles is highly dependent on accurate coregistration and elaborate statistical algorithms, such as statistical parametric mapping.[72]

Much like PET, novel substrates are being developed for SPECT imaging. An example is [^{125}I]iomazenil,[31,73] which binds the benzodiazepine site of the GABA$_A$ receptor.

The major limitation in ictal SPECT imaging is the difficulty in orchestrating the injection. The tracer must be injected rapidly, and is generally only useful for a period of 4 hours. Hence, the facility must generate several vials of the tracer, most of which will be wasted waiting for a seizure to occur. A dedicated individual has to sit at the bedside waiting for a seizure to be able to inject the tracer in a timely fashion. This expense is prohibitive at most centers.

Functional MRI

Functional MRI (fMRI) represents another diagnostic modality based on the acquisition of cerebral blood flow and oxygenation data during ictal or interictal discharges. The premise of the technique lies in the principle of neurovascular coupling, which denotes an expected increase in cerebral blood flow in epileptogenic areas during seizures and alterations in oxygen metabolism.[74] The fMRI data are obtained from the blood oxygenation level–dependent (BOLD) signal, which represents magnetic resonance interference brought about by a decrease in the concentration of deoxyhemoglobin (**Fig. 6**). It is theorized that the increased BOLD signal during seizures reflects an increase in cerebral blood volume and flow without a commensurately

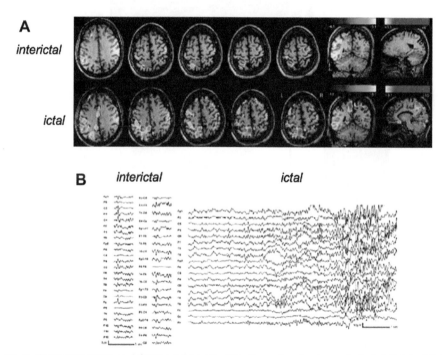

Fig. 6. Concurrent EEG and fMRI lead to identification of epileptogenic foci. (*A*) Interictal and ictal fMRI images demonstrate epileptogenic activity arising from a left parietal cortical dysplasia. (*B*) Scalp EEG data corresponding to the interictal and ictal states in the same patient. (*Adapted from* Tyvaert L, Hawco C, Kobayashi E, et al. Different structures involved during ictal and interictal epileptic activity in malformations of cortical development: an EEG-fMRI study. Brain 2008;13:2042–60; with permission.)

increased rate of oxygen consumption, thereby leading to decreased deoxygenated hemoglobin levels and an increase in the signal. The acquisition of fMRI is often coupled to continuous sEEG recordings in an attempt to correlate fMRI and electrographic information.[75–78] Moreover, fMRI may be used for functional mapping of eloquent brain when planning epilepsy surgery. Even though fMRI is becoming more popular as a diagnostic modality in epilepsy, it is routinely used as one of many sources of information in the patient's workup. However, there are several limitations in its use. First, ictal events are difficult to capture during imaging sessions, and movement artifacts are often prohibitive. Second, the temporal resolution is limited. Hence, ictal onset may be missed, which preferentially favors areas of early ictal

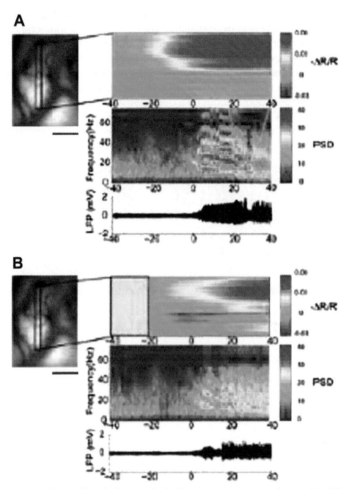

Fig. 7. Optical recordings of intrinsic signals during 2 spontaneous seizures (*A, B*) in a patient. The top panel indicates the optical recordings, the middle panel a color-coded power spectrum of the frequency profile of the local field potentials (LFPs), and the lower panel the raw LFPs over time. Time 0 indicates the electrographic onset of seizures. (*Adapted from* Zhao M, Suh M, Ma H, et al. Focal increases in perfusion and decreases in hemoglobin oxygenation precede seizure onset in spontaneous human epilepsy. Epilepsia 2007;48:2059–67; with permission.)

spread. Data from optical imaging spectroscopy indicate that seizure onset is heralded by increases in oxygen metabolism that are not identified with fMRI.

Optical Recording of Intrinsic Signals

Optical recording of intrinsic signals (ORIS) refers to a novel technique that relies on the recordings of the optical properties of cortical tissue at multiple wavelengths. The premise of the technique lies in the variation in the optical properties of hemoglobin between its oxygenated and deoxygenated state. Such recordings can demonstrate changes in oxygen requirements and cerebral blood volume during an ictal event, in animal models,[79,80] and in humans,[81,82] with a much higher spatial and temporal resolution than with fMRI. It has been shown that interictal spikes and the initial moments of ictal evolution are associated with a dramatic increase in oxygen requirements that initially are not matched by comparable increases in blood flow. The technique has also been used successfully on human brain intraoperatively for the identification of functional cortex (**Fig. 7**).[82,83] Drawbacks include a slow optical signal (hundreds of milliseconds) compared with the electrophysiological events (milliseconds), movement artifacts, difficulty imaging ictal events in the operating room, and the need for signal processing before data can be interpreted. Although optical imaging techniques hold great promise for providing high-resolution hemodynamic data associated with epilepsy, clinical usefulness has been limited to date because of technical limitations.

Invasive EEG

These diagnostic modalities can occasionally provide either nonlocalizing or discordant information. In such cases, invasive EEG with subdural strip and grid electrodes and intraparenchymal depth electrodes can help localize epileptogenic foci (**Fig. 8**). Such electrodes overcome the limitations of scalp electrodes, namely signal

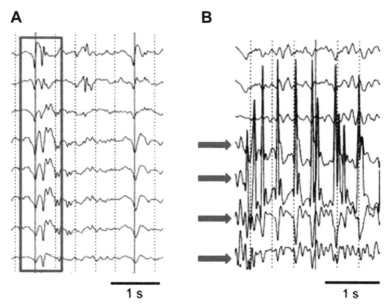

Fig. 8. Examples of interictal spikes (*red box in A*) and seizures (*red arrows in B*) recorded with temporal depth electrodes.

attenuation from the intervening skin, bone, CSF and dura, and muscle artifacts,[84–86] thus representing the most accurate electrophysiological diagnostic technique. The superiority of intracranial electrodes over scalp EEG in localizing seizure foci has been documented in comparisons of simultaneous scalp and intracranial recordings.[86] Invasive electrodes are currently the gold standard in localizing the epileptogenic zone and focus and the IOZ. The major limitations of intracranial electrodes are the risk of implantation (~5% morbidity) and the ability to sample only areas of cortex adjacent to each electrode. Hence, ictal onsets from uncovered regions of brain may not be identified accurately and may even provide falsely localizing information.

SUMMARY

The dynamic spatiotemporal variability in the epileptic focus renders seizure localization a challenge to the clinician. For this reason, a plethora of diagnostic modalities have been developed to identify different aspects of the epileptic focus. Although the clinical semiology and the surface EEG still remain the most widespread methods of localizing seizures, these older techniques are being increasingly supplemented by a variety of anatomic and functional imaging modalities that can help clarify discrepancies when the data are discordant. Identification of a structural lesion, aided by the development of stronger magnets and surface coils is increasing the importance of MRI scans. Novel PET ligands, which can be coregistered with stereotactic MRI scans, are also becoming clinically useful to guide neurosurgical resections. MEG may ultimately be too expensive and may not provide enough ictal data to become a standard of care. Techniques that rely on neurovascular coupling offer increased spatial and temporal resolution but, ultimately, are measuring hemodynamic surrogates of neuronal activity. Whether these will be adequate for surgical planning is still a matter of debate. Ultimately, when the data are equivocal, invasive EEG remains the gold standard for identifying epileptic foci and guiding the surgeon to successful resections. Future research will have to clarify the ideal extent of resection of the epileptogenic lesion, region, focus, and IOZ to achieve the highest rate of freedom from seizures, incorporating a variety of seizure localizing modalities.

REFERENCES

1. Bragin A, Mody I, Wilson CL, et al. Local generation of fast ripples in epileptic brain. J Neurosci 2002;22:2012–21.
2. Fisher RS, Weber WR, Lesser RP, et al. High-frequency EEG activity at the start of seizures. J Clin Neurophysiol 1992;9:441–8.
3. Staba RJ, Wilson C, Bragin A, et al. Quantitative analysis of high-frequency oscillations (80–500 Hz) recorded in human epileptic hippocampus and entorhinal cortex. J Neurophysiol 2002;88:1743–52.
4. Schwartzkroin PA. Epilepsy. Models, mechanisms and concepts. Cambridge (UK): Cambridge University Press; 1993.
5. Pedley TA. Interictal epileptiform discharges: discriminating characteristics and clinical correlations. Am J EEG Technol 1980;20:101–19.
6. Pinto DJ, Patrick SL, Huang WC, et al. Initiation, propagation, and termination of epileptiform activity in rodent neocortex in vitro involve distinct mechanisms. J Neurosci 2005;25:8131–40.
7. Engel J Jr. Functional explorations of the human epileptic brain and their therapeutic implications. Electroencephalogr Clin Neurophysiol 1990;76:296–316.
8. Engel JJ. Intracerebral recordings: organization of the human epileptogenic region. J Clin Neurophysiol 1993;10:90–8.

9. Quesney LF, Olivier A, Andermann F, et al. Preoperative EEG investigation in patients with frontal lobe epilepsy: trends, results and pathophysiological consideration. J Clin Neurophsyiol 1987;4:208–9.

10. Spencer SS, Spencer DD. Entorhinal-hippocampal interactions in medial temporal lobe epilepsy. Epilepsia 1994;35:721–7.

11. Bautista RE, Cobbs MA, Spencer DD, et al. Prediction of surgical outcome by interictal epileptiform abnormalities during intracranial EEG monitoring in patients with extrahippocampal seizures. Epilepsia 1999;40:880–90.

12. Wyllie E, Luders H, Morris HH. Clinical outcome after complete or partial cortical resection for intractable epilepsy. Neurology 1987;37:1634–41.

13. Schwartzkroin PA, Wyler AR. Mechanism underlying epileptiform burst discharge. Ann Neurol 1980;7:95–107.

14. Wyler AR, Burchiel KJ, Ward AA Jr. Chronic epileptic foci in monkeys: correlation between seizure frequency and proportion of pacemaker neurons. Epilepsia 1978;19:475–83.

15. Alarcon G, Guy CN, Binnie CD, et al. Intracerebral propagation of interictal spikes in partial epilepsy: implications for source localization. J Neurol Neurosurg Psychiatry 1994;57:435–49.

16. Berger MS, Ghatan S, Haglund MM, et al. Low-grade gliomas associated with intractable epilepsy: seizure outcome utilizing electrocorticography during tumor resection. J Neurosurg 1993;79:62–9.

17. Cascino GD, Kelly PJ, Sharbrough FW, et al. Long-term follow-up of stereotactic lesionectomy in partial epilepsy: predictive factors and electroencephalographic results. Epilepsia 1992;33:639–44.

18. Haglund MM, Ojemann GA. Extratemporal resective surgery for epilepsy. Neurosurg Clin N Am 1993;4:283–92.

19. Tran TT, Spencer SS, Javidan M, et al. Significance of spikes recorded on intraoperative electrocorticography in patients with brain tumors and epilepsy. Epilepsia 1997;38:1132–9.

20. Tyvaert L, Hawco C, Kobayashi E, et al. Different structures involved during ictal and interictal epileptic activity in malformations of cortical development: an EEG-fMRI study. Brain 2008;13:2042–60.

21. Cascino GD. Epilepsy and brain tumors: implications of treatment. Epilepsia 1990;31(S3):S37–44.

22. Falconer MA, Kennedy WA. Epilepsy due to small focal temporal lesions with bilateral independent spike-discharging foci: a study of seven cases relieved by operation. J Neurol Neurosurg Psychiatry 1961;24:205–12.

23. Fried I, Kim JH, Spencer DD. Limbic and neocortical gliomas associated with intractable seizures: a distinct clinicopathological group. Neurosurgery 1994;34:815–24.

24. Goldring S, Gregorie EM. Surgical management using epidural recordings to localize the seizure focus: review of 100 cases. J Neurosurg 1973;60:457–66.

25. Hirsch JF, Rose CS, Pierre-Kahn A, et al. Benign astrocytic and oligodendrocytic tumors of the cerebral hemispheres in children. J Neurosurg 1989;70:568–72.

26. Jayakar P, Duchowny M, Resnick TJ, et al. Localization of seizure foci: pitfalls and caveats. J Clin Neurophsyiol 1991;8:414–31.

27. Drake J, Hoffman HJ, Kobayashi J, et al. Surgical management of children with temporal lobe epilepsy and mass lesions. Neurosurgery 1987;21:792–7.

28. Penfield W, Jasper H. Epilepsy and the functional anatomy of the human brain. Boston: Little Brown; 1954.

29. Rasmussen T. Surgery of epilepsy associated with brain tumors. In: Purpura DP, Penry JK, Walter RD, editors. Neurosurgical management of the epilepsies. New York: Raven Press; 1975. p. 227–39.

30. Cascino GD. Neuroimaging in epilepsy: diagnostic strategies in partial epilepsy. Semin Neurol 2008;28:523–32.

31. Maehara T. Neuroimaging of epilepsy. Neuropathology 2007;27:585–93.

32. Fish DR, Spencer SS. Clinical correlations: MRI and EEG. Magn Reson Imaging 1995;13:1113–7.

33. Raymond AA, Fish DR, Sisodiya SM, et al. Abnormalities of gyration, heterotopias, tuberous sclerosis, focal cortical dysplasia, microdysgenesis, dysembryoplastic neuroepithelial tumour and dysgenesis of the archicortex in epilepsy. Clinical, EEG and neuroimaging features in 100 adult patients. Brain 1995;118: 629–60.

34. Krautmacher C, Willinek WA, Tschampa HJ, et al. Brain tumors: full- and half-dose contrast-enhanced MR imaging at 3.0 T compared with 1.5 T – initial experience. Radiology 2005;237:1014–9.

35. Griffiths PD, Coley SC, Connolly DJ, et al. MR imaging of patients with localisation-related seizures: initial experience at 3.0 T and relevance to the NICE guidelines. Clin Radiol 2005;60:1090–9.

36. Knake S, Triantafyllou C, Wald LL, et al. 3 T phased array MRI improves the presurgical evaluation in focal epilepsies: a prospective study. Neurology 2005;65: 1026–31.

37. Kuzniecky R, Burgard S, Faught E. Predictive value of magnetic resonance imaging in temporal lobe epilepsy. Arch Neurol 1993;50:65–9.

38. Mosewich RK, So EL, O'Brien TJ, et al. Factors predictive of the outcome of frontal lobe epilepsy surgery. Epilepsia 2000;41:843–9.

39. Cambier DM, Cascino GD, So EL, et al. Video-EEG monitoring in patients with hippocampal atrophy. Acta Neurol Scand 2001;103:231–7.

40. Cascino GD, Trenerry MR, So EL, et al. Routine EEG and temporal lobe epilepsy: relation to long-term EEG monitoring, quantitative MRI, and operative outcome. Epilepsia 1996;37:651–6.

41. Cendes F, Caramanos Z, Andermann F, et al. Proton magnetic resonance spectroscopic imaging and magnetic resonance imaging volumetry in the lateralization of temporal lobe epilepsy: a series of 100 patients. Ann Neurol 1997;42: 737–46.

42. Soares DP, Law M. Magnetic resonance spectroscopy of the brain: review of metabolites and clinical applications. Clin Radiol 2009;64:12–21.

43. So EL. Value and limitations of seizure semiology in localizing seizure onset. J Clin Neurophysiol 2006;23:353–7.

44. Fuchs M, Wagner M, Kastner J. Development of volume conductor and source models to localize epileptic foci. J Clin Neurophysiol 2007;24:101–19.

45. Galicia E, Imai K, Mohamed IS, et al. Changing ictal-onset EEG patterns in children with cortical dysplasia. Brain Dev 2009;31:569–76.

46. Verma A, Radtke R. EEG of partial seizures. J Clin Neurophysiol 2006;23:333–9.

47. Klemm M, Haueisen J, Ivanova G. Independent component analysis: comparison of algorithms for the investigation of surface electrical brain activity. Med Biol Eng Comput 2009;47:413–23.

48. Wongsawat Y. Epileptic seizure detection in EEG recordings using phase congruency. Conf Proc IEEE Eng Med Biol Soc 2008;2008:927–30.

49. Schwartz ES, Dlugos DJ, Storm PB, et al. Magnetoencephalography for pediatric epilepsy: how we do it. AJNR Am J Neuroradiol 2008;29:832–7.

50. Tovar-Spinoza ZS, Ochi A, Rutka JT, et al. The role of magnetoencephalography in epilepsy surgery. Neurosurg Focus 2008;25:E16.
51. Assaf BA, Karkar KM, Laxer KD, et al. Magnetoencephalography source localization and surgical outcome in temporal lobe epilepsy. Clin Neurophysiol 2004;115: 2066–76.
52. Madhavan D, Kuzniecky R. Temporal lobe surgery in patients with normal MRI. Curr Opin Neurol 2007;20:203–7.
53. Lau M, Yam D, Burneo JG. A systematic review on MEG and its use in the presurgical evaluation of localization-related epilepsy. Epilepsy Res 2008;79:97–104.
54. Lee KK, Salamon N. [^{18}F]Fluorodeoxyglucose-positron-emission tomography and MR imaging coregistration for presurgical evaluation of medically refractory epilepsy. AJNR Am J Neuroradiol 2009 [Epub ahead of print].
55. Goffin K, Dedeurwaerdere S, Van Laere K, et al. Neuronuclear assessment of patients with epilepsy. Semin Nucl Med 2008;38:227–39.
56. Patil S, Biassoni L, Borgwardt L. Nuclear medicine in pediatric neurology and neurosurgery: epilepsy and brain tumors. Semin Nucl Med 2007;37:357–81.
57. Uijl SG, Leijten FS, Arends JB, et al. The added value of [^{18}F]fluoro-D-deoxyglucose positron emission tomography in screening for temporal lobe epilepsy surgery. Epilepsia 2007;48:2121–9.
58. Salamon N, Kung J, Shaw SJ, et al. FDG-PET/MRI coregistration improves detection of cortical dysplasia in patients with epilepsy. Neurology 2008;71: 1594–601.
59. Bouvard S, Costes N, Bonnefoi F, et al. Seizure-related short-term plasticity of benzodiazepine receptors in partial epilepsy: a [^{11}C]flumazenil-PET study. Brain 2005;128:1330–43.
60. Goethals I, Van de Wiele C, Boon P, et al. Is central benzodiazepine receptor imaging useful for the identification of epileptogenic foci in localization-related epilepsies? Eur J Nucl Med Mol Imaging 2003;30:325–8.
61. Madar I, Lesser RP, Krauss G, et al. Imaging of delta- and mu-opioid receptors in temporal lobe epilepsy by positron emission tomography. Ann Neurol 1997;41: 358–67.
62. Juhász C, Chugani DC, Muzik O, et al. Alpha-methyl-L-tryptophan PET detects epileptogenic cortex in children with intractable epilepsy. Neurology 2003;60: 960–8.
63. Jung KY, Kang JK, Kim JH, et al. Spatiotemporospectral characteristics of scalp ictal EEG in mesial temporal lobe epilepsy with hippocampal sclerosis. Brain Res 2009;1287:206–19.
64. Natsume J, Bernasconi N, Aghakhani Y, et al. Alpha-[^{11}C]methyl-L-tryptophan uptake in patients with periventricular nodular heterotopia and epilepsy. Epilepsia 2008;49:826–31.
65. Masdeu JC, Arbizu J. Brain single photon emission computed tomography: technological aspects and clinical applications. Semin Neurol 2008;28:423–34.
66. Van Paesschen W. Ictal SPECT. Epilepsia 2004;45(Suppl 4):35–40.
67. Buchhalter JR, So EL. Advances in computer-assisted single-photon emission computed tomography (SPECT) for epilepsy surgery in children. Acta Paediatr Suppl 2004;93:32–5.
68. So EL. Integration of EEG, MRI, and SPECT in localizing the seizure focus for epilepsy surgery. Epilepsia 2000;41(Suppl 3):S48–54.
69. So EL, O'Brien TJ, Brinkmann BH, et al. The EEG evaluation of single photon emission computed tomography abnormalities in epilepsy. J Clin Neurophysiol 2000;17:10–28.

70. O'Brien TJ, So EL, Mullan BP, et al. Subtraction ictal SPECT co-registered to MRI improves clinical usefulness of SPECT in localizing the surgical seizure focus. Neurology 1998;50:445–54.
71. Devous MD Sr, Thisted RA, Morgan GF, et al. SPECT brain imaging in epilepsy: a meta-analysis. J Nucl Med 1998;39:285–93.
72. McNally KA, Paige AL, Varghese G, et al. Localizing value of ictal-interictal SPECT analyzed by SPM (ISAS). Epilepsia 2005;46:1450–64.
73. Sata Y, Matsuda K, Mihara T, et al. Quantitative analysis of benzodiazepine receptor in temporal lobe epilepsy: [^{125}I]iomazenil autoradiographic study of surgically resected specimens. Epilepsia 2002;43:1039–48.
74. Cunningham CJ, Zaamout Mel-F, Goodyear B, et al. Simultaneous EEG-fMRI in human epilepsy. Can J Neurol Sci 2008;35:420–35.
75. Bagshaw AP, Aghakhani Y, Bénar CG, et al. EEG-fMRI of focal epileptic spikes: analysis with multiple haemodynamic functions and comparison with gadolinium-enhanced MR angiograms. Hum Brain Mapp 2004;22:179–92.
76. Bookheimer SY. Functional MRI applications in clinical epilepsy. Neuroimage 1996;4:S139–46.
77. Stefanovic B, Warnking JM, Kobayashi E. Hemodynamic and metabolic responses to activation, deactivation and epileptic discharges. Neuroimage 2005;28:205–15.
78. Warach S, Ives JR, Schlaug G, et al. EEG-triggered echo-planar functional MRI in epilepsy. Neurology 1996;47:89–93.
79. Schwartz TH, Bonhoeffer T. In vivo optical mapping of epileptic foci and surround inhibition in ferret cerebral cortex. Nat Med 2001;7:1063–7.
80. Suh M, Bahar S, Mehta AD, et al. Temporal dependence in uncoupling of blood volume and oxygenation during interictal epileptiform events in rat neocortex. J Neurosci 2005;25:68–77.
81. Haglund MM, Ojemann GA, Hochman DW. Optical imaging of epileptiform and functional activity in human cerebral cortex. Nature 1992;358:668–71.
82. Zhao M, Suh M, Ma H, et al. Focal increases in perfusion and decreases in hemoglobin oxygenation precede seizure onset in spontaneous human epilepsy. Epilepsia 2007;48:2059–67.
83. Schwartz TH, Chen LM, Friedman RM, et al. Intraoperative optical imaging of human face cortical topography: a case study. Neuroreport 2004;15:1527–31.
84. Brekelmans GJ, van Emde Boas W, Velis DN. Comparison of combined versus subdural or intracerebral electrodes alone in presurgical focus localization. Epilepsia 1998;39:1290–301.
85. Engel AK, Moll CK, Fried I, et al. Invasive recordings from the human brain: clinical insights and beyond. Nat Rev Neurosci 2005;6:35–47.
86. Pacia SV, Ebersole JS. Intracranial EEG substrates of scalp ictal patterns from temporal lobe foci. Epilepsia 1997;38:642–54.

Therapeutic Brain Stimulation for Epilepsy

Juliana Lockman, MD, Robert S. Fisher, MD, PhD*

KEYWORDS

- Brain stimulation • Epilepsy • Seizures • Intractable
- Refractory • Treatment

HISTORY

Brain stimulation in people with epilepsy was first explored in the 1940s and 50s by Penfield and Jasper using intraoperative stimulation to map seizure foci in relation to eloquent regions of cortex. Depth electrodes to record epileptiform activity from deep structures became popular after the pioneering works of Bancaud and Talairach.[1] These uses of stimulation were diagnostic.

The first use of electrical stimulation to influence seizures or behavior in people with epilepsy probably was by Robert Heath, a Tulane neurosurgeon. Studies beginning in 1952 implanted electrodes into septal areas, caudate, centromedian (CM) thalamus, mesencephalon, and amygdala. In a patient with complex partial seizures, interictal spikes were recorded from the septal region.[2] With stimulation, "Almost instantly his behavioral state changed from one of disorganization, rage, and persecution to one of happiness and mild euphoria."

Behavioral brain stimulation was continued by Jose Delgado, a Yale physiologist and neurosurgeon, who published several studies on psychobehavioral effects of deep brain stimulation (DBS). The most dramatic of these undoubtedly was his demonstration of stopping a charging bull by radio-controlled stimulation of the internal capsule, causing the bull to circle uncontrollably.[3]

The New York neurosurgeon Irving Cooper is credited with being the first to use electrical stimulation to treat seizures. His first surgical target was the cerebellum, most likely based on decades of physiology findings documenting the inhibitory effects of cerebellar outflow on multiple brain regions and based on animal

The senior author, Robert S. Fisher, was supported by the James and Carrie Anderson Fund for Epilepsy Research, the Susan Horngren Fund, and the Littlefield-DeFreyne Fund. He holds the Maslah Saul, MD Chair.
Department of Neurology and Neurological Sciences, Room A343, 300 Pasteur Drive, Stanford University School of Medicine, Stanford, CA 94305-5235, USA
* Corresponding author.
E-mail address: robert.fisher@stanford.edu (R.S. Fisher).

doi:10.1016/j.ncl.2009.06.005
0733-8619/09/$ – see front matter © 2009 Elsevier Inc. All rights reserved.
neurologic.theclinics.com

experiments showing efficacy in epilepsy models. In 1973, Cooper and colleagues[4] asserted that 6 of 7 patients had marked improvement in seizure control after initiating chronic stimulation of the cerebellar cortex. Cooper also reported seizure reductions after stimulating the anterior thalamus in epilepsy patients (see later discussion).

At least 11 subsequent uncontrolled studies of cerebellar stimulation claimed benefit.[5] In contrast, 2 small controlled studies[6,7] totaling 14 patients showed no benefit. At that point, cerebellar stimulation and DBS in general fell out of favor as a treatment for epilepsy, although some enthusiasm remained among a few practitioners.[8,9] Subsequent success of vagus nerve stimulation for epilepsy and DBS for movement disorders reinvigorated interest in DBS for epilepsy. Currently, only stimulation of the vagus nerve is approved therapy. **Fig. 1** shows sites in the nervous system that have been stimulated for epilepsy.

STIMULATION SITES

A variety of anatomic sites have been targeted for brain stimulation in patients with epilepsy and in laboratory models of epilepsy. In this article, the authors focus on the human studies, but reference may be made to Krauss and Fisher[5] for reviews of early studies in animal models. Clinically based literature consists mainly of case reports with rare randomized controlled trials, making efficacy unclear in many studies. The effect of stimulation is often unable to be investigated independently of other therapies. Furthermore, small uncontrolled studies can be subject to bias created by placebo effect or by regression to the mean—the natural tendency of patients to improve after enrolling in a study when the seizures are under poor control. Finally, many studies predated magnetic resonance imaging (MRI), which is crucial for accurate localization of sites for stimulation. A summary of the available data on sites of brain stimulation for epilepsy is given in the following sections.

Corpus Callosum

Ten patients had electrodes implanted in the corpus callosum as an alternative to callosotomy, but it was reported not to be efficacious.[10]

Brainstem

Locus coeruleus was stimulated unilaterally in 3 patients, 2 with epilepsy.[11] There appeared to be improvement in frequency and severity of seizures in both patients, but small sample size made these results inconclusive.

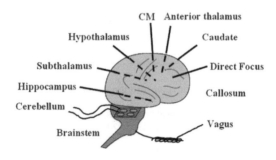

CM=centromedian nucleus of thalamus.

Fig. 1. Sites in the central nervous system (and vagus nerve) for which stimulation has been tried for epilepsy.

Caudate

Research has indicated a role for the caudate in inhibition of the spread of seizure activity. One study showed a beneficial effect of caudate stimulation in monkeys with iatrogenically induced seizures, with subsequent rebound in seizure frequency after discontinuation of stimulation.[12]

In the clinical setting, caudate stimulation was first performed by Sramka and associates[13] in 6 patients, yielding seizure freedom for 2 and reduction in seizures in 4. In a study of 74 patients with intractable epilepsy, focal and generalized interictal electrographic activity appeared to abate with stimulation of the head of the caudate and dentate nucleus of the cerebellum.[14] A report by Gabasvili and coworkers[15] showed cessation of status epilepticus of 4- to 7-day duration in 6 patients with 8 to 10 caudate stimulations at low frequency.

Chkhenkeli and colleagues[16] explored low-frequency (4–8 Hz) stimulation of the ventral aspect of the caudate head in 38 patients. Seizures were eliminated in 21 patients, and there was otherwise worthwhile improvement in 14. Specifically, cessation of ictal patterns arising from the mesial temporal region and neocortex was seen, with improvement in generalized, complex partial, and secondarily generalized seizure types. Another study by the same authors, with similar parameters, demonstrated significant reduction in seizures arising from the mesial temporal region and neocortex.[17]

Centromedian Thalamus

An initial investigation by Velasco and associates[18] explored the CM nucleus in 5 patients with refractory primary generalized or multifocal seizures. Results showed a decline of generalized tonic-clonic seizures by 80% to 100%, complex partial seizures by 60% to 100%, and, in 1 patient, reduction of myoclonic seizures by 100%. After 2 days of stimulation, the authors noted the development of electrographic 2 to 3 Hz rhythmic patterns, outlasting stimulation without an increase in clinical seizure activity. This possible "beneficial kindling" of inhibitory processes may serve as a potential mechanism for the long-lasting effects of stimulation after discontinuation.

A summary of data on 49 patients with follow-up of 6 to 15 years indicated significant benefit for generalized tonic-clonic, absence, tonic, and atonic seizures but no change in frequency of complex partial seizures.[19] Interictal epileptiform activity in the form of generalized spikes, spike-wave complexes, and bilateral synchronous discharges was reduced but without change in focal temporal spikes. In a study of 13 patients with Lennox-Gastaut syndrome, CM stimulation was associated with reduction in seizures by 80%.[20]

A double-blind randomized crossover trial of 7 patients was conducted by Fisher and coworkers[21] in 1992. The first 3 months had the stimulator either on or off, followed by a washout period of 3 months during which all stimulators were off, followed by 3 months with the stimulator in the mode opposite to that of the initial mode. One patient improved substantially from having the stimulator on during the first phase and declined entry into the crossover portion of the trial, making her unable to be included in the statistical analysis. Data indicated reduction in tonic-clonic seizures by 30% during phases with stimulator on versus 8% with stimulator off. The differences were not statistically significant.

Anterior Nucleus of Thalamus

The anterior nucleus of the thalamus, the original target of Cooper, is the only site for which a large randomized controlled trial has been completed. Early investigation involved small studies, with outcomes revealing a range of seizure improvement. Sussman and associates[22] showed substantial reduction in baseline seizure frequency in 3 of 5 patients. Another group of 3 patients demonstrated a reduction in seizures by 75% of baseline frequency.[23] Lim and colleagues[24] showed a reduction in seizure frequency by 49% of baseline frequency in 4 patients with bilateral anterior nucleus of thalamus stimulation, followed for a mean of 43.8 months. Osorio and coworkers[25] showed a mean reduction in seizures by 75% of baseline frequency using a paradigm that delivered stimulation after detecting certain electroencephalographic (EEG) changes.

A pilot study of 10 patients was conducted in preparation for the controlled trial now known as the SANTE (Stimulation of the Anterior Nucleus of Thalamus for Epilepsy) study, and the results were published in 2 separate articles.[26,27] The pilot results indicated seizure reduction to a level between 33% and 47% of baseline, particularly affecting seizure types associated with injury and falls. Hodaie and colleagues[26] in Toronto observed benefit after the stimulator was implanted, but before it was turned on. **Fig. 2** shows positioning of the chest-implantable programmable stimulator and also the electrodes in the thalamus.

The SANTE study was a multicenter, randomized, double-blind parallel group study of 110 implanted patients with refractory partial or secondarily generalized seizures.[28] Stimulation was via a Medtronic implantable programmable pulse generator at 145 pulses per second, with 90-microsecond pulse durations, on for 1 minute and off for 5 minutes. Stimulator cathodes were situated in left and right anterior thalamic nuclei, referential to the anode at the stimulator case. Presentation of preliminary results at the American Epilepsy Society meeting in December 2008 indicated significantly lower median seizure frequencies, compared with baseline, in a group stimulated with 5 V, compared with a placebo controlled group stimulated at 0 V. After 3 months, all patients were transferred to active stimulation at 5 V. Over the 3 years of the trial, median seizure frequencies continued to improve with stimulation. No deaths in the randomized trial were attributed to implantation or stimulation, and no symptomatic hemorrhages occurred. Results are being prepared for publication.

Posterior Hypothalamus

Mammillary bodies of the posterior hypothalamus in patients with epilepsy show epileptiform potentials recorded by depth electrodes.[29] A recent study of posterior

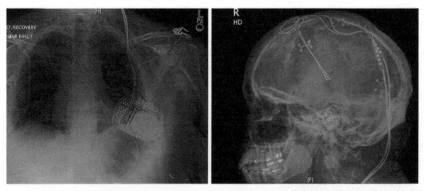

Fig. 2. Radiographs depicting the position of a Medtronic implantable stimulator in the subcutaneous tissue of the chest and connection wires to bilateral deep brain stimulating electrodes in anterior thalamus in a patient with epilepsy.

hypothalamic stimulation in 2 patients with multifocal epilepsy showed reduced seizure frequency by 75% to 80% of preoperative rates, while also mitigating aggressive behaviors at 9 months of follow-up.[30] Stimulation of the mammillothalamic tract was performed in 2 patients with refractory epilepsy due to hypothalamic hamartomas.[31] Results were significant for postoperative decline in baseline seizure frequency, ultimately leading to seizure freedom for 1 patient. Further studies would be required to document the safety of implanting this site, because of its proximity to vessels at the base of the brain.

Subthalamic Nucleus

The subthalamic nucleus is a potentially attractive target for implantation, because tens of thousands of implantations have been done worldwide for treatment of movement disorders. Studies investigating stimulation of the subthalamic nucleus for epilepsy have been limited by small sample sizes, but they have suggested potential benefit for partial seizures. An initial study conducted by Chabardès and coworkers[32] in 2002 showed 67% to 80% reduction in seizure frequency in 3 of 5 patients. Other small studies have shown variable benefit for partial seizures.[33–35] One patient with progressive myoclonic epilepsy had seizures reduced by half.[36] A study by Franzini and colleagues,[30] exploring the zona incerta in 2 patients with frontal lobe seizures, showed reduction in seizures by 85% in one and resolution of status epilepticus in the other.

Hippocampus

A pioneering study by Sramka and colleagues[13] in 1976 primarily evaluated caudate stimulation but also showed benefit in a few patients with direct hippocampal stimulation. Velasco and coworkers[37] conducted a study of 16 patients with partial and secondarily generalized seizures, resulting in complete seizure freedom in 7. Those patients with a grossly normal MRI had greater improvement: 95% reduction in seizure frequency with a normal MRI versus a 50 to 70% reduction with mesial temporal sclerosis.[38] A report by Vonck and associates[39] of 3 patients with medial temporal lobe seizures and normal MRIs showed reduction in complex partial seizures by 50% of baseline rates.

Another study investigating bilateral hippocampal stimulation showed that 4 of 7 patients were responders, with 1 of the 4 ultimately becoming seizure-free for 1.5 years.[40] A study of 12 patients conducted by Boon and associates[41] resulted in 7 responders, 1 of whom ultimately achieved seizure freedom. Osorio and colleagues[42] showed reduction in seizures by 56% in 4 patients, using an algorithm by which stimulation was delivered to bilateral amygdalohippocampal regions in response to automated seizure detection. A trial of 4 patients with double-blind crossover design showed a small, nonsignificant reduction in seizures.[43]

COMPLICATIONS

Much of what is known regarding complications of DBS comes from experience in the treatment of movement disorders. Hardware-related complications, such as infection, paresthesias, and broken leads, are most common. Other adverse events include intracranial hemorrhage, cognitive impairment, and worsening of seizures.

Hamani and Lozano[44] reviewed 254 articles on DBS and identified 10 that principally explored complications. A total of 922 patients were reported to have difficulties, including infection in 6.1%, misplacement/migration in 5.1%, lead fractures in 5%, and skin erosion in 1.3%. Similar complications were observed by Hariz and colleagues[45] in 69 patients with subthalamic nucleus or globus pallidus interna stimulation for Parkinson disease, 7 of whom needed removal or replacement of hardware.

Sensory changes, most commonly paresthesias, were observed in a group of 150 patients who underwent thalamotomy for relief of essential tremor, tremor due to Parkinson disease, multiple sclerosis, or chronic pain.[46]

In 2001, a study of 102 patients having DBS for Parkinson disease found a 3% incidence of symptomatic intracranial hemorrhage in stimulation of the subthalamic nucleus.[47] Subsequent large studies cite a 1.2% to 2.3% risk of clinically significant intracranial hemorrhage.[48,49] Intracranial hemorrhage was found to be a more likely complication in older patients, male patients, those with hypertension, and those with a diagnosis of Parkinson disease. There have been some reports of worsening seizures secondary to hemorrhage.

Cognitive changes have also been noted with DBS. Memory decline has been noted in patients with bilateral independent hippocampal stimulation at low frequency.[50] One child with unilateral stimulation of the hippocampus in the dominant and symptomatic hemisphere showed subsequent decline in verbal and visual memory.[51] In the study by Hariz and associates,[45] memory deficits and psychiatric issues were observed in 18.8% with subthalamic nucleus stimulation and 12.5% with globus pallidus stimulation.

MECHANISMS OF DEEP BRAIN STIMULATION

Several hypotheses have been proposed for the mechanism behind DBS for epilepsy, although research remains limited. Data thus far support mechanisms of disruption at the level of individual neurons, synapses (in the form of increased inhibitory or decreased excitatory potentials), and neuronal networks. The behavior of a neuron in response to stimulation may be somewhat predictable, as estimated by such inherent properties as orientation, membrane resistance, and conductance. However, the activities of a neuronal network appear to be more complex. Network effects rely significantly on stimulation parameters and may ultimately result in either excitation or inhibition at sites remote from the local region of stimulation.

In hippocampal slices, Durand[52] and Gluckman and colleagues[53] found that epileptiform patterns are blocked by electrical stimulation. Associated with this are shifts of potassium from inside neurons to the extracellular space, causing a temporary refractory period for neuronal firing. Vitek[54] demonstrated stimulation of the subthalamic nucleus or ventral intermediate nucleus to act functionally as an inhibitory lesion. However, further studies have shown initial excitation in response to stimulation, followed by inhibition in DBS for patients with Parkinson disease and monkeys with 1-methyl-4-phenyl-1,2,3,6-tetrahydropyridine (MPTP)-induced Parkinson disease.[55,56] Thus, both inhibitory and excitatory components are affected by stimulation of neuronal networks. To date, putative benefits of DBS and the parameters used are empirical, rather than based on an understanding of mechanisms.

RESPONSIVE DEVICES

Vagus nerve stimulation and the previously discussed SANTE trial of the anterior thalamus use stimulation on a timed schedule. Another strategy is to record ongoing EEG and to stimulate in response to a detected correlate of seizure activity—this is called responsive neurostimulation (RNS). Stimulation on schedule is also called "open-loop," to distinguish it from "closed-loop" RNS, which uses a feedback loop. An example of a closed-loop device is the automated cardiac defibrillator. Advances in technology have led to the development of more sophisticated detection algorithms and use of hardware in epilepsy.

A device made by NeuroPace (Mountain View, CA, USA) is implanted into an artificial segment of skull.[57] The hardware is connected to 1 or 2 electrode arrays placed adjacent to a seizure focus or foci. Preset algorithms are designed to detect the onset of EEG patterns associated with seizures. Individual seizure-onset patterns are recorded for each study patient, and the detection algorithm is then modified for optimal detection in each patient. Stimulation can be via subdural strip electrodes or depth electrodes.

A feasibility study of 65 patients showed the device to be well tolerated.[57] The initial 24 patients in the study showed responder rates between 35% and 43%. A pivotal trial of RNS for epilepsy using the Neuropace device is underway, with enrollment of 240 patients (Martha Morrell, personal communication, 2009).

SUMMARY

DBS has been a possible therapy for epilepsy for more than 30 years, and now it is moving to the point of clinical utility. Animal models have shown efficacy of DBS at several brain regions, although not all animal studies have shown efficacy. Clinically, an array of sites have been explored, including the cerebellum, anterior nucleus of the thalamus, CM nucleus, hippocampus, subthalamic nucleus, brainstem, and corpus callosum; direct stimulation of the cortex has also been explored. Interest in evaluating these sites for treatment of epilepsy has been enhanced by the success of vagus nerve stimulation for epilepsy and DBS for movement disorders.

Literature consists of mostly small and uncontrolled studies that are subject to limitations in interpretation. A pivotal large, double-blind controlled trial of anterior nucleus of the thalamus has recently been completed, and it showed efficacy for partial seizures with or without secondary generalization.[28] A controlled trial for RNS is under way.[57] In addition, pilot studies of hippocampal stimulation[41,43] are expected to lead to more definitive trials of this site.

Brain stimulation for epilepsy holds several challenges for the future. Mechanisms of DBS are poorly understood, although investigations are actively being pursued. Little is known about optimal stimulation parameters. DBS has been little examined in cases of intractable generalized epilepsy. Because DBS carries some risk, mainly of hemorrhage and infection, clinicians will need to develop an effective method of identifying the best candidates. DBS is palliative rather than curative, but experience suggests that this relatively new therapy may be of benefit to some people with otherwise untreatable epilepsy.

REFERENCES

1. Bancaud J, Talairach J. Methodology of stereo EEG exploration and surgical intervention in epilepsy. Rev Otoneuroophtalmol 1973;45(4):315–28.
2. Heath RG. Electrical self-stimulation of the brain in man. Am J Psychiatry 1963; 120:571–7.
3. Osmundsen JA. 'Matador' With a Radio Stops Wired Bull: Modified Behavior in Animals Subject of Brain Study. New York Times, May 17, 1965.
4. Cooper IS, Amin I, Gilman S. The effect of chronic cerebellar stimulation upon epilepsy in man. Trans Am Neurol Assoc 1973;98:192–6.
5. Krauss GL, Fisher RS. Cerebellar and thalamic stimulation for epilepsy. Adv Neurol 1993;63:231–45.

6. Van Buren JM, Wood JH, Oakley J, et al. Preliminary evaluation of cerebellar stimulation by double-blind stimulation and biological criteria in the treatment of epilepsy. J Neurosurg 1978;48(3):407–16.
7. Wright GD, McLellan DL, Brice JG. A double-blind trial of chronic cerebellar stimulation in twelve patients with severe epilepsy. J Neurol Neurosurg Psychiatr 1984;47(8):769–74.
8. Davis R, Gray E, Engle H, et al. Reduction of intractable seizures using cerebellar stimulation. Appl Neurophysiol 1983;46(1–4):57–61.
9. Velasco F, Carrillo-Ruiz JD, Brito F, et al. Double-blind, randomized controlled pilot study of bilateral cerebellar stimulation for treatment of intractable motor seizures. Epilepsia 2005;46(7):1071–81.
10. Marino Júnior R, Gronich G. Corpus callosum stimulation and stereotactic callosotomy in the management of refractory generalized epilepsy. Preliminary communication. Arq Neuropsiquiatr 1989;47:320–5.
11. Feinstein B, Gleason CA, Libet B. Stimulation of locus coeruleus in man. Preliminary trials for spasticity and epilepsy. Stereotact Funct Neurosurg 1989;52(1):26–41.
12. Oakley JC, Ojemann GA. Effects of chronic stimulation of the caudate nucleus on a preexisting alumina seizure focus. Exp Neurol 1982;75(2):360–7.
13. Sramka M, Fritz G, Galanda M, et al. Some observations in treatment stimulation of epilepsy. Acta Neurochir (Wien) 1976;(Suppl 23):257–62.
14. Sramka M, Chkhenkeli SA. Clinical experience in intraoperational determination of brain inhibitory structures and application of implanted neurostimulators in epilepsy. Stereotact Funct Neurosurg 1990;54–55:56–9.
15. Gabasvili VM, Chkhenkeli SA, Sramka M. The treatment of status epilepticus by electrostimulation of deep brain structures. Presented at: modern trends in neurology and neurological emergencies. The First European Congress of Neurology. Prague: 1988.
16. Chkhenkeli SA, Sramka M, Lortkipanidze GS, et al. Electrophysiological effects and clinical results of direct brain stimulation for intractable epilepsy. Clin Neurol Neurosurg 2004;106(4):318–29.
17. Chkhenkeli SA, Chkhenkeli IS. Effects of therapeutic stimulation of nucleus caudatus on epileptic electrical activity of brain in patients with intractable epilepsy. Stereotact Funct Neurosurg 1997;69(1–4 Pt 2):221–4.
18. Velasco F, Velasco M, Ogarrio C, et al. Electrical stimulation of the centromedian thalamic nucleus in the treatment of convulsive seizures: a preliminary report. Epilepsia 1987;28(4):421–30.
19. Velasco F, Velasco M, Velasco AL, et al. Electrical stimulation for epilepsy: stimulation of hippocampal foci. Stereotact Funct Neurosurg 2001;77(1–4):223–7.
20. Velasco AL, Velasco F, Jiménez F, et al. Neuromodulation of the centromedian thalamic nuclei in the treatment of generalized seizures and the improvement of the quality of life in patients with Lennox-Gastaut syndrome. Epilepsia 2006; 47(7):1203–12.
21. Fisher RS, Uematsu S, Krauss GL, et al. Placebo-controlled pilot study of centromedian thalamic stimulation in treatment of intractable seizures. Epilepsia 1992; 33(5):841–51.
22. Sussman NM, Goldman HW, Jackel A, et al. Anterior thalamic stimulation in medically intractable epilepsy. Part II. preliminary clinical results. Epilepsia 1988;29(5): 677.
23. Lee KJ, Jang KS, Shon YM. Chronic deep brain stimulation of subthalamic and anterior thalamic nuclei for controlling refractory partial epilepsy. Acta Neurochir Suppl 2006;99:87–91.

24. Lim SN, Lee ST, Tsai YT, et al. Electrical stimulation of the anterior nucleus of the thalamus for intractable epilepsy: a long-term follow-up study. Epilepsia 2007; 48(2):342–7.

25. Osorio I, Overman J, Giftakis J, et al. High frequency thalamic stimulation for inoperable mesial temporal epilepsy. Epilepsia 2007;48(8):1561–71.

26. Hodaie M, Wennberg RA, Dostrovsky JO, et al. Chronic anterior thalamus stimulation for intractable epilepsy. Epilepsia 2002;43(6):603–8.

27. Kerrigan JF, Litt B, Fisher RS, et al. Electrical stimulation of the anterior nucleus of the thalamus for the treatment of intractable epilepsy. Epilepsia 2004;45(4): 346–54.

28. Fisher RS. Release of the "Stimulation of the Anterior Nucleus of the Thalamus in Epilepsy (SANTE)" Trial Results. 2008, American Epilepsy Society meeting, Seattle, Washington.

29. van Rijckevorsel K, Abu Serieh B, de Tourtchaninoff M, et al. Deep EEG recordings of the mammillary body in epilepsy patients. Epilepsia 2005; 46(5):781–5.

30. Franzini A, Messina G, Marras C, et al. Deep brain stimulation of two unconventional targets in refractory non-resectable epilepsy. Stereotact Funct Neurosurg 2008;86(6):373–81 [Epub 2008 Nov 25].

31. Khan S, Wright I, Javed S, et al. High frequency stimulation of the mamillothalamic tract for the treatment of resistant seizures associated with hypothalamic hamartoma. Epilepsia 2009;50(6):1608–11.

32. Chabardès S, Kahane P, Minotti L, et al. Deep brain stimulation in epilepsy with particular reference to the subthalamic nucleus. Epileptic Disord 2002;4(Suppl 3): S83–93.

33. Benabid AL, Vercucil L, Benazzouz A, et al. Deep brain stimulation: what does it offer? Adv Neurol 2003;91:293–302.

34. Neme S, Montgomery EB Jr, Rezai A, et al. Subthalamic nucleus stimulation in patients with intractable epilepsy: the Cleveland experience. In: Hans Lüders, editor. Deep brain stimulation and epilepsy. New York: Martin Dunitz, Inc.; 2004. p. 349–55.

35. Handforth A, DeSalles AA, Krahl SE. Deep brain stimulation of the subthalamic nucleus as adjunct treatment for refractory epilepsy. Epilepsia 2006;47(7): 1239–41.

36. Vesper J, Steinhoff B, Rona S, et al. Chronic high-frequency deep brain stimulation of the STN/SNr for progressive myoclonic epilepsy. Epilepsia 2007;48(10): 1984–9.

37. Velasco AL, Velasco M, Velasco F, et al. Subacute and chronic electrical stimulation of the hippocampus on intractable temporal lobe seizures: preliminary report. Arch Med Res 2000;31(3):316–28.

38. Velasco AL, Velasco F, Velasco M, et al. Electrical stimulation of the hippocampal epileptic foci for seizure control: a double-blind, long-term follow-up study. Epilepsia 2007;48(10):1895–903.

39. Vonck K, Boon P, Achten E, et al. Long-term amygdalohippocampal stimulation for refractory temporal lobe epilepsy. Ann Neurol 2002;52(5):556–65.

40. Vonck K, Boon P, Claeys P, et al. Long-term deep brain stimulation for refractory temporal lobe epilepsy. Epilepsia 2005;46(Suppl 5):98–9.

41. Boon P, Vonck K, De Herdt V, et al. Deep brain stimulation in patients with refractory temporal lobe epilepsy. Epilepsia 2007;48(8):1551–60.

42. Osorio I, Frei MG, Sunderam S, et al. Automated seizure abatement in humans using electrical stimulation. Ann Neurol 2005;57(2):258–68.

43. Tellez-Zenteno JF, McLachlan RS, Parrent A, et al. Hippocampal electrical stimulation in mesial temporal lobe epilepsy. Neurology 2006;66(10):1490–4.
44. Hamani C, Lozano AM. Hardware-related complications of deep brain stimulation: a review of the published literature. Stereotact Funct Neurosurg 2006; 84(5–6):248–51.
45. Hariz MI, Rehncrona S, Quinn NP, et al. Multicentre advanced Parkinson's disease deep brain stimulation group. Multicenter study on deep brain stimulation in Parkinson's disease: an independent assessment of reported adverse events at 4 years. Mov Disord 2008;23(3):416–21.
46. Dostrovsky JO, Davis KD, Lee L, et al. Electrical stimulation-induced effects in the human thalamus. Adv Neurol 1993;63:219–29.
47. Deep-Brain Stimulation for Parkinson's Disease Study Group. Deep-brain stimulation of the subthalamic nucleus or the pars interna of the globus pallidus in Parkinson's disease. N Engl J Med 2001;345(13):956–63.
48. Beric A, Kelly PJ, Rezai A, et al. Complications of deep brain stimulation surgery. Stereotact Funct Neurosurg 2001;77(1–4):73–8.
49. Sansur CA, Frysinger RC, Pouratian N, et al. Incidence of symptomatic hemorrhage after stereotactic electrode placement. J Neurosurg 2007;107(5): 998–1003.
50. Fernández G, Hufnagel A, Helmstaedter C, et al. Memory function during low intensity hippocampal electrical stimulation in patients with temporal lobe epilepsy. Eur J Neurol 1996;3:335–44.
51. Cohen MJ, Holmes GL, Campbell R, et al. Memory performance following unilateral electrical stimulation of the hippocampus in a child with right temporal lobe epilepsy. J Epilepsy 1990;3:115–22.
52. Durand D. Electrical stimulation can inhibit synchronized neuronal activity. Brain Res 1986;382(1):139–44.
53. Gluckman BJ, Neel EJ, Netoff TI, et al. Electric field suppression of epileptiform activity in hippocampal slices. J Neurophysiol 1996;76(6):4202–5.
54. Vitek JL. Mechanisms of deep brain stimulation: excitation or inhibition. Mov Disord 2002;17(Suppl 3):69–72.
55. Dostrovsky JO, Lozano AM. Mechanisms of deep brain stimulation. Mov Disord 2002;17(Suppl 3):S63–8.
56. McIntyre CC, Savasta M, Walter BL, et al. How does deep brain stimulation work? Present understanding and future questions. J Clin Neurophysiol 2004;21(1): 40–50.
57. Sun FT, Morrell MJ, Wharen RE Jr. Responsive cortical stimulation for the treatment of epilepsy. Neurotherapeutics 2008;5(1):68–74.

Advances on the Genetics of Mendelian Idiopathic Epilepsies

Stéphanie Baulac, PhD[a],*, Michel Baulac, MD[a,b]

KEYWORDS

• Epilepsy • Febrile seizures • Idiopathic • Genes • Loci

More than 50 epilepsy syndromes are described and they are broadly divided into generalized and partial syndromes reflecting the evidence that some seizures are generated diffusely and bilaterally in the brain whereas others have a focal onset. Importantly, some syndromes are age specific and begin in the first year of life, whereas others have a later onset in life. It is well known that the age-specific incidence of epilepsy is high during the first year of life and childhood, and declines throughout adulthood. Classifications of epilepsies have often used the terms "idiopathic" and "symptomatic". Idiopathic epilepsies have no evidence of an underlying cause and arise in the absence of neurologic deficits or brain lesions. Most of the idiopathic epilepsies are benign or of moderate severity and are believed to have a genetic etiology. On the other hand, the term symptomatic is used when patients with epilepsy have a known or suspected cause and/or when associated with neurologic deficits. We do not discuss the numerous symptomatic genetic epilepsies (eg, progressive myoclonic epilepsies, encephalopathies, Rett syndrome) where seizure disorders are one part of a complex phenotype; epilepsy resulting from a metabolic or structural defect in the brain.

This article strictly focuses on those Mendelian idiopathic epilepsies in which the causative genes are known (or localized), although these presently account for a small proportion of all epilepsy cases. In autosomal dominant conditions, the presence of a single copy of a mutation (heterozygous state) in one *major* effect gene is sufficient to cause the disease. Penetrance is usually reduced, reflecting the fact that some patients carrying the causal mutation are asymptomatic. The genes for Mendelian diseases are localized by positional cloning in large families with multiple affected family members. Whole genome scans are usually conducted by genotyping a panel

[a] UPMC/Inserm, UMR_S975, Cricm, F-75013, Bâtiment Pharmacie, Hôpital de la Pitié-Salpêtrière, 47 boulevard de l'hôpital, 75013 Paris, France
[b] Center for Epilepsy, AP-HP, Bâtiment Paul Casteigne Hôpital de la Pitié-Salpêtrière, 47 boulevard de l'hôpital, 75013 Paris, France
* Corresponding author.
E-mail address: stephanie.baulac@upmc.fr (S. Baulac).

Neurol Clin 27 (2009) 1041–1061
doi:10.1016/j.ncl.2009.07.001
0733-8619/09/$ – see front matter © 2009 Elsevier Inc. All rights reserved.
neurologic.theclinics.com

of several hundreds of microsatellite markers searching for co-segregation of disease with marker alleles within families. In recent times, genome-wide searches are conducted with either high-density (several thousands) SNPs (single-nucleotide polymorphisms) or DNA microarrays, which provide higher resolution and are less cost-effective. Linkage analysis determines the region of the genome shared by the affected family members. Logarithm of the odds (LOD) scores are calculated to determine the probably of the linkage. This common interval encompasses the mutated epilepsy gene. Sequencing is considered the "gold standard" for mutation detection because it reveals the exact location and the type of mutations. The disease-causing mutation should co-segregate with the disease among family members and should be absent from a control ethnically matched population. For missense mutations (leading to the substitution of an amino acid), it is necessary to demonstrate that the mutation has deleterious effects on the protein function. The functional consequences of each mutation are either the result of a dominant effect of the mutant protein or a loss-of-function because of haploinsufficiency (ie, a loss of 50% of the amount of protein). Notably, the presence of phenotypic heterogeneity in patients harboring the same mutation suggests that modifier genes, which are yet to be identified, also play a significant role.

Multiplex families with autosomal dominant transmission, although not representative of the general population, have been powerful for the elucidation of the molecular basis of Mendelian epilepsies. Since the identification of the first epilepsy gene, *CHRNA4*, in 1995,[1] 10 additional epilepsy genes have been identified. Most of the known genetic culprits in epilepsy are genes encoding components of neuronal ion channels (voltage-gated sodium channels and voltage-gated potassium channels) or neurotransmitter receptors (acetylcholine nicotinic receptor and GABA$_A$ receptor). The latest identified gene, *LGI1* (leucine-rich glioma inactivated 1) is a non-ion channel gene[2,3] which will probably provide new pathways for epileptogenesis.

This review provides a basic overview of idiopathic epilepsy syndromes with their corresponding causal genes. We will first describe neonatal and infancy epilepsies, then childhood and adolescence epilepsies, and last adult-onset epilepsies (**Fig. 1**).

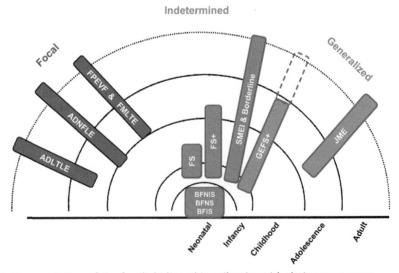

Fig. 1. Representation of the familial idiopathic epilepsies with their age at onset.

For each of these epileptic syndromes, we provide a table recapitulating all epilepsy genes and loci (**Table 1**) and for those for which the gene is known, we provide an illustration of the corresponding protein (**Fig. 2**). We do not discuss the susceptibility genes and loci involved in epilepsies with complex inheritance in which the literature abounds with reports of associations and reports of nonreplication of those association studies.

NEONATAL AND INFANCY EPILEPSY SYNDROMES

Three inherited epilepsy syndromes occur during the first year of life: benign familial neonatal seizures (BFNS), benign familial neonatal-infantile seizures (BFNIS), and benign familial infantile seizures (BFIS). All have similar clinical presentation but differ in age of onset, illustrating the strong age-dependency of these channelopathies. These syndromes arise in healthy neonates or infants and are characterized by afebrile focal motor seizures that can secondarily generalize. Seizures usually remit after weeks or months with administration of standard anti-epileptic drugs. Developmental and intellectual outcome is often normal. All three syndromes show autosomal dominant inheritance with high penetrance. Notably, they are caused by different genes and are genetically heterogeneous.[4]

Benign Familial Neonatal Seizures

BFNS usually start on the second or third day of life and often remit spontaneously after a few weeks or months. Seizures may present several manifestations including tonic attacks, apnea, and clonic, focal, and autonomic features. Most seizures typically remit by 4 months but over the term, febrile seizures occur in 5% and epilepsy in 11% of individuals. BFNS is an autosomal-dominant focal epilepsy in which the vast majority of families have mutations in KCNQ2,[5,6] with a few in KCNQ3[7] encoding respectively the voltage-gated potassium channel subunits Kv7.2 and Kv7.3. Approximately 70 mutations in KCNQ2 (including missense, frameshift, nonsense, splice-site mutations, and whole exon deletions) and 6 in KCNQ3 have been identified in families affected by this epilepsy syndrome (Human Gene Mutation Database).[8] De novo mutations in KCNQ2 have also been reported in sporadic patients with benign neonatal seizures.[9,10] Nearly half of KCNQ2 mutations are predicated to truncate the protein and the remainder are missense mutations. In KCNQ3 gene, only missense mutations have been identified. Studies on the functional consequences of these mutations have been performed for many KCNQ2 and KCNQ3 mutations in heterologous expression systems, with consequences ranging from slight changes in channel properties to a complete loss of channel function.[11] A small proportion of families have no mutations in neither KCNQ2 nor KCNQ3, underlying that at least a third gene needs to be unraveled.

Benign Familial Neonatal-infantile Seizures

The age of onset within families with BFNIS is between 2 days to 7 months with most cases having onset at around 2 to 3 months of age. Most families with BFNIS have mutations in SCN2A, which encodes the α2-subunit of the neuronal voltage-gated sodium channel. To date, 10 missense mutations in SCN2A gene have been reported as the cause of BFNIS.[12–14] The incrimination of SCN2A is interesting as it highlights that whereas BFNS are associated with potassium-channel gene defects; BFNIS are attributable to mutations in a sodium-channel gene. The identification of BFNIS with SCN2A mutations has thus contributed to delineate the benign epilepsy syndromes of the neonatal and infantile periods. The clinical phenotype overlap among families

Table 1
Genes and loci implicated in monogenic idiopathic epilepsies

Epileptic Disorder	Gene or Locus	Protein
Autosomal dominant neonatal and infancy epilepsy syndromes		
Benign familial neonatal seizures (BFNS)	KCNQ2	Neuronal voltage-gated potassium channel Kv7.2
	KCNQ3	Neuronal voltage-gated potassium channel Kv7.3
Benign familial neonatal-infantile seizures (BFNIS)	SCN2A	α2-subunit of the neuronal voltage-gated sodium channel
Benign familial infantile seizures (BFIS)	19q12-q13.11	unknown
	16p12-q12	unknown
Autosomal dominant childhood and adolescence-onset epilepsy syndromes		
Generalized epilepsy with febrile seizures plus (GEFS+)	SCN1B	β1-subunit of the neuronal voltage-gated sodium channel
GEFS+, febrile seizures (FS), Dravet syndrome	SCN1A	α1-subunit of the neuronal voltage-gated sodium channel
GEFS+, FS, childhood absence epilepsy	GABRG2	γ2-subunit of the neuronal GABA$_A$ receptor
GEFS+	2p24	unknown
	8p23-p21	unknown
FS + epilepsy	8q13-q21	unknown
Pure complex FS	19p13.3	unknown
Pure simple FS	6q22-q24	unknown
FS + epilepsy	21q22	unknown
FS + childhood absence epilepsy	3p24.3-p23	unknown
FS + epilepsy	3q26.2-26.3	unknown

Autosomal dominant adolescence and adult-onset epilepsy syndromes

Autosomal dominant nocturnal frontal lobe epilepsy (ADNFLE)	*CHRNA4*	α4-subunit of the neuronal nicotinic acetylcholine receptor
	CHRNA2	α2-subunit of the neuronal nicotinic acetylcholine receptor
	CHRNB2	β2-subunit of the neuronal nicotinic acetylcholine receptor
Autosomal dominant lateral temporal epilepsy (ADLTE)	*LGI1*	Leucine-rich glioma-inactivated 1
Familial mesial temporal lobe epilepsy (FMLTE)	18qter/1q25-q31	unknown
	12q23	unknown
	4q13.2-q21.3	unknown
Familial partial epilepsy with variable foci (FPEVF)	2q	unknown
	22q12	unknown
Juvenile myoclonic epilepsy (JME)	*GABRA1*	α1-subunit of the neuronal GABA$_A$ receptor

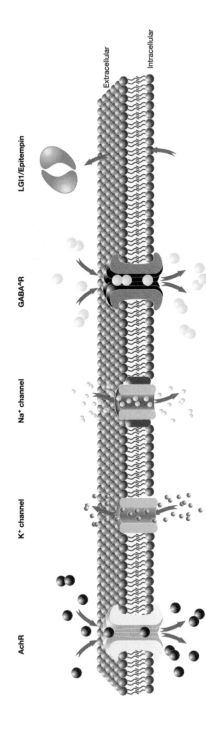

Fig. 2. Illustration of epilepsy-gene products involved in monogenic idiopathic epilepsies.

with BFNIS and other first-year–onset epilepsy syndromes highlights the value of molecular testing.

Benign Familial Infantile Seizures

BFIS is an autosomal dominantly inherited partial epilepsy syndrome of early childhood (starting between 4 and 8 months) with spontaneous remission before the age of 3 years. The seizures often present as a cluster over a few days, raising concern about a more serious condition. They typically present motor features and focal onset on EEG monitoring.[15] Two genetic loci have been reported in BFIS families with autosomal dominant transmission: one on chromosome 19q12-q13.11 in five Italian families[16] and one on 16p12-q12 segregating in several families.[17,18] No causative genes for BFIS have been identified yet. In some families, BFIS later in life co-segregates with paroxysmal choreoathetosis occurring spontaneously or induced by movements, exertion, startling, or anxiety. This syndrome, called infantile convulsions and choreoathetosis, shows linkage to the pericentromeric region of chromosome 16.[19]

CHILDHOOD AND ADOLESCENCE ONSET: FEBRILE SEIZURES WITH EPILEPSY

Febrile seizures (FS) represent the most common form of childhood seizures. They affect 2% to 5% of infants in the Caucasian population[20] and are even more common in the Japanese population, affecting 6% to 9% of infants.[21] FS are not thought of as a true epileptic disease but rather as a special syndrome characterized by its provoking factor (fever) and a typical age of onset between 6 months and 6 years. The outcome is generally very good, but people who have had FS have a higher risk of developing spontaneous afebrile seizures.[22] Familial FS are often associated with a wide variety of afebrile seizures. Among the syndromes associating febrile and afebrile seizures, "Generalized epilepsy with febrile seizures plus (GEFS+)" is a familial context with a spectrum of phenotypes including FS and atypical FS (FS+).[23]

Common forms of FS appear to be multifactorial disorders, believed to be influenced by several susceptibility genes with environmental factors. However, in multigenerational families, the FS susceptibility trait is consistent with a single-major-locus model that best fits with autosomal dominant with reduced penetrance.[24] Although specific genes that affect "pure" autosomal dominant FS cases have not yet been identified, mutations in the genes encoding two subunits of the voltage-gated sodium channel (*SCN1A* and *SCN1B*) and a subunit of the $GABA_A$ receptor (*GABRG2*) have been incriminated in GEFS+ families.

Loci for Febrile Seizures and Epilepsy

Extensive genetic linkage analyses have been performed in multiplex FS families, and here we describe seven genetic loci for autosomal dominant FS. We do not discuss the susceptibility loci involved in FS with complex inheritance (for review, see Nakayama[25]). Although most affected individuals in familial FS only experienced FS, some affected family members later developed afebrile seizures. Only the loci on chromosomes 19p13.3 (FEB2)[26,27] and 6q22-q24[28] appear to be encompassing pure isolated FS. To date, most of the loci incriminated in autosomal dominant FS have not been replicated and the genes for pure FS remain unknown. Because of the genetic heterogeneity, many loci are segregating only in the single family in which they were initially identified. One reason is that genetic mapping in large FS families is complicated by the presence of phenocopies (because of the high incidence of FS in the general population) segregating in the families and that might lead to erroneous linkage. The other hypothesis might be that FS are multigenic, although they seem to have an autosomal dominant transmission. Last, once a locus is identified, the gene is usually identified on behalf of a candidate-gene strategy that consists of sequencing ion channels genes or any other genes involved in neuronal excitability. It is possible that the "FS-genes" do not belong to the neuronal channelopathy family and they are thus not sequenced. Exhaustive search for mutations in all genes of a given interval will soon be available with next-generation sequencing technologies and will probably lead to sorting out of those genes.

- Wallace and colleagues[29] identified a locus on chromosome 8q13-q21 (*FEB1*) for autosomal dominant FS in a three-generation Australian family. Three of the 19 affected subjects had afebrile seizures. Although the LOD score values were significant (maximum pairwise LOD score of 2.53), to date, no other studies have replicated this locus on chromosome 8q13-q21.
- Johnson and colleagues[26] published a second locus for autosomal dominant FS on chromosome 19p13.3 (*FEB2*) by linkage analysis in a large American Midwest family (maximum pairwise LOD score of 4.52). A second putative 19p-linked American family was reported, although LOD scores did not reach the significant threshold value of +3 (maximum pairwise LOD score of 2.30).[27] All patients in both studies experienced only pure FS and none developed concomitant or subsequent epilepsy. The *FEB2* locus appears to be associated with pure, but complex FS (long-lasting FS).
- Peiffer and colleagues[30] identified a locus on chromosome 2q23-q24 (*FEB3*) in a large multigenerational American family with FS segregating an autosomal dominant trait (maximum pairwise LOD score of 8.08). Eighteen of the 21 affected individuals had recurrent FS, all occurring before age 6 years, and 8 also developed afebrile seizures. The phenotype of this family differed substantially from GEFS+ as none of the patients had FS after 6 years of age. This region is also known as a GEFS+ locus, and mutations in the *SCN1A* gene have been reported in GEFS+ families linked to the 2q23-q24 locus.[31] Furthermore, Mantegazza and colleagues[32] reported a missense mutation (M145T) in *SCN1A* segregating in a large Italian family with simple FS. Because no *SCN1A* mutation was reported in this original American family, this locus might represent a distinct genetic entity from the *SCN1A* locus.
- Nabbout and colleagues[28] mapped a locus for FS to chromosome 6q22-q24 in a large five-generation French family and a smaller family in which FS segregated as an autosomal dominant trait (maximum pairwise LOD score of 3.54 and 1.59, respectively). All affected members presented a homogeneous phenotype of simple FS. Among the 29 affected family members, only one patient presented afebrile seizures, and the others did not develop any other form of epilepsy. The locus on 6q22-q24 seems to be exclusive for pure and simple FS.
- Hedera and colleagues[33] identified a locus for FS and afebrile seizures on chromosome 21q22 (maximum pairwise LOD score of 3.35) in a five-generation family with 13 individuals with typical FS and coexisting afebrile seizures in 3 affected individuals. Two patients had documented afebrile generalized tonic-clonic seizures, which coexisted with simple and complex FS, thus meeting criteria for FS+, and potentially suggesting an overlap with the GEFS+ syndrome.
- Nabbout and colleagues[34] reported a locus for FS with childhood absence epilepsy (CAE) on chromosome 3p24.3-p23 in a four-generation French family (maximum pairwise LOD score of 4.64). All 13 affected members had FS, and 5 of these patients subsequently developed CAE and 1 temporal lobe epilepsy (TLE). Another genomic region localized on chromosome 18p could not be excluded (maximum

pairwise LOD score of 1.94) and all patients presenting epilepsy (CAE and TLE) shared a common haplotype at this locus in addition to the haplotype on 3p. Notably, this 18p locus had been reported as a susceptibility locus in a nonparametric whole genome scan performed on a series of nuclear Japanese FS pedigrees.[35]

- Dai and colleagues[36] recently published a four-generation Chinese family with autosomal dominant FS. Two among 12 patients also experienced afebrile seizures. Genome-wide scan detected significant linkage with markers on chromosome 3q26.2-26.3 (maximum pairwise LOD score of 3.77).

Molecular Findings for Generalized Epilepsy with Febrile Seizures Plus

Generalized epilepsy with febrile seizures plus (GEFS+) is an autosomal dominant epilepsy recognized as a distinct clinical entity in 1997 with characteristic, but heterogeneous, seizure phenotypes in affected family members.[23] The most common phenotype is classic FS. Notably, the key feature is FS+, which encompasses either children with FS that occur beyond the age of 6 years or children who have afebrile seizures in addition to FS.[37] The authors recently proposed changing the name of GEFS+ to "genetic epilepsy with febrile seizures plus" instead of "generalized epilepsy with febrile seizures plus" because while generalized epilepsies predominate in GEFS+ families, partial seizures are also encountered.[38] Although GEFS+ syndrome presents a large phenotypic heterogeneity, the clinical concept of GEFS+ has been validated by the identification of single major genes: *SCN1A*, *SCN1B*, and *GABRG2*, described in following paragraphs.

SCN1B

In 1998, the first GEFS+ gene was discovered with the identification of a missense mutation (C121W) in the sodium channel regulatory β1 subunit gene, *SCN1B*, in an Australian family linked to 19q13.1.[39] The mutation C121W was then found to be recurrent in four additional families[40,41] and was shown to disrupt a putative disulfide bridge implicated in the maintenance of the immunoglobulinlike fold and important for interacting with sodium channel subunits.[42] Interestingly, five patients among both families with the C121W mutation had confirmed temporal lobe epilepsy.[40] There have also been different mutations of the same amino acid R85 (R85C and R85H) in two additional Australian families.[40] In a Belgian family with FS and early-onset absence epilepsy, a mutation was identified that predicts a deletion of five amino acids in the extracellular immunoglobulinlike domain of *SCN1B* and potential loss of function.[43] Although *SCN1B* was the first gene incriminated with GEFS+, mutations within this gene remain a rare cause of this familial epileptic context.

SCN1A

In 2000, a tripartite collaboration identified the two first mutations (Thr875Met and Arg1648His) of the sodium channel α1 subunit gene, *SCN1A*, in two French GEFS+ families.[31] In several years, more than 20 missense disease-causing mutations were found and *SCN1A* mutations account for approximately 10% of GEFS+ families.[44] Because fever-induced seizures are known to occur in both GEFS+ families and severe myoclonic epilepsy infancy patients (SMEI, Dravet Syndrome), Claes and colleagues[45] studied seven children with Dravet syndrome for mutations of *SCN1A*. It is now well recognized that the overwhelming majority of known *SCN1A* mutations lead to Dravet syndrome, which is the most severe phenotype in the GEFS+ spectrum. Dravet syndrome is a rare pharmacoresistant epileptic disorder characterized by onset, in the first year of life and by seizures that are commonly, but not exclusively, triggered by fever. FS are clonic, generalized or unilateral, and are often prolonged, resulting in status epilepticus. After 1 year of age, myoclonic seizures and other seizure types appear, psychomotor delay becomes progressively evident from the second year of life, and ataxia frequently develops later.[46] The terms SMEI border-land/borderline (SMEB) is used for a phenotype with individuals sharing many, but not all of the key features of SMEI.[47] Approximately 70% of SMEI and 30% of SMEB patients carry *SCN1A* mutations (including missense, frameshift, nonsense, splice-site mutations, and whole exon or whole gene deletions) that are de novo in most cases.[48] Although this ensemble of catastrophic conditions cannot be regarded as typical idiopathic epilepsies, they share several important features of the other *SCN1A* channelopathies: at the period of disease onset, during the child's develop-ment, the brain MRIs are normal. There is often a familial aggregation of seizures suggestive of a GEFS+ context, and in a few cases the mutation is inherited, with a contribution in some cases of mosaicism to individual and familial phenotypic vari-ation.[48–52] Understanding the functional consequences of *SCN1A* alterations may lead to tremendous progress in some of the mechanisms of epileptogenesis. *SCN1A* is the most relevant epilepsy gene with the largest number of epilepsy-related mutations so far identified.

GABRG2

We identified a missense mutation (K289M) in the $\gamma2$ subunit of the GABA$_A$ receptor gene *GABRG2* in one large French GEFS+ family linked to 5q14.[53] Concomitantly, Wallace and colleagues[54] found a missense mutation (R43Q) in an Australian kindred with childhood absence epilepsy (CAE) and FS. One further mutation (introducing a premature stop codon at Q351) in *GABRG2* was then identified in a second GEFS+ family including an individual with a severe myoclonic epilepsy of infancy,[55] whereas two further mutations have been associated in one family with CAE and FS (IVS6 + 2T→G), and in one family with isolated FS (R139L).[56,57] GABA is the predom-inant brain inhibitory transmitter in adults and its role in epilepsy had been suspected for decades. Nevertheless, mutations in *GABRG2* are apparently rare.

GEFS+ orphan loci

- Audenaert and colleagues[58] described a four-generation Belgian-Dutch family with strong evidence (maximum two-point LOD score of 5.07) for a novel GEFS+ locus on chromosome 2p24. Among the 11 affected family members, 8 had typical FS but none developed epilepsy later in life. Three patients had epileptic seizures without a history of FS. The phenotype of this family did not exactly met the criteria of the GEFS+ syndrome, as none of the patients presented FS+. Linkage to chro-mosome 2p24 was confirmed by the authors in a collection of families with FS and epilepsy using nonparametric linkage approaches.
- We have recently mapped, by genome-wide search, a new gene for GEFS+ on 8p23-p21 in a three-generation French family with 11 affected members, 4 of which were defined as FS+ (maximum pairwise LOD score of 3.00).[59] A second four-generation family with FS and epilepsy was also possibly linked to the 8p23-p21 locus (maximum pairwise LOD score of 2.03). Because no neuronal ion channel genes are located in this interval, identification of the responsible gene will probably reveal a new mechanism of pathogenesis of GEFS+.

In conclusion, the 3 genes, *SCN1B*, *SCN1A,* and *GABRG2*, account for only 15% to 20% of GEFS+ families studied. The most commonly reported GEFS+ gene is *SCN1A*, in which only missense mutations are found. The challenging question is whether the type of channelopathy influences clinical features in GEFS+. We have shown that significantly more patients seem to express isolated FS in association with a mutation in *GABRG2* (46%) than *SCN1A* (17%), whereas many more had FS+ with a mutation in *SCN1A* (57%) than in *GABRG2* (13%).[60] Recently, a study reported that patients with FS and FS+ with *SCN1A* mutations had earlier median onset of FS compared with the population median. Patients with *GABRG2* mutations had a similar early onset in contrast to patients with *SCN1B* mutations where onset was later.[61]

ADOLESCENCE AND ADULT-ONSET EPILEPSY SYNDROMES
Autosomal Dominant Nocturnal Frontal Lobe Epilepsy

Autosomal dominant nocturnal frontal lobe epilepsy (ADNFLE) is an idiopathic focal epileptic syndrome generally beginning in the first 2 decades of life. ADNFLE is characterized by clusters of brief nocturnal motor seizures, with hyperkinetic or tonic manifestations arising from the frontal regions and occurring predominantly during sleep.[62] ADNFLE has been recognized as an autosomal dominant entity with approximately 70% penetrance. Phenotypes among ADNFLE families are relatively homogeneous, with only mild variation between affected family members.[63]

The first gene to be found mutated among monogenic epilepsies was the *CHRNA4* gene, encoding the $\alpha4$ subunit of the nicotinic acetylcholine receptor. Steinlein and colleagues[1] found a missense mutation (Ser248Phe) in a large Australian kindred linked to chromosome 20q. The causative role of *CHRNA4* in ADNFLE was further supported by the report of several mutations in 10 other families (for review, see Marini and Guerrini[64]). It appears that two mutations are recurrent: Ser248Phe and Ser252-Leu. *CHRNA4* mutations have also subsequently been discovered in sporadic nocturnal frontal lobe epilepsy: de novo mutations Ser252Leu[65] and R308H[66] have been reported.

Using a "candidate-gene" approach, two groups have independently identified missense mutations in two ADNFLE families of Italian (V287L)[67] and Scottish origin (V287M)[68] in the *CHRNB2* gene that encodes the $\beta2$ subunit of the nicotinic receptor. The same Val287Met mutation was also found in a four-generation Spanish ADNFLE family.[69] A novel *CHRNB2* mutation (I312M) was recently identified in an additional family.[70] Given the rarity of mutations, the role of *CHRNB2* seems to be minor in ADFNLE.

In 2006, a third nicotinic acetylcholine receptor gene, *CHRNA2*, encoding the $\alpha2$ subunit was reported to be mutated in an Italian family, revealing a novel missense mutation (I279N).[71] The absence of mutations among a cohort of 47 ADNFLE families suggests that a major role of *CHRNA2* in ADNFLE is unlikely.[72]

Interestingly, nicotinic acetylcholine receptor mutations were all located within the first, second, or third transmembrane domain. The one characteristic that all mutations have in common is that they increase the acetylcholine sensitivity of nAChRs, indicating that a gain-of-function effect probably underlies this type of epilepsy.[64] Although over a hundred families are on record, only a minority of them (less than 10%) have been linked to mutations in the *CHRNA4*, *CHRNA2*, and *CHRNB2* genes indicating that ADNFLE is genetically heterogeneous despite a relatively homogeneous clinical picture. A group has illustrated the considerable genetic heterogeneity for ADNFLE by demonstrating the absence of linkage to the *CHRNA4*, *CHRNA2*, and *CHRNB2* loci in three Italian families.[73] Another ADNFLE locus has been mapped to chromosome 15q24 in one family.[74] Although this region is close to a cluster of genes encoding other subunits of the nicotinic acetylcholine receptor, Bonati and colleagues[75] demonstrated that these genes were localized outside the candidate region. The causative gene for ADNFLE in 15q24 remains to be identified.

Autosomal Dominant Lateral Temporal Lobe Epilepsy

Autosomal dominant lateral temporal epilepsy (ADLTE) also named autosomal domi-nant partial epilepsy with auditory features (ADPEAF) is an inherited epileptic syndrome with onset in the first to third decades of life, no hippocampal sclerosis, and no associ-ation with FS.[76] Patients have focal-onset seizures with or without secondarily general-ized tonic-clonic seizures. The hallmark is the auditory component, most often as the aura, sometimes as a triggering factor of the partial seizures. Ictal manifestations may include aphasic, visual, or pseudo vertiginous symptoms, which also point to an involvement of the lateral temporal lobe or adjacent cortical areas. The auditory aura, often compared with a refrigerator noise, a radio sound, or modification of the auditory environment, like sounds in the background coming forward, suggests a very focal onset in the auditory cortex or in its close vicinity.

A locus was mapped to chromosome 10q22-24 in 1995[77] and mutations in the *LGI1* (leucine-rich glioma-inactivated 1) gene have been identified.[2,3] It is now recognized that *LGI1* is mutated in about 50% of ADLTE families.[78,79] In addition, de novo *LGI1* mutations are reported in about 2% of sporadic cases with idiopathic partial epilepsy with auditory features, who are clinically similar to patients with ADLTE but have no family history.[80,81] Nearly half of the 25 *LGI1* mutations so far reported are nonsense and frameshift mutations, suggesting a loss-of-function mechanism, but no obvious genotype-phenotype correlations emerge.[78] In addition, all missense mutations seem to lead to the same common mechanism: an absence of secretion of the mutated LGI1 protein by transfected mammalian cells.[82–86] Little is known about the LGI1 protein also named epitempin. It consists of an N-terminal leucine-rich repeat region and a C-terminal EAR (epilepsy-associated repeat) region,[87] and it is a secreted protein.[84] The function of LGI1 is still debated. Originally identified in glioma studies,[88] the *LGI1* gene is currently considered not to play any important role in brain tumors. LGI1 was first reported to bind and slow the inactivation of the Kv1.1 potassium channel.[89] Second, LGI1 was also suggested to enhance AMPA receptor-mediated synaptic transmission after secretion and binding to ADAM22.[90]

Familial Mesial Temporal Lobe Epilepsy

Familial mesial temporal lobe epilepsy (FMTLE) is a heterogeneous entity. One important subgroup is characterized by a relatively good prognosis, an aura with prominent psychic and autonomic features, absence of antecedent FS, and of hippocampal scle-rosis.[91] Most of the families present an autosomal dominant inheritance pattern with incomplete penetrance. Subsequently, it became apparent that the relationship between FMTLE syndromes, hippocampal sclerosis, and FS is more complex, with the description of TLE families with more severe syndromes, variable association with FS, and hippocampal sclerosis in some of the affected individuals.[60]

We have reported a clinical and genetic study of a French family among whom FS were associated with subsequent TLE in the same individual, without MRI-identifiable hippocampal abnormalities.[92] After scanning the entire genome, first with 380 micro-satellite markers, then with 10 000 SNPs (Stephanie Baulac, PhD, unpublished data), significant LOD scores for markers on 18qter (maximum pairwise LOD score of 3.03) and suggestive LOD scores (maximum pairwise LOD score of 2.33) for markers on 1q25-q31 were obtained supporting the hypothesis that mutations in two genes segregated with the phenotype.

Claes and colleagues[93] have mapped a second locus on chromosome 12q23 (maximum pairwise LOD score of 6.94) in an extended pedigree with familial TLE and FS, where the two disorders of TLE and FS did not systematically co-occur in the same individual.

Hedera and colleagues[94] detected a significant linkage on chromosome 4q13.2-q21.3 (maximum pairwise LOD score of 4.23) in a single large family characterized by a relatively benign course, absence of antecedent FS, and absence of hippocampal sclerosis.

A genetic study of 15 Italian families failed to show any linkage to the previously mentioned loci demonstrating the heterogeneity and the rarity of these genes, which remain to be identified.[95] None of these linkage have been replicated yet.

Familial Partial Epilepsy with Variable Foci

Familial partial epilepsy with variable foci (FPEVF) is an autosomal dominant syndrome characterized by partial seizures where the electroclinical features show that they originate from different brain regions among affected family members in the absence of MRI-detectable structural abnormalities.

Scheffer and colleagues[96] performed a genome-wide search on an Australian family with 10 individuals with partial seizures over four generations and reported a suggestion of linkage on chromosome 2q with a maximum pairwise LOD score of 2.74.

Xiong and colleagues[97] mapped a gene for FPEVF to chromosome 22q12 in two large French-Canadian families characterized by mostly nocturnal seizures arising from frontal, temporal, and occasionally occipital epileptic foci. Linkage was replicated in a four-generation Dutch family with clinical characteristics that fulfilled criteria of both ADNFLE and FPEVF[98] and subsequently in a Spanish and a third French-Canadian family.[99] An Australian family with a similar phenotype did not show any linkage to chromosome 22, indicating genetic heterogeneity of FPEVF.[97]

Juvenile Myoclonic Epilepsy

Juvenile myoclonic epilepsy (JME) accounts for 3% to 12% of all epilepsies. The JME phenotype is characterized by adolescent onset and lifelong grand mal (clonic-tonic-clonic), myoclonic, and absence seizures, and diffuse 3.5- to 6.0-Hz polyspike waves.

Cossette and colleagues[100] conducted a genome scan and found evidence of linkage to chromosome 5q34 in a French-Canadian family with autosomal dominant JME. A missense mutation, A322D, was identified in the *GABRA1* gene, which encodes the $\alpha 1$ subunit of the $GABA_A$ receptor. Ma and colleagues[101] subsequently investigated the contribution of *GABRA1* in a cohort of 54 JME Caucasian families, but failed to detect any disease-causing mutations, suggesting that most autosomal dominant JME is not caused by mutations in the *GABRA1*.

Two other mutation-harboring genes (*CLCN2*[102] and *EFHC1*[103]) have been identified for JME, but only the *GABRA1* gene seems to be a major effect gene, whereas *CLCN2* and *EFHC1* appear to be susceptibility genes.[104]

PERSPECTIVES

The vast majority of inherited idiopathic epilepsies, which occur in individuals with no evident underlying brain disorder before the onset of seizures, belong to the family of channelopathies, with the exception of *LGI1*. To date, idiopathic epilepsies with autosomal dominant inheritance are caused by rare heterozygous mutations in genes encoding potassium and sodium voltage-gated channels, neurotransmitter GABA and acetylcholine receptors and LGI1. These molecular discoveries have also highlighted the increasing complexity of phenotype-genotype correlations in epilepsy channelopathies; the same syndrome can be caused by mutations in different subunit channel genes (eg, *KCNQ2* and *KCNQ3*) or different channel genes (eg, *SCN1A* and *GABRG2*) and different mutations in the same gene can cause distinct phenotypes (eg, *SCN1A*). However, the interest of working on rare Mendelian families has been more than proven by the discovery of *SCN1A* mutations in the devastating Dravet syndrome. Because infants with Dravet syndrome have a strong predilection to seizures with fever, like in the benign GEFS+ syndrome, de novo mutations in *SCN1A* were discovered in more than 70% of children with Dravet syndrome. Early recognition of Dravet syndrome is important, as aggressive control of seizures may improve developmental outcome and *SCN1A* testing is thus essential. However, the phenomenon of parental mosaicism has important implications for genetic counseling in Dravet syndrome.

Identifying New Genes: A Revolution Coming Soon in Genetics

A new generation of high-throughput sequencing technologies promises to transform genetic research, opening up many new possibilities. Sanger sequencing for mutation detection in genes located in the morbid loci is expansive and time-consuming. Now, selective capture of sequence fragments from patient DNA, coupled with next-generation sequencing, will revolutionize the search for mutations in targeted genes located within the morbid loci. Sequence capture arrays will allow exhaustive mutational screening in all coding sequences of a region of several megabases. Analysis by high-throughput sequencing represents a flexible and cost-effective approach for large-scale resequencing of complex genomes. In addition, structural variant duplications, small insertions and deletions, and larger structural rearrangements that are likely to be important contributors to disease will be detected by next-generation sequencing. Detection of a tremendous number of variants is expected, and strategies for validation of these changes will need to be elaborated.

The most frequent etiologic assumption for choosing the candidate gene is that epilepsy belongs to the "channelopathy" family; thus, ion channel and neurotransmitter receptor genes are frequent candidates. These genes have usually already been sequenced and excluded for each loci associated with epilepsy, through traditional polymerase chain reaction sequencing methods. Exhaustive sequencing will allow an etiologic assumption–free approach and will probably lead to the discovery of epilepsy-genes with novel functions.

Approaching Some Mechanisms of Epileptogenesis

When a variant is identified in a gene encoding an ion channel, a modification of the function of the channel must be shown to prove causality of the mutation. Several cellular or animal models suggest that mutations in the various ion channels or their receptors may change the properties of the channel in several distinct ways. For instance, several of the *SCN1A* mutations found in epilepsy seem to increase excitability, although the opposite effect has also been reported. The functional result, even for a single *SCN1A* mutation, may vary between different model systems, and depending on the neural network, the alteration may induce a loss or a gain of function at the synaptic level. In addition, mutations introducing a premature stop, like most of the *SCN1A* alterations in Dravet syndrome, result in haploinsufficiency that would theoretically reduce neuronal excitability. Recently, the study of a knock-in mouse line with an *SCN1A* loss-of-function nonsense mutation recapitulating the human Dravet syndrome suggested that *SCN1A* haploinsufficiency causes a loss of cellular excitability in inhibitory cells predominantly, and not in the excitatory pyramidal cells.[105] This failure of GABAergic interneurons produces an increase in overall cortical excitability. A wide range of functional in vitro experiments in heterologous systems have studied the consequences of the SCN1A mutations causing GEFS+ mutations; no common mechanism of ion channel dysfunction underpinning the epilepsy phenotype has been identified.

Identification of further epilepsy genes will also allow uncovering of novel actors involved in epileptogenesis. Study of the function of LGI1, the only non-ion channel gene so far identified in monogenic idiopathic epilepsy, will probably lead to new pathways for the understanding of temporal lobe epilepsies.

Finding New Drug Targets

How can epilepsy gene hunting lead to better care for patients with epilepsy? Most of the presently available antiepileptic drugs appear to be directed against ion channel targets or other components of the synaptic machinery.[106] An example is provided by the parallel between the discovery of the implication of KCNQ2 and KCNQ3 genes in BFNS, and the development of retigabine, a potent KCNQ channel opener, a novel anticonvulsant with a broad but distinctive efficacy profile in animal studies. The efficiency of retigabine has been recently confirmed in phase III clinical trials.[107] This development suggests that KCNQ channels may be an important new class of targets for anticonvulsant therapies. The importance of M-channel function in reducing neuronal excitability has been increased by the finding that KCNQ2/3 mutations causing mild reduction of M-channel activity are linked to neonatal epilepsy. The M-channel has thus emerged as a promising target for treating epilepsy.

SV2A, a synaptic vesicle protein, has recently been identified as the likely target for levetiracetam[108] and potential follow-on structural analogs. Mice in which the protein has been deleted by gene targeting exhibit seizures.[109] It seems reasonable that the SV2A ligands could protect against seizures through effects on synaptic release mechanisms. Although SV2A is directly linked to the synaptic machinery, this illustrates that non-ion channel proteins may be important targets for antiepileptics. In certain idiopathic epilepsies, the causative genes do not encode subunits of ion channels or neurotransmitter receptor, but unknown proteins like LGI1. Understanding the physiology of such proteins may lead to defining new targets for anticonvulsant and antiepileptogenic therapeutic agents.

ACKNOWLEDGMENTS

We thank Dr. Richard Miles for critical reading of the manuscript and Luce Follea for design of figure 2 figures. This paper was supported in part by Sanofi-Aventis.

REFERENCES

1. Steinlein OK, Mulley JC, Propping P, et al. A missense mutation in the neuronal nicotinic acetylcholine receptor alpha 4 subunit is associated with autosomal dominant nocturnal frontal lobe epilepsy. Nat Genet 1995;11:201–3.
2. Kalachikov S, Evgrafov O, Ross B, et al. Mutations in LGI1 cause autosomal-dominant partial epilepsy with auditory features. Nat Genet 2002;30:335–41.
3. Morante-Redolat JM, Gorostidi-Pagola A, Piquer-Sirerol S, et al. Mutations in the LGI1/Epitempin gene on 10q24 cause autosomal dominant lateral temporal epilepsy. Hum Mol Genet 2002;11:1119–28.
4. Deprez L, Jansen A, De Jonghe P, et al. Genetics of epilepsy syndromes starting in the first year of life. Neurology 2009;72:273–81.

5. Biervert C, Schroeder BC, Kubisch C, et al. A potassium channel mutation in neonatal human epilepsy. Science 1998;279:403–6.
6. Singh NA, Charlier C, Stauffer D, et al. A novel potassium channel gene, KCNQ2, is mutated in an inherited epilepsy of newborns. Nat Genet 1998;18:25–9.
7. Charlier C, Singh NA, Ryan SG, et al. A pore mutation in a novel KQT-like potassium channel gene in an idiopathic epilepsy family. Nat Genet 1998;18:53–5.
8. Soldovieri MV, Miceli F, Bellini G, et al. Correlating the clinical and genetic features of benign familial neonatal seizures (BFNS) with the functional consequences of underlying mutations. Channels (Austin) 2007;1:228–33.
9. Claes LR, Ceulemans B, Audenaert D, et al. De novo KCNQ2 mutations in patients with benign neonatal seizures. Neurology 2004;63:2155–8.
10. Ishii A, Fukuma G, Uehara A, et al. A de novo KCNQ2 mutation detected in non-familial benign neonatal convulsions. Brain Dev 2009;31:27–33.
11. Singh NA, Westenskow P, Charlier C, et al. KCNQ2 and KCNQ3 potassium channel genes in benign familial neonatal convulsions: expansion of the functional and mutation spectrum. Brain 2003;126:2726–37.
12. Berkovic SF, Heron SE, Giordano L, et al. Benign familial neonatal-infantile seizures: characterization of a new sodium channelopathy. Ann Neurol 2004;55:550–7.
13. Herlenius E, Heron SE, Grinton BE, et al. SCN2A mutations and benign familial neonatal-infantile seizures: the phenotypic spectrum. Epilepsia 2007;48:1138–42.
14. Heron SE, Crossland KM, Andermann E, et al. Sodium-channel defects in benign familial neonatal-infantile seizures. Lancet 2002;360:851–2.
15. Vigevano F. BM: idiopathic and/or benign localization-related epilepsies in infants and young children. In: Roger JBM DC, Genton P, Tassinari CA, et al, editors. Epileptic syndromes in infancy, childhood and adolescence. 3rd edition. Eastleigh (UK): John Libbey & Co Ltd; 2002.
16. Guipponi M, Rivier F, Vigevano F, et al. Linkage mapping of benign familial infantile convulsions (BFIC) to chromosome 19q. Hum Mol Genet 1997;6:473–7.
17. Callenbach PM, van den Boogerd EH, de Coo RF, et al. Refinement of the chromosome 16 locus for benign familial infantile convulsions. Clin Genet 2005;67:517–25.
18. Caraballo R, Pavek S, Lemainque A, et al. Linkage of benign familial infantile convulsions to chromosome 16p12-q12 suggests allelism to the infantile convulsions and choreoathetosis syndrome. Am J Hum Genet 2001;68:788–94.
19. Szepetowski P, Rochette J, Berquin P, et al. Familial infantile convulsions and paroxysmal choreoathetosis: a new neurological syndrome linked to the pericentromeric region of human chromosome 16. Am J Hum Genet 1997;61:889–98.
20. Hauser WA. The prevalence and incidence of convulsive disorders in children. Epilepsia 1994;35(Suppl 2):S1–6.
21. Tsuboi T. Epidemiology of febrile and afebrile convulsions in children in Japan. Neurology 1984;34:175–81.
22. Annegers JF, Hauser WA, Elveback LR, et al. The risk of epilepsy following febrile convulsions. Neurology 1979;29:297–303.
23. Scheffer IE, Berkovic SF. Generalized epilepsy with febrile seizures plus. A genetic disorder with heterogeneous clinical phenotypes. Brain 1997;120(Pt 3):479–90.
24. Johnson WG, Kugler SL, Stenroos ES, et al. Pedigree analysis in families with febrile seizures. Am J Med Genet 1996;61:345–52.

25. Nakayama J. Progress in searching for the febrile seizure susceptibility genes. Brain Dev 2009;31:359–65.
26. Johnson EW, Dubovsky J, Rich SS, et al. Evidence for a novel gene for familial febrile convulsions, FEB2, linked to chromosome 19p in an extended family from the Midwest. Hum Mol Genet 1998;7:63–7.
27. Kugler SL, Stenroos ES, Mandelbaum DE, et al. Hereditary febrile seizures: phenotype and evidence for a chromosome 19p locus. Am J Med Genet 1998;79:354–61.
28. Nabbout R, Prud'homme JF, Herman A, et al. A locus for simple pure febrile seizures maps to chromosome 6q22-q24. Brain 2002;125:2668–80.
29. Wallace RH, Berkovic SF, Howell RA, et al. Suggestion of a major gene for familial febrile convulsions mapping to 8q13-21. J Med Genet 1996;33:308–12.
30. Peiffer A, Thompson J, Charlier C, et al. A locus for febrile seizures (FEB3) maps to chromosome 2q23-24. Ann Neurol 1999;46:671–8.
31. Escayg A, MacDonald BT, Meisler MH, et al. Mutations of SCN1A, encoding a neuronal sodium channel, in two families with GEFS+2. Nat Genet 2000;24:343–5.
32. Mantegazza M, Gambardella A, Rusconi R, et al. Identification of an Nav1.1 sodium channel (SCN1A) loss-of-function mutation associated with familial simple febrile seizures. Proc Natl Acad Sci U S A 2005;102:18177–82.
33. Hedera P, Ma S, Blair MA, et al. Identification of a novel locus for febrile seizures and epilepsy on chromosome 21q22. Epilepsia 2006;47:1622–8.
34. Nabbout R, Baulac S, Desguerre I, et al. New locus for febrile seizures with absence epilepsy on 3p and a possible modifier gene on 18p. Neurology 2007;68:1374–81.
35. Nakayama J, Yamamoto N, Hamano K, et al. Linkage and association of febrile seizures to the IMPA2 gene on human chromosome 18. Neurology 2004;63:1803–7.
36. Dai XH, Chen WW, Wang X, et al. A novel genetic locus for familial febrile seizures and epilepsy on chromosome 3q26.2-q26.33. Hum Genet 2008;124:423–9.
37. Singh R, Scheffer IE, Crossland K, et al. Generalized epilepsy with febrile seizures plus: a common childhood-onset genetic epilepsy syndrome. Ann Neurol 1999;45:75–81.
38. Scheffer I. BS: generalized (genetic) epilepsy with febrile seizures plus. In: Engel JJ PT, editor. Philadelphia: Lippincott, Williams &Wilkins; 2008. p. 2553–8.
39. Wallace RH, Wang DW, Singh R, et al. Febrile seizures and generalized epilepsy associated with a mutation in the Na+-channel beta1 subunit gene SCN1B. Nat Genet 1998;19:366–70.
40. Scheffer IE, Harkin LA, Grinton BE, et al. Temporal lobe epilepsy and GEFS+ phenotypes associated with SCN1B mutations. Brain 2007;130:100–9.
41. Wallace RH, Scheffer IE, Parasivam G, et al. Generalized epilepsy with febrile seizures plus: mutation of the sodium channel subunit SCN1B. Neurology 2002;58:1426–9.
42. Meadows LS, Malhotra J, Loukas A, et al. Functional and biochemical analysis of a sodium channel beta1 subunit mutation responsible for generalized epilepsy with febrile seizures plus type 1. J Neurosci 2002;22:10699–709.
43. Audenaert D, Claes L, Ceulemans B, et al. A deletion in SCN1B is associated with febrile seizures and early-onset absence epilepsy. Neurology 2003;61:854–6.

44. Lossin C. A catalog of SCN1A variants. Brain Dev 2009;31:114–30.
45. Claes L, Del-Favero J, Ceulemans B, et al. De novo mutations in the sodium-channel gene SCN1A cause severe myoclonic epilepsy of infancy. Am J Hum Genet 2001;68:1327–32.
46. Dravet C, Bureau M, Oguni H, et al. Severe myoclonic epilepsy in infancy: Dravet syndrome. Adv Neurol 2005;95:71–102.
47. Scheffer IE, Harkin LA, Dibbens LM, et al. Neonatal epilepsy syndromes and generalized epilepsy with febrile seizures plus (GEFS+). Epilepsia 2005; 46(Suppl 10):41–7.
48. Depienne C, Trouillard O, Saint-Martin C, et al. Spectrum of SCN1A gene mutations associated with Dravet syndrome: analysis of 333 patients. J Med Genet 2009;46:183–91.
49. Depienne C, Arzimanoglou A, Trouillard O, et al. Parental mosaicism can cause recurrent transmission of SCN1A mutations associated with severe myoclonic epilepsy of infancy. Hum Mutat 2006;27:389.
50. Gennaro E, Santorelli FM, Bertini E, et al. Somatic and germline mosaicisms in severe myoclonic epilepsy of infancy. Biochem Biophys Res Commun 2006; 341:489–93.
51. Marini C, Mei D, Helen Cross J, et al. Mosaic SCN1A mutation in familial severe myoclonic epilepsy of infancy. Epilepsia 2006;47:1737–40.
52. Morimoto M, Mazaki E, Nishimura A, et al. SCN1A mutation mosaicism in a family with severe myoclonic epilepsy in infancy. Epilepsia 2006;47:1732–6.
53. Baulac S, Huberfeld G, Gourfinkel-An I, et al. First genetic evidence of GABA(A) receptor dysfunction in epilepsy: a mutation in the gamma2-subunit gene. Nat Genet 2001;28:46–8.
54. Wallace RH, Marini C, Petrou S, et al. Mutant GABA(A) receptor gamma2-subunit in childhood absence epilepsy and febrile seizures. Nat Genet 2001; 28:49–52.
55. Harkin LA, Bowser DN, Dibbens LM, et al. Truncation of the GABA(A)-receptor gamma2 subunit in a family with generalized epilepsy with febrile seizures plus. Am J Hum Genet 2002;70:530–6.
56. Audenaert D, Schwartz E, Claeys KG, et al. A novel GABRG2 mutation associated with febrile seizures. Neurology 2006;67:687–90.
57. Kananura C, Haug K, Sander T, et al. A splice-site mutation in GABRG2 associated with childhood absence epilepsy and febrile convulsions. Arch Neurol 2002;59:1137–40.
58. Audenaert D, Claes L, Claeys KG, et al. A novel susceptibility locus at 2p24 for generalised epilepsy with febrile seizures plus. J Med Genet 2005;42: 947–52.
59. Baulac S, Gourfinkel-An I, Couarch P, et al. A novel locus for generalized epilepsy with febrile seizures plus in French families. Arch Neurol 2008;65:943.
60. Baulac S, Gourfinkel-An I, Nabbout R, et al. Fever, genes, and epilepsy. Lancet Neurol 2004;3:421–30.
61. Sijben AE, Sithinamsuwan P, Radhakrishnan A, et al. Does a SCN1A gene mutation confer earlier age of onset of febrile seizures in GEFS+? Epilepsia 2009;50:953–6.
62. Scheffer IE, Bhatia KP, Lopes-Cendes I, et al. Autosomal dominant frontal epilepsy misdiagnosed as sleep disorder. Lancet 1994;343:515–7.
63. Scheffer IE, Bhatia KP, Lopes-Cendes I, et al. Autosomal dominant nocturnal frontal lobe epilepsy. A distinctive clinical disorder. Brain 1995;118(Pt 1):61–73.
64. Marini C, Guerrini R. The role of the nicotinic acetylcholine receptors in sleep-related epilepsy. Biochem Pharmacol 2007;74:1308–14.

65. Phillips HA, Marini C, Scheffer IE, et al. A de novo mutation in sporadic nocturnal frontal lobe epilepsy. Ann Neurol 2000;48:264–7.
66. Chen Y, Wu L, Fang Y, et al. A novel mutation of the nicotinic acetylcholine receptor gene CHRNA4 in sporadic nocturnal frontal lobe epilepsy. Epilepsy Res 2009;83:152–6.
67. De Fusco M, Becchetti A, Patrignani A, et al. The nicotinic receptor beta 2 subunit is mutant in nocturnal frontal lobe epilepsy. Nat Genet 2000;26:275–6.
68. Phillips HA, Favre I, Kirkpatrick M, et al. CHRNB2 is the second acetylcholine receptor subunit associated with autosomal dominant nocturnal frontal lobe epilepsy. Am J Hum Genet 2001;68:225–31.
69. Diaz-Otero F, Quesada M, Morales-Corraliza J, et al. Autosomal dominant nocturnal frontal lobe epilepsy with a mutation in the CHRNB2 gene. Epilepsia 2008;49:516–20.
70. Cho YW, Yi SD, Lim JG, et al. Autosomal dominant nocturnal frontal lobe epilepsy and mild memory impairment associated with CHRNB2 mutation I312M in the neuronal nicotinic acetylcholine receptor. Epilepsy Behav 2008;13:361–5.
71. Aridon P, Marini C, Di Resta C, et al. Increased sensitivity of the neuronal nicotinic receptor alpha 2 subunit causes familial epilepsy with nocturnal wandering and ictal fear. Am J Hum Genet 2006;79:342–50.
72. Gu W, Bertrand D, Steinlein OK, et al. A major role of the nicotinic acetylcholine receptor gene CHRNA2 in autosomal dominant nocturnal frontal lobe epilepsy (ADNFLE) is unlikely. Neurosci Lett 2007;422:74–6.
73. De Marco EV, Gambardella A, Annesi F, et al. Further evidence of genetic heterogeneity in families with autosomal dominant nocturnal frontal lobe epilepsy. Epilepsy Res 2007;74:70–3.
74. Phillips HA, Scheffer IE, Crossland KM, et al. Autosomal dominant nocturnal frontal-lobe epilepsy: genetic heterogeneity and evidence for a second locus at 15q24. Am J Hum Genet 1998;63:1108–16.
75. Bonati MT, Asselta R, Duga S, et al. Refined mapping of CHRNA3/A5/B4 gene cluster and its implications in ADNFLE. Neuroreport 2000;11:2097–101.
76. Winawer MR, Ottman R, Hauser WA, et al. Autosomal dominant partial epilepsy with auditory features: defining the phenotype. Neurology 2000;54:2173–6.
77. Ottman R, Risch N, Hauser WA, et al. Localization of a gene for partial epilepsy to chromosome 10q. Nat Genet 1995;10:56–60.
78. Nobile C, Michelucci R, Andreazza S, et al. LGI1 mutations in autosomal dominant and sporadic lateral temporal epilepsy. Hum Mutat 2009;30:530–6.
79. Ottman R, Winawer MR, Kalachikov S, et al. LGI1 mutations in autosomal dominant partial epilepsy with auditory features. Neurology 2004;62:1120–6.
80. Bisulli F, Tinuper P, Scudellaro E, et al. A de novo LGI1 mutation in sporadic partial epilepsy with auditory features. Ann Neurol 2004;56:455–6.
81. Michelucci R, Mecarelli O, Bovo G, et al. A de novo LGI1 mutation causing idiopathic partial epilepsy with telephone-induced seizures. Neurology 2007;68:2150–1.
82. Chabrol E, Popescu C, Gourfinkel-An I, et al. Two novel epilepsy-linked mutations leading to a loss of function of LGI1. Arch Neurol 2007;64:217–22.
83. de Bellescize J, Boutry N, Chabrol E, et al. A novel three base-pair LGI1 deletion leading to loss of function in a family with autosomal dominant lateral temporal epilepsy and migraine-like episodes. Epilepsy Res 2009;85:118–22.
84. Senechal KR, Thaller C, Noebels JL, et al. ADPEAF mutations reduce levels of secreted LGI1, a putative tumor suppressor protein linked to epilepsy. Hum Mol Genet 2005;14:1613–20.

85. Sirerol-Piquer MS, Ayerdi-Izquierdo A, Morante-Redolat JM, et al. The epilepsy gene LGI1 encodes a secreted glycoprotein that binds to the cell surface. Hum Mol Genet 2006;15:3436–45.
86. Striano P, de Falco A, Diani E, et al. A novel loss-of-function LGI1 mutation linked to autosomal dominant lateral temporal epilepsy. Arch Neurol 2008;65:939–42.
87. Staub E, Perez-Tur J, Siebert R, et al. The novel EPTP repeat defines a superfamily of proteins implicated in epileptic disorders. Trends Biochem Sci 2002;27:441–4.
88. Chernova OB, Somerville RP, Cowell JK, et al. A novel gene, LGI1, from 10q24 is rearranged and downregulated in malignant brain tumors. Oncogene 1998;17: 2873–81.
89. Schulte U, Thumfart JO, Klocker N, et al. The epilepsy-linked Lgi1 protein assembles into presynaptic Kv1 channels and inhibits inactivation by Kvbeta1. Neuron 2006;49:697–706.
90. Fukata Y, Adesnik H, Iwanaga T, et al. Epilepsy-related ligand/receptor complex LGI1 and ADAM22 regulate synaptic transmission. Science 2006;313:1792–5.
91. Berkovic SF, McIntosh A, Howell RA, et al. Familial temporal lobe epilepsy: a common disorder identified in twins. Ann Neurol 1996;40:227–35.
92. Baulac S, Picard F, Herman A, et al. Evidence for digenic inheritance in a family with both febrile convulsions and temporal lobe epilepsy implicating chromosomes 18qter and 1q25-q31. Ann Neurol 2001;49:786–92.
93. Claes L, Audenaert D, Deprez L, et al. Novel locus on chromosome 12q22-q23.3 responsible for familial temporal lobe epilepsy associated with febrile seizures. J Med Genet 2004;41:710–4.
94. Hedera P, Blair MA, Andermann E, et al. Familial mesial temporal lobe epilepsy maps to chromosome 4q13.2-q21.3. Neurology 2007;68:2107–12.
95. Striano P, Gambardella A, Coppola A, et al. Familial mesial temporal lobe epilepsy (FMTLE): a clinical and genetic study of 15 Italian families. J Neurol 2008;255:16–23.
96. Scheffer IE, Phillips HA, O'Brien CE, et al. Familial partial epilepsy with variable foci: a new partial epilepsy syndrome with suggestion of linkage to chromosome 2. Ann Neurol 1998;44:890–9.
97. Xiong L, Labuda M, Li DS, et al. Mapping of a gene determining familial partial epilepsy with variable foci to chromosome 22q11-q12. Am J Hum Genet 1999; 65:1698–710.
98. Callenbach PM, van den Maagdenberg AM, Hottenga JJ, et al. Familial partial epilepsy with variable foci in a Dutch family: clinical characteristics and confirmation of linkage to chromosome 22q. Epilepsia 2003;44:1298–305.
99. Berkovic SF, Serratosa JM, Phillips HA, et al. Familial partial epilepsy with variable foci: clinical features and linkage to chromosome 22q12. Epilepsia 2004;45:1054–60.
100. Cossette P, Liu L, Brisebois K, et al. Mutation of GABRA1 in an autosomal dominant form of juvenile myoclonic epilepsy. Nat Genet 2002;31:184–9.
101. Ma S, Blair MA, Abou-Khalil B, et al. Mutations in the GABRA1 and EFHC1 genes are rare in familial juvenile myoclonic epilepsy. Epilepsy Res 2006;71:129–34.
102. Haug K, Warnstedt M, Alekov AK, et al. Mutations in CLCN2 encoding a voltage-gated chloride channel are associated with idiopathic generalized epilepsies. Nat Genet 2003;33:527–32.
103. Suzuki T, Delgado-Escueta AV, Aguan K, et al. Mutations in EFHC1 cause juvenile myoclonic epilepsy. Nat Genet 2004;36:842–9.
104. Greenberg DA, Pal DK. The state of the art in the genetic analysis of the epilepsies. Curr Neurol Neurosci Rep 2007;7:320–8.

105. Ogiwara I, Miyamoto H, Morita N, et al. Na(v)1.1 localizes to axons of parvalbumin-positive inhibitory interneurons: a circuit basis for epileptic seizures in mice carrying an Scn1a gene mutation. J Neurosci 2007;27: 5903–14.
106. Rogawski MA, Loscher W. The neurobiology of antiepileptic drugs. Nat Rev Neurosci 2004;5:553–64.
107. Porter RJ, Partiot A, Sachdeo R, et al. Randomized, multicenter, dose-ranging trial of retigabine for partial-onset seizures. Neurology 2007;68:1197–204.
108. Lynch BA, Lambeng N, Nocka K, et al. The synaptic vesicle protein SV2A is the binding site for the antiepileptic drug levetiracetam. Proc Natl Acad Sci U S A 2004;101:9861–6.
109. Janz R, Goda Y, Geppert M, et al. SV2A and SV2B function as redundant Ca2+ regulators in neurotransmitter release. Neuron 1999;24:1003–16.

Sudden Unexpected Death in Epilepsy (SUDEP): Update and Reflections

Lina Nashef, MBCHB, MD, FRCP[a],*, Philippe Ryvlin, MD, PhD[b,c]

KEYWORDS

- Epilepsy • SUDEP • Definitions • AEDs
- Mortemus • Supervision

Although initially well known to specialists in the nineteenth and early twentieth centuries, later in the twentieth century intrinsic dangers associated with epilepsy were denied. Gradually, however, acceptance replaced denial, and the subject has been "topical" for some years. Yet, despite significant strides, there has been little translational research and virtually no advance in prevention. Instead, an almost fatalistic attitude has been adopted in some quarters. Unselected epidemiologic studies with similar designs in different populations, reviews, and repetition dominate the literature, and, with notable exceptions, with little sense of direction. Those seeking yet another comprehensive review of the subject will not find it in this article, and are advised to read one of the many texts available.[1–6] This article reflects on current knowledge, and on how we may seek answers to what we need to know to quantify, monitor, and reduce risk. A brief overview is followed by a discussion of definitions, drug treatment, genetic susceptibility, mechanisms in relation to seizure monitoring and supervision, with some suggestions for the way forward.

OVERVIEW

There is excess mortality in epilepsy compared with the general population. Most of the excess is due to underlying disease, but some is epilepsy related, including accidental trauma, drowning, status epilepticus, suicide, and sudden unexpected

[a] Neurology Department, King's College Hospital, Denmark Hill, London, United Kingdom, SE5 9RS
[b] Department of Functional Neurology and Epileptology and CTRS-IDEE (Institut des Epilepsies de l'Enfant et de l'Adolescent), Hospices Civils de Lyon, INSERM U821, France
[c] Université Claude Bernard Lyon 1, Lyon, France
* Corresponding author.
E-mail address: lina.nashef@kch.nhs.uk (L. Nashef).

Neurol Clin 27 (2009) 1063–1074
doi:10.1016/j.ncl.2009.08.003
0733-8619/09/$ – see front matter © 2009 Elsevier Inc. All rights reserved.

death in epilepsy (SUDEP), which constitutes a significant proportion of epilepsy-related deaths. In young people, in whom background mortality is low, SUDEP is noticeable, but amongst older people, any excess is hidden by high background mortality and other competing causes. Incidence rates observed vary depending on the population studied. A population-based study by Ficker and colleagues[7] reported an incidence of 0.35 per 1000, based on a small number of cases. The risk of sudden death was 24 times higher in the epilepsy population compared with the general population. SUDEP incidence is higher in selected cohorts, with a wide spread of reported incidence rates up to 1 in 100 in intractable surgical series.[1] Different risk factors and mechanisms may operate with a final common pathway of cardiorespiratory failure, likely to be periictal. Respiratory compromise and hypoxia occur frequently in seizures and are caused not only by direct central mechanisms but also, in the absence of someone capable of giving assistance, by position and airway obstruction, during periictal coma, when self-adjustment of body position is impaired. Cardiac changes are also frequent during seizures, with ictal sinus tachycardia most commonly recorded. Bradycardia/sinus arrest also occur, albeit infrequently, as do rare malignant dysrrhythmias. Functional cardiac changes such as apical ballooning may also occur. Case control studies, with different methodologies, control groups, and case ascertainment,[1,8–16] have identified some associated risk factors, the clearest of which is a history of generalized tonic-clonic seizures and uncontrolled epilepsy. It remains to be elucidated which factors make one individual more susceptible to this outcome than another with comparable epilepsy severity. Factors of particular interest, primarily because they are potentially amenable to modification, relate to aspects of treatment, lifestyle, and the likely protective effect of supervision.

WHAT'S IN A NAME? REVIEW OF DEFINITIONS

The definition of sudden death in epilepsy differs from that of sudden death in general, as the latter includes deaths with and without an identified pathologic cause. Sudden death in epilepsy refers to deaths without an identified pathologic or toxicologic cause of death, understandably leading to the use by some investigators of the adjective "unexplained," which evokes a sense of mystery. These deaths are not generally speaking unexplained, however, given that evidence favors that the majority of SUDEP cases occuring as a consequence of terminal seizures, but influenced by functional rather than structural mechanisms.

Earlier epidemiologic studies of mortality in epilepsy applied different definitions of SUDEP with regard to case ascertainment. In particular, although some were inclusive, other studies excluded cases where an epileptic seizure was "known" to have occurred around the time of death. It became quickly apparent, however, that it was not possible to classify most deaths into those with a definite terminal seizure and those without, even when detailed interviews looking at circumstances of death were performed.[17] Among the minority of witnessed events, there are some with observed habitual seizures, presumed epileptic, and others without, but in which epileptic activity cannot be excluded. Among unwitnessed events (the majority in most studies), there is often circumstantial evidence suggesting, but not unequivocally proving, an epileptic seizure, and others in which such evidence is lacking but in which a seizure, nevertheless, could have occurred. For example, clinical practice shows that although tongue bite is a good indicator of a generalized tonic-clonic seizure, as supported by an autopsy study,[18] absence of tongue bite does not exclude tonic-clonic seizure. The definition proposed was therefore a pragmatic workable definition that grouped these together (**Box 1**) and refers to a category not a condition, within which different mechanisms and circumstances may apply.

An area of ambiguity is the use of the terms asphyxiation and suffocation. Historically, deaths in epilepsy were frequently attributed to such mechanisms (**Box 2**) and asphyxiation was certified as a cause of death in epilepsy, at least in the United Kingdom. Although impediments to breathing and hypoxia, whether caused by the environment or body position, are likely contributory factors, it is too simplistic to ascribe the death to asphyxia or suffocation, in that the ictal and postictal coma may prevent correction in response to rising carbon dioxide or falling oxygen levels through self-adjustment of body position. Furthermore, it is not possible on pathologic grounds to differentiate categorically between deaths caused by asphyxia and deaths from other causes. The presence of petechial hemorrhages, for example, considered a sign of asphyxiation, has been shown not to be specific. Subpericardial, subpleural and subendothelial hemorrhages may develop spontaneously after death. Subconjunctival petechiae occur with hypoxia and an acute increase in vascular cephalic pressure (with obstruction or right heart failure), and petechial hemorrhages can also occur after attempted resuscitation.[19] It is thus neither possible nor appropriate to create a separate category. Nevertheless, the finding of a significantly increased incidence of the prone position in SUDEP cases than would be expected by chance is of interest,[15] and provides one mechanism by which supervision may be protective. In the study of circumstances of death already referred to,[17] 11/26 patients were found in a position that could have compromised breathing.

As autopsy is not always performed, and if performed may be limited, researchers in the United States suggested levels of probability with cases classified as definite (with autopsy), probable (without autopsy), possible, and not SUDEP.[21] SUDEP would be considered only if the death was sudden and unexpected and occurred in benign circumstances. Although the concept behind this classification is helpful, particularly in epidemiologic studies, the "possible SUDEP" category, is unsatisfactory, in that it combines cases with insufficient information to classify the death with those in whom there is a competing cause for death. The late Dr. Annegers suggested that future criteria could consider subdividing the "possible" category. He suggested that, particularly where autopsy rates are low, definite and probable SUDEP cases are grouped together. For epidemiologic studies, he also suggested that an upper range of incidence rates is calculated to include possible cases.[22]

A limitation, from an epidemiologic point of view, of the definition given in **Box 1** is its focus on "pure" SUDEP cases. There are situations in which a death may be due to the combined or additive effect of the epilepsy and a concomitant condition. For example, in one study, in two patients aged 34 and 63 years with long-standing epilepsy, excluded from the SUDEP category, death occurred when witnessed habitual convulsive seizures ended abruptly, and autopsy revealed significant coronary atheroma.[17] In these cases epileptic seizures precipitated death in the presence of heart disease. Perhaps deaths caused by likely epileptic seizures with a concomitant cause of death could be classified as SUDEP Plus.

Box 1
SUDEP definition

Sudden, unexpected, witnessed or unwitnessed, nontraumatic and nondrowning death in an individual with epilepsy, with or without evidence for a seizure and excluding documented status epilepticus where postmortem examination does not reveal a cause for death.[19]

> **Box 2**
> **Delasiauve 1854**
>
> "La mort est due souvent à une suffocation mécanique spéciale. Atteints d'accès dans leur lit, les malades se retournent instinctivement sur le ventre le paroxysme les surprend dans cette position et les cloue, en quelque sorte, la face contre les oreiller ou le traversin. L'interruption de l'air ne tarde pas, si tous secours fait défaut, à provoquer l'asphyxie. On constate alors la bouffissure violacée du visage, du cou, et quelquefois de la partie supérieure de la poitrine; l'aplatissement des lèvres collées à la lange, qui se présente a leur ouverture; l'écrasement des narines et différents signes de congestion cérébrale et pulmonaire."[20]

MORTALITY IN EPILEPSY: THE BROAD VIEW

Research on SUDEP has largely failed to take a broad view, hence the interest generated by the publication of the results of the Ransom study in 2008.[23] The study looked at the medication possession ratio (MPR) in people on antiepileptic drug (AED) treatment through Medicaid. Quarters (i.e. Periods of 3 month each or 1/4 of the year) were labeled as "adherent" and "nonadherent", the latter if MPR was less than 80% of the prescribed dose. In this large study, in terms of patients (33,658) and quarters (388,564, 26% nonadherent), there was significantly increased overall mortality in the nonadherent quarters with narrow confidence intervals. This finding also applied to visits to emergency units, fractures, hospital admissions, and motor vehicle accident injuries. Although there may be unknown variables that could have influenced the findings, this study suggests that factors relating to AED treatment have clear bearing on mortality associated with epilepsy.

Mortality trends in epilepsy have also been studied in England in relation to geographic profile[24] using data from national statistics. Large differences are seen in mortality across regions and there is some relationship between mortality rate and deprivation index (a surrogate for social deprivation). Although interpretation requires further analysis, the data again suggest that there is some variation in mortality that may be amenable to intervention related to lifestyle, medical treatment, or compliance.

The reason for highlighting these 2 datasets is that in focusing on the detail, the bigger picture may have been missed. Some consistency is needed in death certification and national monitoring. In selected geographic areas, where various national medical and social records are already well developed, registers of SUDEP cases would allow for data to be analyzed in relation to other variables such as demographics, drug treatment, epilepsy services, deprivation, and lifestyle. These data could not only provide clues on risk factors but also allow for monitoring of trends, essential if any future interventions are to be tested, be they strictly medical or through a focus on lifestyle, self-management, adherence to treatment, and supervision. Furthermore, changes in SUDEP and in mortality in general may be affected by different patterns of prescribing, which need to be detected. As most cohorts are reported from tertiary centers with few population-based cohorts, the emphasis has been on severe intractable focal epilepsy. Yet it is clear from the literature and from those who make contact with the self-help group Epilepsy Bereaved that those with infrequent seizures and untreated epilepsy also die suddenly. Although their relative risk may be lower, given that most people with epilepsy are not at the severe end of the spectrum, their numbers may still be significant. They may constitute a category in which the potential for prevention is greater. Without large SUDEP registers or large-scale studies, their numbers could remain unknown.

AEDS: MORE FOCUS IS NEEDED

As alluded to earlier in this article, because AED prescribing and adherence to treatment are amenable to intervention, better understanding is needed of how AED prescribing may influence the risk of SUDEP. Initial studies looked at postmortem drug levels as a surrogate for adherence to treatment. Methodological problems, however, made it difficult to draw definitive conclusions and results of studies were contradictory.[2] Nevertheless, it is by no means excluded that lack of adherence to treatment may be a risk factor in some SUDEP cases. In case control studies, several drug-related factors emerged as significant in some studies. These factors include never having been treated,[9] number of previous AEDs tried,[9] polytherapy,[12,16] frequent change in medication,[16] and association with carbamazepine use or high levels thereof.[9,11] Caution is needed in the interpretation of these findings and association should not be equated with causality.

AEDs are likely to provide some protection against SUDEP by preventing seizures, an effect directly dependent on their antiepileptic efficacy. The finding in the largest case control study, that never having been treated is a risk factor, supports this view.[9] This remains an important starting premise. In a minority of patients, AEDs could have the opposite effect. AEDs may worsen seizures in some patients, particularly those with idiopathic generalized epilepsy if they are prescribed narrow-spectrum drugs. There are other theoretic considerations. An AED or AED combination could influence risk, not only by giving insufficient protection from severe seizures but also by altering risk through various potential mechanisms, perhaps stabilizing or destabilizing autonomic, cardiac, or brainstem function, either as a direct effect or if withdrawn abruptly. Some combinations or overmedication may affect the severity of the postictal phase. Some drugs may introduce more instability with medication changes or with lack of adherence to treatment than others. There could be trends in SUDEP incidence with changing trends in prescribing.

As an example, the article by Aurlien and colleagues[25] allows us to consider some of these issues. In discussing this in some detail, it is not the authors' intention specifically to implicate this particular AED. Aurlien and colleagues[25] reported on 4 consecutive young adult female SUDEP patients with idiopathic epilepsy treated with lamotrigine monotherapy. One was unclassified (focal aura, normal magnetic resonance imaging, generalized discharges on electroencephalogram [EEG]) and the others had idiopathic generalized epilepsy (one with juvenile myoclonic epilepsy [JME]). Last documented seizure frequency was: 1.5 simple partial seizures/month; seizure free for 6 and 7 months; two seizures during the last week (previously seizure-free for 3 months). The investigators considered the following possible explanations: an insufficient effect of lamotrigine leading to fatal seizures; a direct effect of lamotrigine on vital functions, such as cardiac rhythmicity; a combination of drug-induced effects and seizures; or coincidence. At autopsy, lamotrigine levels were as follows: not performed; none detectable (previously 7 μmol/L); 15 μmol/L (previously 24.4 μmol/L); 3.2 μmol/L (previously 27.5 μmol/L, when also on carbamazepine). Which of the possible explanations suggested is true is unknown. There may have been selection bias in preferential prescribing of lamotrigine to women of child-bearing age with idiopathic epilepsy. Valproate, although more effective,[26] may have been avoided because of potential teratogenicity. Notwithstanding reservations about accuracy of postmortem blood levels, another possible explanation is suggested by the absent or lower levels measured. Could there be a differential SUDEP risk associated with AED withdrawal, prescribed or otherwise, through an effect on seizure severity or autonomic function? Some people believe, for example, that the full effect of starting and stopping valproate in idiopathic epilepsy is not all immediate, with a delayed effect observed. Effective control may be lost less quickly with some drugs than others.

In a study elsewhere in this issue,[17] several drug factors were reported, some prescribed. At least some of these were likely to be relevant, although without a control group it is difficult to be certain. Examples of reported drug factors are as follows. Two of 26 SUDEP cases had never been prescribed treatment. Compliance was considered poor in one and unknown in another. A third, usually compliant, omitted a phenytoin dose 3 days before death. One had discontinued medication independently, whereas another, in remission, had spoken of drug reduction but it is not known if that had taken place. In another, medication was being withdrawn. Other prescribed reductions within 4 weeks of death included two with phenytoin withdrawal. In one, because of ongoing partial seizures, phenytoin was being substituted by carbamazepine in a crossover regime, with phenytoin reduced as carbamazepine was introduced. A witnessed tonic-clonic seizure occurred, the first in 9 months, the evening before an unwitnessed nocturnal death.

There are thus many aspects to drug prescribing that could affect risk but that have not begun to be unravelled. Some relate to drug prescribing, whereas others relate to adherence to treatment, and all need further exploration.

GENETIC SUSCEPTIBILITY

This topic is discussed in detail by Ghali and Nashef.[27] A synopsis is presented in this article. That a family history of sudden death has not generally been reported in SUDEP does not exclude a genetic tendency. Inheritance may be complex and penetrance reduced. To investigate a possible tendency, studies need to focus on specific syndromes, for example, idiopathic epilepsy, and look for possible overlap between SUDEP, cardiac syncope, sudden infant death syndrome (SIDS), intrauterine death, or premature sudden cardiac death. Although mortality data are limited in specific syndromes, there is a suggestion that mortality differs between epileptic syndromes over and above that expected from the severity of the epilepsy. There are examples of reported increased mortality in genetic symptomatic epilepsies, in which there is often multisystem involvement and more than one possible cause. Examples include the X-linked Rett syndrome, Lafora disease, mitochondrial encephalomyopathy, lactic acidosis and strokelike episodes (MELAS) and reportedly the inv dup15 chromosomal anomaly.[28,29]

The observation that most known genetic mutations in epilepsies affect ion channel genes, as in genetic long QT syndromes (LQTS), which cause increased susceptibility to sudden death, raised the possibility that epileptic channelopathies might favor sudden cardiac death. There is an increased mortality in Dravet syndrome or severe myoclonic epilepsy of infancy (SMEI) caused by *SCN1A* mutations. Mutations in the same gene account for 5% to 10% of families with generalized epilepsy with febrile seizures plus (GEFS+) and also cause familial hemiplegic migraine. A family with GEFS+ caused by a novel *SCN1A* mutation with 2 SUDEP cases in individuals with more severe epilepsy was reported.[30] *SCN1A* mutations may result in brainstem autonomic dysfunction and there is also evidence in animals of a role for Nav1.1 in sinoatrial pacemaker function. The *SCN1B* gene, implicated in GEFS+, absence epilepsy, and temporal lobe epilepsy, has now been reported in Brugada syndrome.[31] Aurlien and colleagues[32] reported a SUDEP case in which a novel missense mutation was found in the LQTS-associated gene *SCN5A* coding for the cardiac sodium channel and discussed whether the mutation may explain the epilepsy and sudden death.

Cases with idiopathic generalized epilepsies (IGE), but no known genetic mutations, with a history of generalized tonic seizures, are also well represented in SUDEP cohorts. In one case control study from Stockholm,[16] no increase in risk was associated with any particular type of epilepsy, although a lower risk was associated with localization-related symptomatic epilepsy compared with generalized idiopathic epilepsy, especially among men, but numbers were small and confidence intervals wide. The largest case control study by Langan and colleagues[9] from the United Kingdom did not find an association with syndromic classification; however, information on this variable was incomplete. In the study referred to earlier in this article on circumstances of death, 9/26 SUDEP cases were classified as having idiopathic primary generalized epilepsy.[17] This cohort was largely identified through the self-help group Epilepsy Bereaved rather than specialized services. Of these IGE cases, 1 with JME in remission on valproic acid had been considering medication reduction in the months before death, although it was not known if this had taken place. Two others had only ever been treated with carbamazepine or phenytoin. Two, both with a positive photoparoxysmal response on EEG, were found dead near visual display units. One was known to have discontinued medication independently and was found with a bitten tongue; the other, having only had a small number of convulsions in similar settings previously, had never been treated. Genton and Gelisse[33] reported 3 cases of premature death among 170 consecutive JME cases, 2 of whom would be classified as probable SUDEP cases (death rate of 0.9/1000). Overall, the available, although limited, evidence raises the possibility that in idiopathic epilepsy, with a history of generalized tonic-clonic seizures, SUDEP may occur more often than in other syndromes with comparable epilepsy severity. At present, this is only a suggestion, but it needs to be explored further. AED choices may be particularly important in this subgroup, as suggested by Aurlien and colleagues.[25]

The above refers to possible overlap in phenotype (epilepsy and cardiac) in genetic ion channel disorders, whereby a mutation primarily presents as epilepsy but also causes a predisposition to sudden death in those in whom convulsive seizures are uncontrolled. Another hypothesis is that there may be an unrelated coexisting "mild" susceptibility to sudden death, which would manifest itself in the presence of uncontrolled seizures.[34] To identify genetic susceptibility variants, a SUDEP clinical/DNA cohort needs to be established. Such work can be aided by identification and clarification of susceptibility variants to sudden cardiac deaths or SIDS using genome-wide association studies. Despite the dramatic success in reducing SIDS by altering sleeping position from prone to supine, and the focus on respiration, cardiac factors have also been found to be relevant. Around 5% to 10% of SIDS cases are now known to be linked to ion channelopathies. Schwartz and colleagues[35] first found evidence for this by performing a study of neonatal electrocardiograms (ECGs) for a period of 18 years and correlating this with SIDS. Other reported/studied genetic risk factors in SIDS include genes involved in inflammatory and infectious processes such as interleukin-10 (IL-10), genes pertinent to the development of the autonomic nervous system, and the serotonin transporter gene.[27,36]

The 5-HTT gene-linked polymorphic region (5-HTTLPR), whose various alleles (S, L_A, L_G) translate into functional differences in 5-HTT expression, is of particular interest because of the multiple link between epilepsy, serotonin, and respiration. The serotonergic caudal raphe nucleus plays a major role in the central control of respiration,[37] in particular in the context of repeated hypoxia, through so-called long-term facilitation,[38] which might account for the relation between 5-HTTLPR and SIDS, and could likewise play a role in the respiratory dysfunction often observed during or following a seizure. Serotonin also seems to have antiepileptic and antiepileptogenic properties in animal models of partial epilepsy[39,40] and possibly in humans,[41] although it might aggravate absence seizures. Some AEDs, including carbamazepine, may exert their antiepileptic action by promoting serotonin release.[42] The high rate of depression in patients with uncontrolled epilepsy suggests an altered central serotonergic balance, which might be partly related to 5-HTTLPR polymorphism. The latter has been associated with a higher risk of developing major depression. One could thus speculate whether depressed patients with epilepsy might be at higher risk of SUDEP, although this has not been reported. Of relevance is the observation of a protective effect of fluoxetine, a selective serotonin reuptake inhibitor, in reducing ictal respiratory arrest in DBA/2 mice with audiogenic seizures, at doses that did not reduce seizure severity.[43] Whether this translates to a protective effect with similar agents in humans is at present speculative, but suggests a novel avenue by which prevention can be explored. This suggestion has prompted a pilot study by one of the investigators (P.R.) to research the impact of fluoxetine on the severity of ictal and postictal apnea.

RECORDED SUDEP AND NEAR-SUDEP

The few reported cases of SUDEP and near-SUDEP occurring during EEG video telemetry should be scrutinized because they provide the most detailed evidence of the mechanisms leading to death. Near SUDEP is a cardiac or respiratory arrest that required active resuscitation to prevent death. The first SUDEP case described by Bird and colleagues[44] occurred in a patient with focal epilepsy undergoing presurgical work-up with intracranial recordings. After drug reduction, 5 seizures occurred and the patient died during the fifth seizure (complex partial seizure with secondary generalization). The head turned to the left, the body followed, and the patient was face down, the head slightly to the left. EEG showed focal then generalized discharges followed by "brief complete flattening, alternating with spindling spike discharges, before activity ceased". This was seen first on the side of seizure onset then bilaterally. A pulse artifact, observed with one of the intracranial electrodes, lasted a further 120 seconds at 46 beats/min and faded gradually, indicating perfusion well beyond EEG suppression. Respiration and oximetry were not recorded, but the pattern was not that typically seen secondary to anoxia. EEG suppression postictally is not infrequently seen on a video EEG telemetry unit but has not yet been studied systematically. This pattern, seen in other cases (see review[1]), has been referred to as "CNS electrical shutdown", and reported in another 2 case reports of monitored SUDEP.[45,46] This phenomenon may reflect mechanisms involved in cessation of seizures and may underlie respiratory or cardiac failure. Caution is required, however, in not equating forebrain with hindbrain shut down, as the two may be dissociated. A few monitored near-SUDEP cases have also been reported, pointing to central or obstructive apnea as the primary mechanism.[47,48]

MORTEMUS, which stands for the MORTality in Epilepsy Monitoring Unit (EMU) Study, aims at auditing cases of deaths, near-SUDEP, and ictal asystole that have occurred in patients undergoing long-term video EEG monitoring (http://www.mortemus.org). The primary aim is to gather more reliable cardiac, respiratory, and EEG data from patients who suffer such incidents while being monitored, to better understand the pathophysiology of SUDEP. Another aim of MORTEMUS is to evaluate the incidence and risk factors of death, SUDEP, and near-SUDEP in patients admitted to EMUs for recording seizures, in an attempt to optimize the safety of these procedures. A case control study of the identified SUDEP, near-SUDEP, and ictal asystole will be performed. MORTEMUS was initially based in Europe, but now includes Australia in the evaluation of SUDEP incidence in EMUs. Centers from other countries, including the United States and India, are also contributing to the database of monitored SUDEP cases. Preliminary findings suggest that the risk of death in EMUs is comparable to that observed in cohorts of drug-resistant epilepsy, indicating that all EMUs should be aware of this infrequent but still significant risk. Continuous supervision and EKG are mandatory, and Spo_2 monitoring coupled with appropriate alarms are recommended. More than 100 ictal asystoles have been identified so far. Preliminary data suggest that these are self-limiting.

Another possible source of useful information, at least in relation to recording electrographic activity before SUDEP, is from new implantable, closed-loop, intracranial neurostimulation devices,[49] which are currently undergoing clinical trials in the treatment of intractable epilepsy.

SUPERVISION AND SEIZURE DETECTION

Although there may be alternative explanations, the observation that most SUDEP cases are unwitnessed or occur in bed at night has always raised the possibility that a witnessed seizure is less likely to be fatal. Although there may be other possible physiologic explanations, this suggestion may also partly explain the lower incidence of SUDEP in children. One case control study looked at supervision and found that the use of special precautions (eg, listening devices) or sharing a bedroom with someone capable of giving assistance was protective.[9] This finding, although self-evident, needs to be replicated. Simple interventions include adjusting body position during postictal coma or stimulating respiration. Studies of cardiorespiratory parameters during seizures[50] with prolonged video EEG monitoring in localization-related epilepsy have demonstrated hypoxia, hypercapnea, and hypoventilation during seizures. Such studies can also document the effect of simple interventions. Clearly, witnessed SUDEP cases do occur and not all deaths are preventable by simple measures, but some may be. To recommend supervision goes against the goal of independence for people with epilepsy, and decisions relating to lifestyle can be made only by the informed patient. To minimize intrusion on privacy, adequate seizure alarms would be helpful. Performance of available products in tests reportedly falls short. More work is needed in this area. The idea of an apnea alarm, based on an acoustic respiratory signal, is appealing and one will soon be undergoing clinical trials (John Duncan, FRCP, London, UK, personal communication, 2009). Reliable seizure prediction seems some way into the future.

SUMMARY

SUDEP remains a significant clinical problem, which, in the authors' opinion, is to some extent potentially preventable. Research needs to focus on interventions that may alter risk. Some wide-ranging suggestions for future developments that in time can translate to clinical practice have been presented. These suggestions, the authors believe, give rise to cautious optimism.

REFERENCES

1. Tomson T, Nashef L, Ryvlin P. Sudden unexpected death in epilepsy: current knowledge and future directions. Lancet Neurol 2008;7(11):1021–31.

2. Rugg-Gunn F, Nashef L. Sudden unexpected death in epilepsy. The epilepsies 3. In: Shorvon S, Pedley T, editors. Blue books of neurology. Philadelphia: Saunders Elsevier; 2009. p. 211–40.

3. Tomson T, Walczak T, Sillanpaa M, et al. Sudden unexpected death in epilepsy: a review of incidence and risk factors. Epilepsia 2005;46(Suppl 11):54–61.

4. Camfield P, Camfield C. Sudden unexpected death in people with epilepsy: a pediatric perspective. Semin Pediatr Neurol 2005;12(1):10–4.

5. Stöllberger C, Finsterer J. Cardiorespiratory findings in sudden unexplained/unexpected death in epilepsy (SUDEP). Epilepsy Res 2004;59(1):51–60.

6. Hughes JR. A review of sudden unexpected death in epilepsy: prediction of patients at risk. Epilepsy Behav 2009;14(2):280–7.

7. Ficker DM, So EL, Shen WK, et al. Population-based study of the incidence of sudden unexplained death in epilepsy. Neurology 1998;51(5):1270–4.

8. Vlooswijk MC, Majoie HJ, De Krom MC, et al. SUDEP in the Netherlands: a retrospective study in a tertiary referral center. Seizure 2007;16(2):153–9.

9. Langan Y, Nashef L, Sander JW. Case-control study of SUDEP. Neurology 2005; 64(7):1131–3.

10. Opeskin K, Berkovic SF. Risk factors for sudden unexpected death in epilepsy: a controlled prospective study based on coroners cases. Seizure 2003;12(7):456–64.

11. Nilsson L, Bergman U, Diwan V, et al. Antiepileptic drug therapy and its management in sudden unexpected death in epilepsy: a case-control study. Epilepsia 2001;42(5):667–73.

12. Walczak TS, Leppik IE, D'Amelio M, et al. Incidence and risk factors in sudden unexpected death in epilepsy: a prospective cohort study. Neurology 2001; 56(4):519–25.

13. Langan Y. Sudden unexpected death in epilepsy (SUDEP): risk factors and case control studies. Seizure 2000;9(3):179–83 [Review].

14. Opeskin K, Burke MP, Cordner SM, et al. Comparison of antiepileptic drug levels in sudden unexpected deaths in epilepsy with deaths from other causes. Epilepsia 1999;40(12):1795–8.

15. Kloster R, Engelskjøn T. Sudden unexpected death in epilepsy (SUDEP): a clinical perspective and a search for risk factors. J Neurol Neurosurg Psychiatr 1999; 67(4):439–44.

16. Nilsson L, Farahmand BY, Persson PG, et al. Risk factors for sudden unexpected death in epilepsy: a case-control study. Lancet 1999;353(9156):888–93.

17. Nashef L, Garner S, Sander JW, et al. Circumstances of death in sudden death in epilepsy: interviews of bereaved relatives. J Neurol Neurosurg Psychiatr 1998; 64(3):349–52.

18. Ulrich J, Maxeiner H. Tongue bite injuries–a diagnostic criterium for death in epileptic seizure? Arch Kriminol 2003;212(1–2):19–29.

19. Nashef L. Sudden unexpected death in epilepsy: terminology and definitions. Epilepsia 1997;38:S6–8.

20. Le Docteur Delasiauve. Terminaisons. Traité de l'épilepsie. Paris: Victor Masson; 1854. 165–73 [in French].

21. Annegers JF, Coan SP. SUDEP: overview of definitions and review of incidence data. Seizure 1999;8(6):347–52.

22. Annegers JF. United States perspectives on definitions and classifications. Epilepsia 1997;38(s11):S9–12.

23. Faught E, Duh MS, Weiner JR, et al. Nonadherence to antiepileptic drugs and increased mortality: findings from the RANSOM Study. Neurology 2008;71(20): 1572–8.

24. Unit of Health Care Epidemiology, Oxford University and South East England Public Health Observatory. Epilepsy in England 1996 to 2004. A geographical profile of mortality. Available at: www.sepho.org.uk/. Accessed 2008.
25. Aurlien D, Leren TP, Taubøll E, et al. Lamotrigine in idiopathic epilepsy – increased risk of cardiac death? Acta Neurol Scand 2007;115(3):199–203.
26. Marson AG, Al-Kharusi AM, Alwaidh M, et al. (SANAD Study group). The SANAD study of effectiveness of valproate, lamotrigine, or topiramate for generalised and unclassifiable epilepsy: an unblinded randomised controlled trial. Lancet 2007; 369(9566):1016–26.
27. Ghali N, Nashef L. Genetics of sudden death in epilepsy. In: Lathers C, Schreider PL, Bungo MW, et al, editors. Sudden death in epilepsy. Forensic and clinical issues. Boca Raton (FL): CRC Press; 2010.
28. Hogart A, Leung KN, Wang NJ, et al. Chromosome 15q11-13 duplication syndrome brain reveals epigenetic alterations in gene expression not predicted from copy number. J Med Genet 2009;46(2):86–93.
29. IDEAS IsoDicentric 15 Exchange, Advocacy & Support. Available at: http://www.idic15.org/dr_physicianadvisory.php. 2009.
30. Hindocha N, Nashef L, Elmslie F, et al. Two cases of sudden unexpected death in epilepsy in a GEFS+ family with an SCN1A mutation. Epilepsia 2008;49:360–5.
31. Watanabe H, Koopmann TT, Le Scouarnec S, et al. Sodium channel beta1 subunit mutations associated with Brugada syndrome and cardiac conduction disease in humans. J Clin Invest 2008;118:2260–8.
32. Aurlien D, Leren TP, Taubøll E, et al. New SCN5A mutation in a SUDEP victim with idiopathic epilepsy. Seizure 2009;18(2):158–60.
33. Genton P, Gelisse P. Premature death in juvenile myoclonic epilepsy. Acta Neurol Scand 2001;104:125–9.
34. Nashef L, Hindocha N, Makoff A. Risk factors in sudden death in epilepsy (SUDEP): the quest for mechanisms. Epilepsia 2007;48:859–71.
35. Schwartz PJ, Stramba-Badiale M, Segantini A, et al. Prolongation of the QT interval and the sudden infant death syndrome. N Engl J Med 1998;338:1709–14.
36. Moon RY, Horne RS, Hauck FR. Sudden infant death syndrome. Lancet 2007; 370(9598):1578–87.
37. Richter DW, Manzke T, Wilken B, et al. Serotonin receptors: guardians of stable breathing. Trends Mol Med 2003;9(12):542–8.
38. Mahamed S, Mitchell GS. Simulated apnoeas induce serotonin-dependent respiratory long-term facilitation in rats. J Physiol 2008;586(8):2171–81.
39. Raju SS, Noor AR, Gurthu S, et al. Effect of fluoxetine on maximal electroshock seizures in mice: acute vs chronic administration. Pharm Res 1999;39(6):451–4.
40. Wada Y, Hirao N, Shiraishi J, et al. Pindolol potentiates the effect of fluoxetine on hippocampal seizures in rats. Neurosci Lett 1999;267(1):61–4.
41. Favale E, Rubino V, Mainardi P, et al. Anticonvulsant effect of fluoxetine in humans. Neurology 1995;45(10):1926–7.
42. Dailey JW, Reith ME, Yan QS, et al. Anticonvulsant doses of carbamazepine increase hippocampal extracellular serotonin in genetically epilepsy-prone rats: dose response relationships. Neurosci Lett 1997;227(1):13–6.
43. Tupal S, Faingold CL. Evidence supporting a role of serotonin in modulation of sudden death induced by seizures in DBA/2 mice. Epilepsia 2006;47:21–6.
44. Bird JM, Dembney KAT, Sandeman D, et al. Sudden unexplained death in epilepsy: an intracranially monitored case. Epilepsia 1997;38:S52–6.
45. Lee HW, Hong SB, Tae WS, et al. Partial seizures manifesting as apnea only in an adult. Epilepsia 1999;40:1828–31.

46. McLean BN, Wimalaratna S. Sudden death in epilepsy recorded in ambulatory EEG. J Neurol Neurosurg Psychiatr 2007;78:1395–7.

47. So EL, Sam MC, Lagerlund TL. Postictal central apnea as a cause of SUDEP: evidence from near-SUDEP incident. Epilepsia 2000;41:1494–7.

48. Thomas P, Landré E, Suisse G, et al. Syncope anoxo-ischémique par dyspnée obstructive au cours d'une crise partielle complexe temporale droite. Epilepsies 1996;8:339–46.

49. Skarpaas TL, Morrell MJ. Intracranial stimulation therapy for epilepsy. Neurotherapeutics 2009;6(2):238–43.

50. Bateman LM, Li CS, Seyal M. Ictal hypoxemia in localization-related epilepsy: analysis of incidence, severity and risk factors. Brain 2008;131(Pt 12):3239–45 (3):199–203.

Index

Note: Page numbers of article titles are in **boldface** type.

Neurol Clin 27 (2009) 1075–1085
doi:10.1016/S0733-8619(09)00076-0
0733-8619/09/$ – see front matter © 2009 Elsevier Inc. All rights reserved.

neurologic.theclinics.com

Moving?

Make sure your subscription moves with you!

To notify us of your new address, find your **Clinics Account Number** (located on your mailing label above your name), and contact customer service at:

Email: journalscustomerservice-usa@elsevier.com

800-654-2452 (subscribers in the U.S. & Canada)
314-447-8871 (subscribers outside of the U.S. & Canada)

Fax number: 314-447-8029

Elsevier Health Sciences Division
Subscription Customer Service
3251 Riverport Lane
Maryland Heights, MO 63043

*To ensure uninterrupted delivery of your subscription, please notify us at least 4 weeks in advance of move.